Surgical Infections

Guest Editor

John E. Mazuski, MD, PhD

SURGICAL CLINICS
OF NORTH AMERICA

www.surgical.theclinics.com

Consulting Editor
RONALD F. MARTIN, MD

April 2009 • Volume 89 • Number 2

SAUNDERS an imprint of ELSEVIER, Inc.

W.B. SAUNDERS COMPANY

A Division of Elsevier Inc.

1600 John F. Kennedy Blvd., Suite 1800, Philadelphia, PA 19103-2899

http://www.theclinics.com

SURGICAL CLINICS OF NORTH AMERICA Volume 89, Number 2

April 2009 ISSN 0039-6109, ISBN-10: 1-4377-0544-8, ISBN-13: 978-1-4377-0544-7

Editor: Catherine Bewick

Surgical Clinics of North America (ISSN 0039-6109) is published bimonthly by Elsevier Inc., 360 Park Avenue South, New York, NY 10010-1710. Months of publication are February, April, June, August, October, and December. Business and Editorial Offices: 1600 John F. Kennedy Blvd., Suite 1800, Philadelphia, PA 19103-2899. Customer Service Office: 6277 Sea Harbor Drive, Orlando, FL 32887-4800. Periodicals postage paid at New York, NY and additional mailing offices. Subscription prices are $269.00 per year for US individuals, $432.00 per year for US institutions, $134.00 per year for US students and residents, $330.00 per year for Canadian individuals, $537.00 per year for Canadian institutions, $371.00 for international individuals, $537.00 per year for international institutions and $185.00 per year for Canadian and foreign students/residents. To receive student/resident rate, orders must be accompanied by name of affiliated institution, date of term, and the *signature* of program/residency coordinator on institution letterhead. Orders will be billed at individual rate until proof of status is received. Foreign air speed delivery is included in all *Clinics* subscription prices. All prices are subject to change without notice. POSTMASTER: Send address changes to *Surgical Clinics*, Elsevier Periodicals Customer Service, 11830 Westline Industrial Drive, St. Louis, MO 63146. **Customer Service: 1-800-654-2452 (US). From outside of the United States, call 1-314-453-7041. Fax: 1-314-453-5170. E-mail: JournalsCustomerService-usa@elsevier.com (for print support),** journalsonlinesupport-usa@elsevier.com (for online support).

Reprints. For copies of 100 or more, of articles in this publication, please contact the Commercial Reprints Department, Elsevier Inc., 360 Park Avenue South, New York, New York 10010-1710. Tel. (212) 633-3812, Fax: (212) 462-1935, e-mail: reprints@elsevier.com.

The *Surgical Clinics of North America* is also published in Spanish by McGraw-Hill Interamericana Editores S.A., P.O. Box 5-237 06500 Mexico D.F. Mexico; and in Portuguese by Interlivros Edicoes Ltda., Rua Comandante Coelho 1085, CEP 21250, Rio de Janeiro, Brazil; and in Greek by Paschalidis Medical Publications, Athens Greece.

The *Surgical Clinics of North America* is covered in *MEDLINE/PubMed (Index Medicus)*, *EMBASE/Excerpta Medica*, *Current Contents/Clinical Medicine*, *Current Contents/Life Sciences*, *Science Citation Index*, and *ISI/BIOMED*.

Printed and bound by CPI Group (UK) Ltd, Croydon, CR0 4YY

Transferred to Digital Print 2011

Contributors

CONSULTING EDITOR

RONALD F. MARTIN, MD
Staff Surgeon, Marshfield Clinic, Marshfield; and Clinical Associate Professor, University of Wisconsin School of Medicine and Public Health, Madison, Wisconsin; Lieutenant Colonel, Medical Corps, United States Army Reserve

GUEST EDITOR

JOHN E. MAZUSKI, MD, PhD
Associate Professor of Surgery, Washington University School of Medicine, St. Louis, Missouri

AUTHORS

GREG J. BEILMAN, MD
Professor of Surgery and Anesthesia, Division of Surgical Critical Care, University of Minnesota, Minneapolis, Minnesota

MATTHEW C. BYRNES, MD
Assistant Professor of Surgery, Division of Surgical Critical Care, University of Minnesota, Minneapolis; and North Memorial Medical Center, Robbinsdale, Minnesota

WILLIAM G. CHEADLE, MD
Professor of Surgery, Veterans Affairs Medical Center, Department of Surgery, University of Louisville, Louisville, Kentucky

CRAIG M. COOPERSMITH, MD
Associate Professor of Surgery and Anesthesiology, Department of Surgery, Washington University School of Medicine, St. Louis, Missouri

PHILIP A. EFRON, MD
Surgical Critical Care Fellow, Department of Surgery, Washington University School of Medicine, St. Louis, Missouri

HEATHER L. EVANS, MD, MS
Assistant Professor, Department of Surgery, University of Washington; Director of Surgical Infectious Disease, Harborview Medical Center, Seattle, Washington

DONALD E. FRY, MD
Executive Vice President, Michael Pine and Associates; Adjunct Professor of Surgery, Northwestern University Feinberg School of Medicine, Chicago, Illinois; and Emeritus Professor of Surgery, University of New Mexico School of Medicine, Albuquerque, New Mexico

MATTHEW R. GOEDE, MD
Fellow, Surgical Critical Care, Barnes-Jewish Hospital/Washington University School
of Medicine, St. Louis, Missouri

BARBARA HAAS, MD
Department of Surgery, University of Toronto, Toronto, Ontario, Canada

GABRIEL HERSCU, MD
Surgical Resident, Department of Surgery, University of California, Irvine Medical Center,
Orange, California

ALICIA N. KIENINGER, MD
Instructor, Department of Surgery, Johns Hopkins University School of Medicine,
Baltimore, Maryland

JOHN P. KIRBY, MS, MD
Assistant Professor of Surgery, Department of Surgery, Washington University School
of Medicine, Saint Louis, Missouri

MICHAEL F. KSYCKI, DO
Assistant Professor of Surgery, Miller School of Medicine, University of Miami,
Miami, Florida

PAMELA A. LIPSETT, MD
Professor, Department of Surgery, Anesthesiology and Critical Care Medicine, and
Nursing, Johns Hopkins University Schools of Medicine and Nursing, Baltimore, Maryland

STEPHEN F. LOWRY, MD, FACS, FRCS(Edin) (Hon)
Professor and Chair, Department of Surgery, University of Medicine and Dentistry of New
Jersey-Robert Wood Johnson Medical School, New Brunswick, New Jersey

MARK A. MALANGONI, MD, FACS
Case Western University School of Medicine; Department of Surgery, MetroHealth
Medical Center, Cleveland, Ohio

ADDISON K. MAY, MD
Professor of Surgery and Anesthesiology, Division of Trauma and Surgical Critical Care,
Department of Surgery, Vanderbilt University Medical Center, Nashville, Tennessee

JOHN E. MAZUSKI, MD, PhD
Associate Professor of Surgery, Washington University School of Medicine, St. Louis,
Missouri

NICHOLAS NAMIAS, MD, MBA
Professor of Surgery and Anesthesiology, Miller School of Medicine, University of Miami,
Miami, Florida

AVERY B. NATHENS, MD, PhD, MPH
Department of Surgery, University of Toronto, Toronto, Ontario, Canada

NILAM P. PATEL, PharmD, BCPS
Department of Pharmacy, MetroHealth Medical Center, Cleveland, Ohio

MOTAZ QADAN, BSc (Hons), MBChB, MRCS(Ed)
Price Fellow, Price Institute of Surgical Research, Department of Surgery, University of Louisville, Louisville, Kentucky

ROBERT G. SAWYER, MD, FACS
Professor, Departments of Surgery and Public Health Sciences, University of Virginia School of Medicine; Chief, Division of Acute Care Surgery, and Co-Director, Surgical Trauma and Burn Intensive Care Unit, UVA Health System, Charlottesville, Virginia

JOSEPH S. SOLOMKIN, MD
Professor of Surgery, Department of Surgery, University of Cincinnati College of Medicine, Cincinnati, Ohio

SAMUEL ERIC WILSON, MD
Professor of Surgery, Department of Surgery, University of California, Irvine Medical Center, Orange, California

Contents

The history of adjunctive treatments for severe sepsis has been fraught with more failures than successes. To date, there have been few interventions that have been demonstrated to be efficacious by multiple large, well-designed, multicenter randomized clinical trials. However, recent research into treatment strategies using drotrecogin alfa (activated), effective blood glucose management, early goal-directed therapy, protocolization of care, and intensivist management has demonstrated positive results. Further research is being conducted to verify the success of these initial trials. This article summarizes some of the available adjunctive treatments for severe sepsis.

Surgical site infections are a frequent cause of morbidity following surgical procedures. Gram-positive cocci, particularly staphylococci, cause many of these infections, although gram-negative organisms are also frequently involved. The risk of developing a surgical site infection is associated with a number of factors, including aspects of the operative procedure itself, such as wound classification, and patient-related variables, such as preexisting medical conditions. Both nonpharmacologic measures and antimicrobial prophylaxis for selected procedures are used to prevent development of these infections. Compliance with these generally accepted preventive principles may lead to overall decreases in the incidence of these infections.

Surgical prosthetics provide unquestioned benefit to patients in maintenance of life and limb. However, complications associated with prosthetic devices continue to represent a significant source of morbidity and mortality. Even as the surgeon becomes more adept at management of infections, the bacterial characteristics change in favor of increased virulence and greater resistance to antimicrobials. Excision or retention of the prosthesis depends on the time of presentation, the microbial isolates recovered, and the extent of surrounding tissue destruction. Recent work shows improving results with in situ replacement.

Skin and soft tissue infections are a common cause of hospitalization and use of antibiotic therapy, and may result in significant disability. Infections managed by surgeons may vary from simple, noncomplicated cellulitis to severe necrotizing soft tissue infections. The differentiation of necrotizing infections from nonnecrotizing infections is critical to achieving adequate surgical therapy. An understanding of the changing epidemiology of all complicated skin and soft tissue infections is required for selection of appropriate empiric antibiotic therapy.

bacteriuria may be treated with catheter removal only, and do not necessarily require antibiotic therapy. Patients with symptomatic infections should receive effective antimicrobial therapy, but removal of the catheter is also fundamental to clearing the urinary tract of infection. Antibiotic therapy of urinary tract infections is facilitated by the renal concentration of many antibiotics, permitting very high antibiotic concentrations to be achieved in the urine.

Clostridium difficile is the most common cause of infectious diarrhea in hospitalized patients. Its effects are mediated by *C difficile* toxins A and B. Recent outbreaks of severe colitis have been associated with a new strain of the bacterium that produces large amounts of the toxins. Although oral metronidazole and oral vancomycin can be used to treat *C difficile*–associated disease, intraluminal vancomycin is preferable for more severe *C difficile* colitis. Early surgical intervention can improve outcomes with fulminant colitis, although overall mortality remains high.

The development of antimicrobial resistant pathogens in surgical patients is a significant problem, and infections caused by these organisms are associated with increased morbidity and mortality. Programs to prevent the spread of resistant organisms emphasize standard infection control practices and appropriate antibiotic prescribing practices. Antibiotic restriction and selective reporting of bacterial susceptibilities have had limited success in decreasing development of resistance, and are difficult to maintain effectively in the absence of widespread clinician acceptance. Potentially more promising are integrated decision support tools, which can support optimal antibiotic selection while preserving the sense of clinician autonomy. The use of antibiotic cycling programs for critically ill patients may be another approach to preserving the efficacy of the currently antimicrobial against the continued pressure of increasing bacterial resistance.

Infection after surgery continues to be a major source of morbidity and expense despite extensive efforts with educational programs, guidelines, and hospital-based policies and procedures. The public and the government are demanding better performance and greater accountability. Our system operations within our institutions have failed. We need to adopt a culture dedicated to quality control through better information technology and data-driven initiatives to achieve improved clinical outcomes from infectious complications in surgery.

Despite ongoing efforts to standardize therapy and improve management, the morbidity and mortality associated with surgical infections remain high. Continued innovation is required to improve outcomes further, particularly in the face of the increasing prevalence of multidrug resistant organisms. Although they remain in the experimental stages, a number of recent advances have the potential to have significant impact on the management and outcomes of surgical infections. These include novel diagnostic strategies, antimicrobials targeting microbial virulence factors, novel vaccines, and risk stratification based on genetic profiling.

THE CLINICS ARE NOW AVAILABLE ONLINE!

Access your subscription at:
www.theclinics.com

Foreword

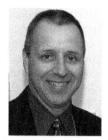

Ronald F. Martin, MD
Consulting Editor

A chance to cut is a chance to cure—at least that what I was taught. At the time it seemed like a great catch phrase that empowered us surgeons with supernatural abilities. Then one day I was conversing with a neurosurgeon friend of mine who told me that in neurosurgery (according to him, of course) they don't actually "fix" their patients—they make them different. To be fair, for many of these patients different is markedly better. This conversation did, however, cause me to rethink my previous notions regarding cutting and curing and the like. After a while I came to the conclusion that a chance to cut is a chance to improve someone (hopefully), but to cure someone is something else altogether. To cure someone we would have to put him back the way he was, perhaps, as if we had never been there. If one accepts this logical leap then possibly the best chance we have to "cure" somebody is to eradicate an infection.

History is replete with examples of the operative management of infection. Some of the earliest descriptions of medical care are of the drainage of pus. Also, there has been much misunderstanding and propagation of falsehoods regarding the management and prevention of infection over the centuries. Today it would seem as if we have a more complete understanding of what constitutes infections and how to treat or prevent them.

Yet, we don't really use what we already know.

Despite the large amount of published material on infection control and prophylaxis, we often don't change our behaviors. Perhaps it is inertia. Perhaps it is autonomy. Perhaps it is ignorance. Perhaps it is a consequence of adult learning behavior. Be that as it may, we are currently well armed with existing information that would allow us to significantly reduce the incidence and spread of perioperative and nosocomial infections and we don't use the information to its fullest extent.

As of the writing of this Foreword, we citizens of the United States have just inaugurated a new President. Among the greatest challenges we face at present is to try to decide what we each must sacrifice in order to ensure better days ahead for a country that is foundering a bit. For some it will be monetary loss (or investment if you prefer). For some it will be a change in lifestyle or job choice. But for us in medicine it will most likely be a significant loss of autonomy and a significant increase in accountability and transparency. Parenthetically, that will come with a monetary hit also.

Surg Clin N Am 89 (2009) xiii–xv
doi:10.1016/j.suc.2009.02.002
0039-6109/09/$ – see front matter © 2009 Elsevier Inc. All rights reserved.

surgical.theclinics.com

Physicians and surgeons in many circumstances hate transparency. I do. I'll confess. Personally, I don't like it because it seems to me that the metrics we use when being "transparent" seem to be half-baked many times and rarely take into account many of the non-measured factors that make a difference. Data acquisition is often incomplete, which further aggravates the analysis. Also, we tend to take problems within a system and assign the fault to somebody who really can't control the situation. In case I am being obtuse I will give you an example: a primary care physician is paid on a pay-for-performance platform. She asks her patient who has diabetes to eat properly, take her insulin, and watch her glucose. When the patient returns to see her physician she has gained weight and skipped her insulin for multiple days since her last visit. Her hemoglobin A_{lc} is now 9.6 and as a result, the physician takes a pay cut. I'll leave the philosophy to you, dear reader, as to the fairness of this, but this is what happens. Rather than find the system disconnect and address that, we find an easy target and micro-penalize that person. In effect, it reduces cost slightly overall to the payer (maybe), marginally improves quality for those who do comply, and cost shifts within the system, all without addressing the weakest link in the chain.

Regardless of my reticence to like transparency, I accept and embrace it and commend it to you. In the end there are many reasons to do so. First, because it won't go away. Second, because it will probably help our patients and us, especially if we actively participate. Our participation and feedback will, it is hoped, correct some of the deficiencies in data collection and analysis and identify the system failures written of earlier. If we don't participate, others are unlikely to help those who remain mute.

Surgeons have been at the forefront of quality control and transparency historically. Morbidity and mortality conferences are transparent to us but no one else—that may be why we accept it. The National Safety Quality Improvement Project is an excellent example of "voluntary" data-gathering that seems to be working. In my opinion, surgeons are excellent at cooperating when all other options have been exhausted.

One of our brethren, Dr. Atul Gawande, and his colleagues recently published a report in the New England Journal of Medicine detailing how the simple use of a checklist in multiple countries with widely disparate resources reduced adverse outcome by a substantial and significant percentage.[1] The study may not have been perfect but it does clearly illustrate one thing: when we function as part of a system as opposed to a collection of individuals we seem to get better results. And get this–in Dr Gawande's study, they weren't even able to ensure that the checklist was being adhered to and it still worked! One could say that weakens the report but I submit that it tells us that the Hawthorne effect isn't all bad. Just getting people to participate, or think they are participating, in a system of quality improvement probably improves outcomes compared to sheer anonymous and autonomous behavior.

Back to infection.

We surgeons have to deal with infection on two major fronts: treatment of existing infection and prevention of nosocomial infection. We are pretty good at the former and not as good as we could be at the latter. Most of us adhere to the best operative techniques we can but data suggest we aren't as good at the use of evidence-guided prophylaxis as we can be. Many of these lapses can be traced to systems problems in the identification of the right choice and timely delivery of antibiotics for each patient. Yet some of these lapses are a stubborn adherence to either unproved choices or, worse yet, choices that have been disproved.

Our hospital systems don't necessarily adhere to best current practices either. It remains absolutely curious to me that there is any kind of hospital room other than a private room. Also, I cannot think of why there is not a sink for health care providers in every entrance to every patient room. I know it costs money to renovate and re-plumb but it seems cheaper to do that than to treat a series of patients in the ICU whose aggressive *Clostridium difficile* colitis has required colectomy. How many of you have walked through an ICU and seen intubated patients lying flat—under the poster on the wall that reads, "keep head of bed at 30 degrees at all times." Some hospitals embrace central line teams, others don't.

Surgeons will always be integral in the management of infection for many patients. And we will always put our patients at some risk for developing infection. We can also participate to our fullest to reduce that risk. We as a group have an excellent history of taking quality control measures seriously. We now have to consider our role in a larger sense and advocate as best as possible for a systems approach to infection prevention and treatment.

For those of you who have followed the previous Forewords, the theme of this series is to try to define where and how surgeons fit into to the larger system and advance the knowledge for those matters in which we surgeons should be expert. In this case we may have a head start but we still have a long way to go. Dr. Mazuski and his colleagues have assembled an excellent collection of reviews on matters that are applicable to all of us who practice surgery. Understanding these topics allows us individually to better care for patients who have infection and help us function better within our systems in the broader sense as public advocate. We are indebted to Dr. Mazuski and his contributors for their efforts. Whether a chance to cut is a chance to cure is true, I'll leave to your judgment. But a gram of prevention is worth several kilograms of cure when it comes to infectious disease. As always, your feedback, comments, and criticism are welcome on this or any other matter related to the *Surgical Clinics of North America*.

Ronald F. Martin, MD
Department of Surgery
Marshfield Clinic
1000 North Oak Avenue
Marshfield, WI 54449

E-mail address:
martin.ronald@marshfieldclinic.org

REFERENCE

1. Haynes AB, Weiser TG, Berry WR, et al. A surgical safety checklist to reduce morbidity and mortality in a global population. N Eng J Med 2009;360:491–9.

Preface

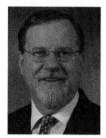

John E. Mazuski, MD, PhD
Guest Editor

Men at some time are masters of their fates:
The fault, dear Brutus, is not in our stars,
But in ourselves, that we are underlings.
                    Shakespeare, Julius Caesar, Act I, Scene 2
We have met the enemy and he is us.
                    Walt Kelly

Since antiquity, the problem of infection has been inextricably linked with surgical therapy. Egyptian papyri describe infectious complications of traumatic wounds and use of drainage for abscesses. Galen taught that "laudable pus" was essential for the healing of wounds, thereby setting back surgical therapy for nearly two millennia, even though some surgeons, such as Ambrose Paré, questioned the wisdom of this theory. In the middle of the nineteenth century, Semmelweis and Lister developed simple measures to decrease postpartum and postoperative infections, finally putting to rest the notion that infection was somehow a beneficent aspect of surgical therapy.[1]

Today, the surgical practitioner confronts the problem of infection every day. Even with the twentieth-century miracle of antimicrobial chemotherapy, surgeons need to drain abscesses, débride infected wounds, and otherwise attend to patients presenting with various acute infectious problems. In addition to treating established infections, however, the surgeon often encounters infection as the undesirable consequence of a surgical intervention. It was estimated that more than 290,000 surgical site infections developed in hospitalized surgical patients in 2002, leading directly to 8205 deaths. These surgical site infections represented only about 20% of the more than 1,700,000 health care–associated infections estimated to have occurred that year, many if not most of which arose in surgical patients. These nosocomial infections, including hospital-acquired pneumonia, urinary tract infections, and catheter-related bloodstream infections, led to nearly 100,000 deaths.[2]

What, then, is a surgical infection, the subject of this issue? Is it an infection for which a surgical procedure is indicated, such as a large soft tissue abscess? Is it an infection that develops after an operation, such as a surgical site infection? Should

Surg Clin N Am 89 (2009) xvii–xix
doi:10.1016/j.suc.2009.02.001
0039-6109/09/$ – see front matter
surgical.theclinics.com

a remote infection, such as pneumonia following an operation, also be considered a surgical infection? Is a surgical infection all of these and more? One could probably identify some form of surgical intervention as appropriate for virtually any type of infectious disease. The patient who has endocarditis may need a cardiac valve replacement, the patient who has a joint infection may need open drainage and débridement, and the patient who has meningitis may need a cerebrospinal fluid shunt because of noncommunicating hydrocephalus. Rather than attempting to rigidly define surgical infections, it is probably easier to operationally describe them as infections that the surgical practitioner encounters frequently during the course of his or her practice.

Even with that restriction, a full discussion of all topics related to surgical infections would consume multiple volumes, rather than this single issue of *Surgical Clinics of North America*. The subject matter for this issue has therefore focused on those areas believed to be most relevant to the practicing general surgeon on a day-to-day basis. However, many of these topics will be of interest to specialty surgeons and other medical practitioners also.

The individual articles of this issue are grouped into three general areas. The first four articles concern complex interactions of pathogens, host, and therapeutic modalities relevant to surgical infections. Motaz and Cheadle provide an overview of the microorganisms responsible for most surgical infections, Lowry describes the host response to infection, Patel and Malangoni summarize antimicrobial chemotherapy, and Byrnes and Beilman discuss other therapeutic modalities for the treatment of patients who have surgical infections.

The next series of articles focuses on specific infections of interest to surgical practitioners. Kirby and Mazuski outline measures to prevent surgical site infections, and Herscu and Wilson specifically discuss infections occurring after implantation of prosthetic materials. May elaborates on the diagnosis and management of skin and soft tissue infections. Mazuski and Solomkin describe both community-acquired and nosocomial intra-abdominal infections. There follows a series of articles focusing on other infectious complications of surgical therapy: Kieninger and Lipsett, Goede and Coopersmith, and Ksycki and Namias provide detailed information regarding postoperative pneumonia, catheter-related bloodstream infections, and urinary tract infections, respectively. The final article in this section, by Efron and Mazuski, describes *Clostridium difficile* colitis, a modern pestilence directly related to use and misuse of antibiotics.

Numerous interventions can be used to prevent and treat infections associated with surgical therapy. The ultimate section of this issue attempts to bring together some of those themes. Evans and Sawyer summarize measures to avoid development of resistant bacteria and Fry delineates systems approaches for prevention of surgical infections. Finally, Haas and Nathens describe potential future approaches for the management of surgical infections.

In the end, we, as surgeons, share responsibility for creating many of the modern-day plagues of nosocomial infections. Nevertheless, we also possess tools that can help thwart or ameliorate these infections. What is required is effective use of existing evidence-based practices for the prevention and management of surgical infections. Future investigations will lead to new approaches to control these infections, but these scientific advances will only be of value if they can be integrated into surgical practice. Ultimately, we are indeed our own worst enemies if we choose to ignore the importance of appropriately preventing and treating these infections, which can counteract even our best surgical skills. By conscientiously applying the principles outlined in this issue for managing surgical infections, we can protect our patients from the adverse consequences of these infections, and thereby improve the overall quality of surgical care.

John E. Mazuski, MD, PhD
Department of Surgery
Washington University School of Medicine
660 South Euclid Avenue
Campus Box 8109
Saint Louis, MO 63110-1093, USA

E-mail address:
mazuskij@wustl.edu

REFERENCES

1. Rutkow IM. Surgery: An Illustrated History. Saint Louis: Mosby; 1993.
2. Klevens RM, Edwards JR, Richards CL Jr, et al. Estimating health care-associated infections and deaths in U.S. hospitals, 2002. Public Health Rep 2007;122:160–6.

Common Microbial Pathogens in Surgical Practice

Motaz Qadan, BSc (Hons), MBChB, MRCS(Ed)[a], William G. Cheadle, MD[b,*]

KEYWORDS

• Bacteria • Fungi • Infection • Surgery • Post-operative

The process of inflammation as applied to surgical wounds was discussed by Hippocrates, who coined the term laudable pus as a sign of eventual wound healing, as opposed to erysipelas, a spreading inflammation that often meant the death of the patient. Although many scholars suspected microorganisms, it would take the development of the compound microscope to allow the microbiologists of the nineteenth century to describe the multitude of bacterial and fungal organisms and their relationship to infection. Pasteur developed the germ theory of disease by demonstrating that bacteria did not contaminate culture medium in curved flasks and Koch described the postulates by which infection from a particular microorganism would be defined. He was awarded the Nobel Prize in 1905 for his description of the *Mycobacterium tuberculosis* bacillus.

The Hungarian obstetrician Ignaz Semmelweis, who practiced in Austria in the mid-nineteenth century, demanded that his residents and students wash their hands in sodium hypochlorite before touching patients and also had his obstetric instruments soaked in the same solution. This eventually ushered in the era of asepsis, and although his contemporaries failed to adopt these measures, the prevailing rate of post-partum endometritis, which had been extremely high, decreased markedly in his patients, to an estimated 5%.[1]

Lord Lister, a general surgeon who did mostly orthopedics, was the first to use an antiseptic agent, carbolic acid, in 1865, to reduce the risk of surgical site infection

Conflict of Interest Statement: W.G. Cheadle had full access to all the data and had final responsibility for the decision to submit the manuscript for publication. There were no personal relationships or financial conflicts to disclose. This article is an original contribution that has neither been published before nor is under consideration for publication elsewhere. Dr. Motaz Qadan holds the Joint Royal College of Surgeons of Edinburgh (RCSEd)/James and Emmeline Ferguson Research Fellowship.

[a] Price Institute of Surgical Research, Department of Surgery, University of Louisville, Louisville, KY 40202, USA
[b] Veterans Affairs Medical Center, Department of Surgery, University of Louisville, Louisville, KY 40202, USA
* Corresponding author. Veterans Affairs Medical Center (151), 800 Zorn Avenue, Louisville, KY 40206.
E-mail address: wg.cheadle@louisville.edu (W.G. Cheadle).

(SSI). This treatment revolutionized the treatment of open fractures in which the extremity was salvaged. These early measures have been refined to the modern aseptic and antiseptic techniques used today, and with appropriate use of prophylactic antibiotics, the overall SSI rate has been reduced to approximately 5%.[2] The National Surgical Quality Improvement Program (NSQIP) identified that pneumonia, urinary tract infection (UTI), and sepsis respectively occurred in 3.6%, 3.5%, and 2.1% of surgical patients in the database.[3] Since infection rates are not zero, significant improvements with additional knowledge of local wound conditions and the infecting microbes can still be made.

ANATOMIC CONSIDERATIONS OF BACTERIAL AND FUNGAL PATHOGENS

Apart from viruses and prions, which are beyond the scope of this report, all pathogenic organisms are made up of cells. Cells are distinct entities of cytoplasm that are bound by a cell membrane and consist of genetic (DNA) material. Bacterial cells are referred to as prokaryotes and all other cells are eukaryotes. Prokaryotes lack a distinct nuclear compartment, have DNA in the form of a single circular chromosome (additional bacterial DNA may be carried in plasmids), and are able to undergo simultaneous transcription and translation without mRNA. They also lack any membrane-bound organelles within their cellular boundaries. Interestingly, eukaryotic membrane-bound organelles, such as mitochondria, are thought to share common evolutionary pathways with entire prokaryotic cells, a fundamental hypothesis in the endosymbiosis theory. In fact, the term "pro-karyote" literally translates to "before the nucleus" and refers to the evolutionary origin of prokaryotic cells preceding more complex eukaryotes.

Bacterial cell walls are complex and divide bacteria into two classes: gram-positive and gram-negative cells. Gram staining, developed by the Danish scientist Hans Christian Gram in 1884, tests the ability of bacteria to retain a violet stain after washing with iodine and alcohol, with purple indicating a positive Gram stain and pink indicating a negative one. In gram-positive bacteria, the outer wall is made of peptidoglycan, whereas gram-negative species have little peptidoglycan but possess an additional outer layer rich in polysaccharides. Bacterial cell wall layers provide complex protective defense shields against immune cells and antimicrobial agents. Potentially, they may stimulate certain pathogenic responses on degradation and systemic spread.

Some prokaryotes possess flagella (tails), which permit motility, and fimbriae or pili, which aid in adhesion to various surfaces. Bacterial ribosomes (denoted 70S), although similar to eukaryotic ribosomes (80S), are the specific target of antimicrobial agents such as aminoglycosides. **Fig. 1** provides a schematic representation of the generalized structure of a prokaryotic cell.

Classification of prokaryotes is complex. Based on a mixture of size, shape, color, and immunohistochemical and biologic markers, bacteria are classified into genera (*singular – genus*), which are further subdivided into species (capable of interbreeding). Examples include *Escherichia coli* and *Staphylococcus aureus*. Differences within a genus depend on immunologic and phenotypic properties, including the presence of flagella, the type of toxins produced, the ability to hemolyze blood, and so forth. Direct genomic studies are also employed today to accurately identify organisms based on genome size, ratio of bases within DNA, and the presence of certain DNA sequences.

Fungi are eukaryotes that are very different from human and plant cells. They are multicellular multinucleate organisms that grow either in filaments (hyphae) to form a mycelium, or as mononuclear spherical organisms that replicate by budding and

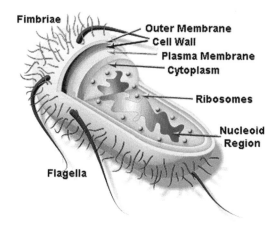

Fimbriae
Outer Membrane
Cell Wall
Plasma Membrane
Cytoplasm
Ribosomes
Nucleoid
Region
Flagella

Fig. 1. Structure of a prokaryotic cell. (*Courtesy of* T. Sheppard, BSc., London. Copyright © 2005 Tim Sheppard. Available at www.blobs.org; used with permission.)

division (yeast). Although some may exist as commensals on human skin and hair, several are important human pathogens both superficially and deeper in tissues, where they invade and digest surrounding material by releasing digestive enzymes and absorb available nutrients for survival.

Gram-Positive Cocci

Staphylococcus

Staphylococcus aureus is a catalase and coagulase-producing gram-positive organism that frequently occurs in human nasal passages, mucous membranes, or skin of carriers. It is traditionally identified by its characteristic golden yellow grapelike clumped colonies on culture (*staphule* – Greek for grapes; *aureus* – Latin for gold) (**Fig. 2**). This organism is arguably the most important pathogenic organism in evolving surgical infections, and thus, receives considerable attention below.

S aureus constitutes the majority of skin and soft tissue infections encountered in the surgical population, accounting for up to 20% of SSI isolates but also 13% of all nosocomial infections (**Table 1**).[4] This facultatively anaerobic organism was first reported in 1880 in Aberdeen, Scotland, by the surgeon Sir Alexander Ogston, in pus drained from infected abscesses. Since then, an estimated 500,000 patients a year

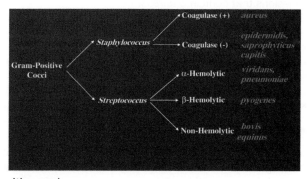

Fig. 2. Gram-positive cocci.

Table 1
National Nosocomial Infections Surveillance top 10 most common isolates (percentage distribution) in surgical site infections and nosocomial infections

Pathogen	Surgical Site Infections (n = 17,671)	All Sites (n = 101,821)
Staphylococcus aureus	20	13
Escherichia coli	8	12
Coagulase-negative Staphylococci	14	11
Enterococcus spp	12	10
Pseudomonas aeruginosa	8	9
Enterobacter spp	7	6
Candida albicans	3	5
Klebsiella pneumoniae	3	5
Gram-positive anaerobes	1	4
Proteus mirabilis	3	3

Data from National Nosocomial Infections Surveillance (NNIS) report, data summary from October 1986–April 1996, issued May 1996. A report from the National Nosocomial Infections Surveillance (NNIS) System. Am J Infect Control 1996;24(5):380–8.[4]

are thought to contract S aureus in US hospitals.[5] Superficial carriage is arguably commensal in nature and often nonpathogenic but deep-seated S aureus penetration is associated with significant morbidity and mortality and requires intensive therapy. In the nonsurgical population, it is the cause of pneumonia, endocarditis, disseminated bacteremia, toxic shock syndrome, and food poisoning among many other disease entities in adult and pediatric populations.

S aureus is capable of producing several exotoxins, including enterotoxins and superantigens, which result in the organism's virulence.[6] These include the following:

- Alpha-toxin (hemolysin), which binds to susceptible cells such as monocytes and platelets and results in leakage of contents. When released systemically, septic shock ensues.
- Beta-toxin, which classically binds, and is tested for, using sheep erythrocytes and is not usually encountered in human disease states.
- Delta-toxin, which is produced by S aureus as well as other staphylococcal species but its function remains largely unknown.
- Leucocidin, which is a hemolytic toxin (less so than alpha-toxin) that acts on polymorphonuclear leukocytes and helps S aureus evade phagocytosis. It is expressed in only 2% of S aureus isolates but is identified in over 90% of necrotizing lesions that contain S aureus.
- ET_A and ET_B exfoliation toxin, which results in widespread epidermal loss and skin blistering in neonates via protease- and esterase-mediated degradation of important integrity-maintaining epidermal proteins.
- Enterotoxins and toxic shock syndrome toxin (TSST), which possess superantigenic properties and may cause toxic shock syndrome. Enterotoxins, when ingested, result in the most common form of food poisoning. Activation of T cells and cytokine release account for the actions of these toxins.

Mildly pathogenic products include:

- Coagulase, which binds to prothrombin, and, in turn, converts fibrinogen to fibrin, thereby resulting in clot formation. It is thought to deter immune cells from arriving at the site of S aureus action.

- Staphylokinase, which degrades fibrin, much like streptokinase, and may aid in bacterial spreading.
- Proteases, lipases, DNase and fatty-acid modifying enzyme (FAME), which degrade various components and may aid in S aureus spread within abscesses.

Following the introduction of penicillin by Sir Alexander Fleming in 1943, antibacterial sensitivity of S aureus to penicillin has been gradually replaced by resistance. By the 1960s, resistance was thought to near 80%.[7] Resistance to penicillin is mediated by penicillinase (beta-lactamase), an enzyme that degrades the beta-lactam ring of penicillin. The emergence of penicillinase-resistant penicillins such as methicillin in 1959 and flucloxacillin shortly after were a welcomed discovery, until less than 2 years later, when, in 1961, the first reported case of resistance to methicillin was observed!

Following initial identification, methicillin-resistant S aureus (MRSA) has risen to endemic rates in US and UK hospitals, with a sharp rise in incidence occurring in the 1990s. Incidence rates published by the US Centers for Disease Control and Prevention (CDC) have demonstrated a greater than twofold increase from 127,000 reported cases to 278,000 between 1999 and 2005.[8] Risk factors include previous antibiotic administration, prolonged hospitalization, and multiple patient comorbidities.[9]

Despite evasion of methicillin to bacterial penicillinase, the organism was able to acquire new-found resistance, encoded for in the mec operon coding region, which is part of the staphylococcal cassette chromosome mec (SCCmec) within bacterial plasmids. Resistance conferred via the mecA gene alters penicillin binding properties and thus also implies automatic resistance to penicillinase-sensitive antibiotics such as penicillin and cephalosporins.

MRSA is now understood to consist of two exclusive subtypes: a nosocomial, or hospital-acquired, type (HA-MRSA) and a community-acquired type (CA-MRSA). Although originally defined according to source of origin, the apparently clear-cut distinction between these subtypes is more complex. Both types are equally resistant to traditional beta-lactam antibiotics although HA-MRSA appears to have a larger resistance profile, with sensitivity restricted to vancomycin, teicopleinin, or the newer oxazolidinones such as linezolid. HA-MRSA appears to affect patients in hospitals with open wounds, those who undergo invasive procedures, and ones with weakened immune systems. Transfer is predominantly staff- and instrument-related, awareness of which has resulted in the development of strict hand-washing and barrier-oriented infection control policies that are now in place.

Although most MRSA infections remain health care–associated, a rising incidence of community-acquired infection is apparent. Community-acquired infection incidence rates in the United States in 2005 were estimated at 13.7% in a recently published large series.[10] Consequently, community-acquired MRSA (CA-MRSA) is gaining increased attention among microbiologists and health care workers today. It was first noted in the early 1990s and was associated with a number of different skin and soft tissue syndromes (furuncles, impetigo, and cellulitis) in individuals who were previously healthy and had not been hospitalized within 1 year of infective episodes.[11–13] Originally thought to be similar in origin to its nosocomial counterpart, community-acquired strains have been shown to be genetically diverse with unique microbiologic properties, rendering them a separate entity.[13] Areas of aggregation have included army bases, jails, and among inner-city children, where close individual contact and poor hygiene, and hence transmission, are most likely. The community-acquired strain is associated with virulence factors thought to promote transmissibility and likelihood of disease. CA-MRSA is specifically associated with carriage of

SCCmec Type IV and panton-valentine leucocidin (PVL) virulence factor. In a study of patients from the San Francisco Bay Area, 70% of MRSA isolates from prison inmates and clinics specializing in soft and skin tissue infections were positive for PVL carriage.[14] Of 671 isolates collected over a 5-year period, most could be traced back to only two clonal groups, both of which carried the SCCmec type IV resistance determinate and both more likely to be recovered from skin. This pattern indicated the likelihood of rapid clonal supplantation within community-based transmission, probably attributable to the aforementioned virulence factors. In another study of over 800 soldiers from Brook Army Medical Center, it was found that 3% (24) of soldiers were colonized with CA-MRSA, 9 of whom developed soft tissue infections in the 8- to 10-week observation that followed.[15] PVL genes were detected in all nine cases. In contrast, of 28% who were colonized with the methicillin-sensitive S aureus (MSSA) strain, only 3% went on to develop soft tissue infections in the same observation period, highlighting very clearly the increased virulence potentially associated with carriage of the PVL gene in community evolving species.

MRSA has recently been treated with newer antimicrobial agents such as clindamycin and linezolid. These new agents are available in the oral form, thereby avoiding complex administration issues associated with intravenous delivery. More serious invasive MRSA infection, which is typically hospital-acquired, requires intravenous vancomycin treatment, a glycopeptide that is associated with toxic side effects and poorly absorbed in the oral form. Alarmingly, a rising vancomycin minimum inhibitory concentration (MIC) in the hospital-acquired strain is well documented, confirming the emergence of vancomycin-intermediate-resistant S aureus (VISA) and vancomycin-resistant S aureus (VRSA) species.[11] The former was first identified in Japan in 1996 and the latter in the United States in 2002. These organisms have since affected specific populations, such as hemodialysis patients, but incidence rates are nevertheless rising.[16] Preliminary reports of S aureus resistance to linezolid are available and pose serious future concern.[17]

Another frequently encountered bacterium in surgical infections is the skin commensal Staphylococcus epidermidis. This facultatively anaerobic, catalase-positive and coagulase-negative organism, along with Staphylococcus saprophyticus and Staphylococcus capitis, are collectively referred to as Staphylococcal albus, because of the formation of white spherical colonies on culture (albus – Latin for white).

Although less virulent than S aureus, S epidermidis is able to form a teichoic acid slime, derived from the staphylococcal cell wall, which results in the formation of a resilient biofilm that protects the bacterium against host and chemotherapeutic defense mechanisms, and thus, renders the organism more virulent.[18,19] Furthermore, in a recent study by El-Azizi and colleagues,[20] the authors were able to show that bacteria isolated from disrupted prosthetic biofilm were significantly less resistant to antimicrobial therapy than those in the biofilm itself.

Classically, S epidermidis is isolated from infected surgical wounds, particularly sternal wounds, where it is the most common isolate.[21,22] Other common operations where this organism is implicated include that that use prostheses, such as joint replacement and vascular graft procedures. It is commonly recovered from the site of infected indwelling catheters, where it is usually associated with the formation of bacterial biofilm.[18,19]

Little else is known about the pathogenesis of S epidermidis. Treatment is complex with resistance reported to both penicillin and methicillin. In 2003, approximately 90% of all coagulase-negative staphylococcal species were resistant to methicillin.[23]

Streptococcus

These gram-positive, facultatively anaerobic cocci play a significant role in surgical infections such as erysipelas and type II necrotizing fasciitis (streptococcal fasciitis), despite being commensal organisms of the mouth, throat, skin, and human intestine. Their name is derived from their twisted chain-like pattern of growth following cellular division (*strepto* – Greek for twisted).

An organized approach to classification of these organisms yields a better understanding of their various roles in disease (see **Fig. 2**). They are first divided into their ability to break down red blood cells in the laboratory, which yields three types: alpha-hemolytic, beta-hemolytic, and nonhemolytic.

Alpha-hemolytic species cause partial breakdown of blood, which results in an impartially degraded green haem halo surrounding the streptococcal colony in blood agar. Within this group, there are two dominant species, *Streptococcus viridans* (*viridans* – Latin for green) and *Streptococcus pneumoniae*, the causative organisms for endocarditis and pneumococcal pneumonia respectively. Their role in surgical disease is limited.

Beta-hemolytic organisms cause complete hemolysis of red cells in agar, and, therefore, form a white area surrounding the colony. They are further divided into Lancefield Types A-T, named after the prominent work of the late American microbiologist, Rebecca Craighill Lancefield. Surgically relevant are *Streptococcus pyogenes*, a Lancefield group A organism, and *Enterococcus* (formerly *Streptococcus* group D – reclassified in 1984).[24] These organisms play a large pathogenic role in surgical microbial disease and are discussed below.

Non-hemolytic streptococcal species, often referred to as gamma-hemolytic (a misnomer), rarely account for serious human disease. Enterococcal species, which cause a variable degree of hemolysis, must not be confused with nonhemolytic streptococci, an entirely different bacterial genus.

Streptococcus pyogenes, also known as group A *Streptococcus* (GAS), was traditionally regarded as the main pathogen of complicated skin and soft tissue infection. Its presence in cellulitis, and more specifically, erysipelas, which primarily affects the upper dermis, is well documented. It has also been reported in infected abdominal wounds, bites, and complicated poly-microbial diabetic disease. Its most notable role, however, remains its etiologic role in type II necrotizing fasciitis, or streptococcal gangrene, where it is the dominant organism along with few other Streptococcal group B, C, and G species.[25] The organism's ability to multiply and spread laterally in deep dermal tissue is often life-threatening. Early recognition and aggressive treatment is imperative in this disease. In a recently published series of 165 patients with necrotizing fasciitis, overall mortality was reported at 17% with 25% requiring amputation of the affected extremity in addition to surgical debridement.[26]

Central to pathogenic mechanisms is the production of extracellular toxins, of which two are hemolytic and three pyrogenic. There are various other nucleases, DNAses, and proteolytic enzymes that are also secreted. Hemolytic toxins include Streptolysin O and S, the former usually used as an antigenic serum marker of recent streptococcal infection. These degrade red blood cells as well as platelets and polymorphonuclear leukocytes. Pyrogenic toxins are classified from A to C and are responsible for the development of scarlet fever. Common sequelae of streptococcal exotoxins include streptococcal toxic shock syndrome (TSS), glomerulonephritis, and, less commonly today, acute rheumatic fever. Interestingly, streptokinase, an enzyme produced by the bacteria, is used as a cardiovascular thrombolytic agent following myocardial infarction (MI), more often than its staphylococcal counterpart.[6,27]

Treatment is with penicillin and its various derivates. However, appreciation that this organism often coexists in polymicrobial disease indicates that additional broad-spectrum coverage is frequently required. For example, type I necrotizing fasciitis often includes highly virulent clostridial anaerobes among other organisms.

Enterococcal species include both *Enterococcus faecalis* and *Enterococcus faecium*, commensals in the adult gastrointestinal tract (90% and 5%, respectively).[28] These partially hemolytic organisms frequently account for SSIs, particularly following clean-contaminated and contaminated surgery of the bowel. Enterococcal organisms have gained recent attention because of their intrinsic resistance to a variety of antimicrobial agents, including semisynthetic penicillinase-resistant penicillins, cephalosporins, trimethoprim-sulfamethoxazole, aminoglycosides, and clindamycin.[29] These organisms are also capable of acquiring resistance to other agents including chloramphenicol, macrolides, tetracycline, and fluoroquinolones.

Interestingly, enterococcal organisms were the first to exhibit resistance against vancomycin in 1986.[30,31] The mechanism of resistance involves alteration of vancomycin-binding targets. Vancomycin binds to [d-alanine – d-alanine] targets, which are either replaced with [d-lactate] or the entire synthesis of cell wall precursors with vancomycin-binding targets are inhibited. Several subtypes of vancomycin resistance are described and are denoted VanA to VanE.[32]

Since the emergence of vancomycin-resistant enterococcus (VRE), incidence has steadily increased in the United States (although not the United Kingdom) until, in 2004, the National Nosocomial Infections Surveillance (NNIS) reported that 30% of all ICU enterococcal infections were vancomycin resistant.[23] Currently, almost 75% of E faecium and 5% of E faecalis are resistant to vancomycin, with the latter fortunately accounting for the vast majority of recovered isolates.[33,34] Alarmingly, recent evidence shows this resistance could be transferred to other organisms, such as MRSA.[35,36]

Sensitive enterococcal organisms may be treated with ampicillin or vancomycin. Vancomycin-resistant *E faecium* is treated generally with linezolid, or can be treated with daptomycin or quinupristin/dalfopristin. For vancomycin-resistant *E faecalis* infections, ampicillin may be used if the organism is sensitive. Quinupristin/dalfopristin should not be used to treat *E faecalis*, since this organism is intrinsically resistant to this antibiotic.[37,38]

Gram-Positive Bacilli

These Gram-positive rod-shaped bacteria are obligate anaerobes that are capable of spore formation, and include *Clostridium perfringens*, *Clostridium difficile*, *Clostridium tetani*, and *Clostridium botulinum* (*Kloster – Greek* for rods). The latter two are known for producing tetanus and botulinum toxins respectively but otherwise have a limited role in surgical disease.

C perfringens causes the rare surgical disease known as gas gangrene, a rapidly spreading surgical emphysema mediated by the enterotoxin alpha-toxin. Its ability to form gaps between cells results in the characteristic formation of gas pockets below the dermis. Untreated, it results in life-threatening sequelae. It is most commonly encountered in type I polymicrobial cases of necrotizing fasciitis. Its presence has been shown to be an independent predictor of mortality and limb loss among affected cases in the recently published series described earlier.[26] Although *C perfringens* is often implicated in monobacterial gas gangrene, it is not exclusively associated with this disease. Other clostridial species, such as C *septicum*, may also cause gas gangrene.

C difficile is frequently seen on surgical wards in patients on prolonged antibiotic therapy. This organism has recently gained attention in public health circles because of increasing incidence rates and severity of the symptomatic pathognomic disease, pseudomembranous colitis.[39] Eradication of the normal colonic flora with previously administered antibiotics combined with *C difficile* ingestion may result in the formation of pseudomembranes. A severe hemorrhagic inflammation often ensues, resulting in a profound and rapidly transmissible diarrheal state in hospitalized patients.[40] In the elderly, frail, and immunocompromised, sequelae may be life-threatening. Classically, abdominal radiographs fail to demonstrate evidence of obstruction. Risk factors for disease development include antimicrobial therapy and proton pump inhibitors (PPIs).[41–44] Symptoms are often compounded by narcotics prescribed for associated pain, which inhibit colonic peristalsis and may potentially cause toxic megacolon, a surgical emergency.[45,46] Inflammation, mucosal secretion, and cell damage in the colon are mediated via the secretion of two toxins, known as toxin A and toxin B.[47] It is unclear as to why certain individuals will develop symptomatic disease but production of these toxins is essential for disease to occur.[39] Furthermore, recent strains associated with increased severity of disease, such as the North American pulsed-field gel electrophoresis type 1 (NAP 1), have been shown to produce up to 16 times more toxin A and 23 times more toxin B than standard less virulent strains of *C difficile*. NAP 1 also exhibits resistance to moxifloxacin and gatifloxacin, a phenomenon not encountered in previous *C difficile* strains.[39]

Effective treatment of clostridial species is with metronidazole, although, once again, special attention should be paid to individual circumstances; for example broad-spectrum antimicrobial coverage may be required for other organisms likely to coexist (type I necrotizing fasciitis) or discontinuing original culprit antimicrobial agents that may have permitted uncontrolled growth of the clostridial species (*C difficile* pseudomembranous colitis). Oral vancomycin is also effective in the treatment of symptomatic *C difficile*. Appropriate stool culture and sensitivities will guide the treating surgeon and careful liaison with hospital microbiologists is essential to ensure adequate isolation and disinfection protocols are followed.

Other Gram-Positive Species

There are several other Gram-positive bacilli such as *Bacillus*, *Cornyebacterium*, *Lactobacilli*, and *Listeria*, which may cause serious disease in humans but are less relevant to surgical readers. Additional details are not provided in this article.

Gram-Negative Cocci

The most notable gram-negative cocci are the *Neisseria* species, *Neisseria meningitides* and *Neisseria gonorrhoeae*, which commonly cause meningitis and gonorrhea respectively and do not feature in surgical disease. The discussion therefore moves on to the more relevant gram-negative bacilli, which are frequently encountered in surgical patients.

Gram-Negative Bacilli

Almost all surgically relevant gram-negative bacilli are aerobes, apart from *Bacteroides fragilis*, an anaerobe that frequently affects surgical patients. Generally speaking, gram-negative bacterial species tend to occur as intestinal commensals in humans, and, as such, infection related to these organisms usually follows abdominal bowel surgery, particularly colonic surgery, where there is breach of an abdominal viscus. Gram-negative bacteria account for a significant proportion of SSI isolates and all nosocomial infections. *Enterobacter* spp, *Escherichia coli*, *Klebsiella pneumoniae,* and *Proteus mirabilis* account for 21% of all SSIs alone.[4]

Enterobacteriaceae

This is a large family of gram-negative bacterial rods, which, for classification purposes, are divided into lactose fermenters, and nonlactose fermenters (NLF). Lactose fermenters are able to ferment sugars to produce lactic acid, and include *Enterobacter* spp, *E coli*, *K pneumoniae* and *Proteus* spp, which are discussed in the following paragraphs. NLFs include *Salmonella*, *Shigella,* and *Yersinia* species and account for the nonsurgical, but, nevertheless, important disease entities such as typhoid (*Salmonella typhii*), bacillary dysentery (*Shigella dysenteriaea*), food poisoning (*Salmonella entiridis*), and historically, the Plague (*Yersinia pestis*).

E coli is arguably is the most intensively studied bacterial organism since its discovery in 1885. Simple growth requirements and an easily manipulated genetic make-up have resulted in an important biotechnological role today, via the creation of recombinant DNA for the mass production of a variety of proteins. Without acquiring virulence factors, it is an unharmful colonic commensal that often protects bowel against overgrowth of pathogenic species. However, virulent strains of *E coli* account for several types of gastroenteritis and often result in food product recalls and considerable media attention. Easily transmissible through the fecal-oral route, contamination of food products with harmful strains occurs mostly through unhygienic food preparation and include enterotoxigenic, enteropathogenic, enteroinvasive, enterohemorrhagic (0157), and enteroaggregative strains, all of which cause profound diarrhea, with or without fever, and which may be life-threatening. Toxins produced by the various subtypes mediate many of the pathogenic gastroenteritic features. The enterohemorrhagic 0157 strain also causes hemolytic-uremic syndrome in children around 5% of the time, where spread of the 0157 "Vera-toxin" classically results in the triad of microangiopathic hemolytic anemia, acute renal failure, and thrombocytopenia.

Following colonic surgery, *E coli* may result in SSI and/or peritonitis, where illness may be profound. Fortunately the organism remains very sensitive to gentamicin as well as other antimicrobial agents such as cephalosporins, carbapenems, aztreonam, ciprofloxacin, trimethoprim-sulfamethoxazole, and nitrofurantoin. *E coli* resistance to antimicrobial therapy is a growing problem since adaptive mutations in the genome were found to occur at an alarmingly faster rate than previously anticipated.[48] Furthermore, as a common bacterium in polymicrobial biofilm, *E coli* carries multiresistant drug plasmids, which it is able to transfer to other neighboring species, such as *S aureus*, thereby acting as a reservoir of transferable resistance.[49]

Beta-lactam resistance is also on the rise and results in multidrug resistance to a large variety of penicillins and cephalosporins, rendering treatment more difficult.[50] The extensive and empiric use of third generation cephalosporins in surgical intensive care units is etiologic to growing *E coli* antibiotic resistance. The concepts of beta-lactamase resistance and plasmid transference apply similarly to K pneumoniae and other *Enterobacteriaceae* species.

Extended-spectrum beta-lactamase production by gram-negatives resulting in multidrug resistance has been shown to significantly increase mortality, length of hospitalization, and associated costs.[16,51,52]

Pseudomonads

Pseudomonas aeruginosa is a gram-negative rod generally associated with opportunistic infections and most commonly accounts for infections of the urinary tract, ventilator-associated pneumonias (VAP), and wound infections. It is thought to account for up to 8% of SSIs.[4] It plays a role in the formation of bacterial biofilm and is the most frequent colonizer of medical devices and catheters. Community-acquired disease is only rarely caused by *P aeruginosa*.

As a commensal colonizer, superficial culture does not always provide grounds for treatment but blood-borne and deep-seated infections are indications for urgent intervention. This organism has recently gained microbiological attention because of emerging multidrug resistance, thought to occur via complex multistep genetic mutations, drug efflux mechanisms, and horizontal transfer within colonies. The 2004 NNIS report documented rising resistance rates of *P aeruginosa* to both quinolones and imipenem, although imipenem has remained widely effective in many units in the past decade.[23,25] Aminoglycosides and third-generation cephalosporins also remain effective at this time.

Curved, Spiral, or Helical Organisms

Campylobacter jejuni
Via the production of a cholera-like enterotoxin, *Campylobacter jejuni* is now recognized as the most common cause of food-borne gastroenteritis in the developed world, and results in epithelial cell damage in jejunal and ileal segments of affected patients. Postinfection, this organism will rarely result in the Guillain-Barré neuropathy several weeks following gastroenteritic symptoms in affected individuals.

Helicobacter pylori
Helicobacter pylori is a classic helical organism that was only identified as late as 1982 by the Australian Nobel Prize winners Robin Warren and Barry Marshall. Their discovery paved the way for the production of highly effective drug therapy and simple cures, reducing surgical treatment of peptic ulcer disease to a relative rarity. *H pylori* is currently thought to infect half of the world's population and is a recognized risk factor for gastric carcinogenesis.[53] Through its ability to produce urease, this organism is able to evade the hostile acidic environment of the stomach where it most commonly resides and contributes to 90% of peptic ulcer disease. Mucinase production, evasion of the host IgG response, and the potential production of IL-10 to counteract T-lymphocyte cytokine production are all mechanisms that contribute to the organism's virulence.[54] *H pylori* was originally classified as a *Campylobacter* organism, which was subsequently modified to a *Campylobacter*-like organism (CLO). It was reclassified again as a separate entity altogether. "CLO tests" may still ring familiar among surgeons who biopsy gastric mucosa in search of this organism. Peptic ulcer disease therapy was modified to include antibiotics with antacid treatments following successful isolation of the organism and classically includes two of amoxicillin, clarithromycin, tetracycline, or metronidazole with the newer and more potent PPIs.

Other Gram-Negative Species

Acinetobacter spp
This strictly aerobic nonfermenting cocco-bacillus is a nosocomial organism that accounts for serious life-threatening infection in debilitated patients. Sources include hospital surfaces and medical devices because this bacterium is able to survive on wet and dry surfaces alike. Rising resistance among the species along with inherent resistance to antimicrobial agents including penicillin and, occasionally, aminoglycosides has provided cause for concern. Like *Pseudomonas* species, drug efflux and horizontal transfer of resistance play key roles in rising resistance rates. Last resort carbapenems, which were previously highly effective against this organism, are now

susceptible to evolving resistance mechanisms as reported by the CDC. Recent promise has been shown using Polymyxin B in highly resistant species.[55]

Bacteroides fragilis

Bacteroides fragilis is a normal component of the human bowel flora, and the most common anaerobic species involved in intra-abdominal infections. *B fragilis*, an obligate anaerobe, has a polysaccharide capsule that retards phagocytosis and is thus able to evade innate host defense mechanisms.[56] The capsular material is important in the organism's ability to form abscesses, even after the organism has been heat-killed, and is thought to account for its common etiologic role in the formation of appendicitic abscesses. This anaerobic organism is typically associated with other aerobic pathogens in a synergistic relationship, causing mixed infection but prolonging its survival in aerobic conditions. This requires special attention for therapy and in terms of awareness of transference of resistance. This organism is inherently resistant to many antibiotics including aminoglycosides and beta-lactams with recent acquired resistance reported for erythromycin, clindamycin and tetracycline. Current sensitivities include metronidazole, carbapenems, and penicillinase-resistant penicillins.

Fungi

Although these organisms are not typical surgical pathogens, they are seen in surgical patients who are debilitated as a result of comorbid disease, prolonged hospitalization, or extensive antibiotic treatment, where protective commensal flora are eliminated, allowing for pathogenic species of all types to freely differentiate and multiply. Even commensal fungi develop pathogenic properties during times of suboptimal host defense capabilities. Infection caused by fungal organisms is known as mycosis.

Fungal mycoses are broadly divided into superficial and deep infections. Superficial infections include skin, hair, and subcutaneous tissue layers, such as nails and deeper skin planes. Spread usually occurs following direct contact. Deep infection involves internal organs and the bloodstream, where infection is normally restricted to opportunistic fungi affecting immunocompromised individuals. This type of infection is often life-threatening, particularly in debilitated individuals.

In the context of surgical disease, fungal infection is best divided into *C albicans*–related disease (candidiasis) and non–*C albicans* disease, since *C albicans* is the most frequently encountered fungal pathogen in surgical patients. Non–*C albicans* fungi are rarely encountered in surgical patients and are summarized in **Table 2**.

C albicans is a yeastlike fungus that is able to grow in filaments (hyphae and pseudohyphae), a factor that contributes to the organism's potential virulence. Surgical patients who receive potent antimicrobial or chemotherapeutic agents are most susceptible, as well as immunocompromised individuals with nonsurgical diseases such as leukemia and AIDS. Infection in surgical patients occurs in two ways:

- It may occur at sites of normal commensal growth, where elimination of other protective commensals by antimicrobial agents provides an opportunity for unrestricted growth of the fungus. Sites include the mouth, skin, nails, vagina, and bowel.
- Infection may also occur in areas of skin breach, where loss of integrity of the protective defense layer occurs. These areas frequently include blood-catheter sites, where the catheter then acts as a transport medium for the organism from the skin into the circulation. Life-threatening blood-borne candidiasis may ensue. Other areas of skin breach include surgical wounds, where *C albicans* is infrequently involved.

Table 2 Important fungal pathogens[57]	
Superficial Infection	**Deep Infection**
Epidermophyton	Aspergillus
Microsporum	Blastomyces
Trichophyton	Candida
Sporothrix	Coccidioides
	Cryptococcus
	Histoplasma
	Paracoccidioides

Data from Mims C, Dockrell H, Goering R, et al. Medical microbiology. 3rd edition. Mosby; 2004.

Diagnosis may often be made by clinical examination; the appearance of oral candidiasis (thrush) for example is characteristic. However, cultures of blood, wounds, or catheters are usually required. Interpretation of such culture results is problematic, because, except in the case of fungemia, positive culture results may indicate only colonization rather than a true invasive candidal infection.

Antifungal agents are used to treat C albicans infections. These are applied topically in the case of superficial infections, or administered intravenously in the case of deep-seated organ infections or fungal septicemic states. Drug resistance has not been an issue when treating these relatively uncommon pathogens, probably because of the lack of empiric, oversubscribed, and unnecessary prescription of chemotherapy. An appreciation by the treating surgeon that serious fungal infections are likely to coexist with overwhelming bacterial sepsis, especially in the debilitated host, provides grounds for urgent bacterial culture and empiric therapy.

FUTURE IMPLICATIONS

Fundamental research into resistance mechanisms and the genome of the microbe will be required to lower the risk of surgical infections even further. However, an integral understanding of local conditions and the early innate immune response will also be required, as it is doubtful that microbe contamination can ever be eliminated. Definition of the host defense response for a particular individual, particularly those prone to repetitive infections, will eventually lead to targeted therapy augmentation before surgical treatment if infections are to be eliminated. The potential genetic mechanisms that cause only some individuals to spiral into full-fledged septic shock while others are able to fully recover following a microbial insult remain unclear. The heterogeneity of the innate immune cell performance remains poorly defined, but when further understood, will ultimately provide novel avenues for future immune therapy.

University and private sector funding into research dedicated to the intensive study of bacterial genomics and the comprehensive understanding of mechanisms by which resistance is acquired will lead to the development of new and effective antimicrobial agents with previously unrecognized targets. The rapid rise of resistance and acquired adaptive mutations to last-resort chemotherapeutic agents warrants an urgent understanding of the issues at stake. A willingness to contribute through the adequate, accurate, timely, and nonprolonged prescribing of antibiotics is the first step to halting the rapid progression in microbial resistance and is the shared responsibility of all treating surgeons today.

REFERENCES

1. Turina M, Cheadle WG. The management of established surgical site infections. Surg Infect (larchmt) 2006;7(S3):33–41.
2. Polk HC Jr, Lopez-Mayor JF. Postoperative wound infection: a prospective study of determinant factors and prevention. Surgery 1969;66(1):97–103.
3. Khuri SF, Daley J, Henderson W, et al. The National Veterans Administration Surgical Risk Study: risk adjustment for the comparative assessment of the quality of surgical care. J Am Coll Surg 1995;180(5):519–31.
4. National Nosocomial Infections Surveillance (NNIS) report, data summary from October 1986–April 1996, issued May 1996. A report from the National Nosocomial Infections Surveillance (NNIS) System. Am J Infect Control 1996;24(5):380–8.
5. Bowersox J. Experimental staph vaccine broadly protective in animal studies. 1999. Available at: http://www3.niaid.nih.gov/news/newsreleases/1999/staph.htm. Accessed October 20, 2008.
6. Todar K. Todar's online textbook of bacteriology. Online edition 2008. Available at: http://www.textbookofbacteriology.net/. Accessed October 20, 2008.
7. Chambers HF. The changing epidemiology of *Staphylococcus aureus*? Emerg Infect Dis 2001;7(2):178–82.
8. Klein E, Smith DL, Laxminarayan R. Hospitalizations and deaths caused by methicillin-resistant *Staphylococcus aureus*, United States, 1999–2005. Emerg Infect Dis 2007;13(12):1840–6.
9. Crum NF, Lee RU, Thornton SA, et al. Fifteen-year study of the changing epidemiology of methicillin-resistant *Staphylococcus aureus*. Am J Med 2006; 119(11):943–51.
10. Klevens RM, Morrison MA, Nadle J, et al. Invasive methicillin-resistant *Staphylococcus aureus* infections in the United States. JAMA 2007;298(15):1763–71.
11. Awad SS, Elhabash SI, Lee L, et al. Increasing incidence of methicillin-resistant *Staphylococcus aureus* skin and soft-tissue infections: reconsideration of empiric antimicrobial therapy. Am J Surg 2007;194(5):606–10.
12. Naimi TS, LeDell KH, Como-Sabetti K, et al. Comparison of community- and health care-associated methicillin-resistant *Staphylococcus aureus* infection. JAMA 2003;290(22):2976–84.
13. Department of Health and Human Services, Centers for Disease Control and Prevention. Community-Associated MRSA Information for Clinicians. 2008. Available at: http://www.cdc.gov/ncidod/dhqp/ar_mrsa_ca_clinicians.html. Accessed October 20, 2008.
14. Diep BA, Sensabaugh GF, Somboona NS, et al. Widespread skin and soft-tissue infections due to two methicillin-resistant *Staphylococcus aureus* strains harboring the genes for Panton-Valentine leucocidin. J Clin Microbiol 2004;42(5):2080–4.
15. Ellis MW, Hospenthal DR, Dooley DP, et al. Natural history of community-acquired methicillin-resistant *Staphylococcus aureus* colonization and infection in soldiers. Clin Infect Dis 2004;39(7):971–9.
16. Siegel JD, Rhinehart E, Jackson M, et al. The Healthcare Infection Control Practices Advisory Committee. Management of multidrug-resistant organisms in healthcare settings 2006. Available at: http://www.cdc.gov/ncidod/dhqp/pdf/ar/mdroguideline2006.pdf. Accessed October 20, 2008.
17. Hentschke M, Saager B, Horstkotte MA, et al. Emergence of linezolid resistance in a methicillin resistant *Staphylococcus aureus* strain. Infection 2008;36(1):85–7.
18. Vadyvaloo V, Otto M. Molecular genetics of *Staphylococcus epidermidis* biofilms on indwelling medical devices. Int J Artif Organs 2005;28(11):1069–78.

19. von EC, Arciola CR, Montanaro L, et al. Emerging *Staphylococcus* species as new pathogens in implant infections. Int J Artif Organs 2006;29(4):360–7.
20. El-Azizi M, Rao S, Kanchanapoom T, et al. In vitro activity of vancomycin, quinupristin/dalfopristin, and linezolid against intact and disrupted biofilms of staphylococci. Ann Clin Microbiol Antimicrob 2005;4:2–11.
21. Gardlund B, Bitkover CY, Vaage J. Postoperative mediastinitis in cardiac surgery—microbiology and pathogenesis. Eur J Cardiothorac Surg 2002;21(5): 825–30.
22. Tegnell A, Aren C, Ohman L. Coagulase-negative staphylococci and sternal infections after cardiac operation. Ann Thorac Surg 2000;69(4):1104–9.
23. National Nosocomial Infections Surveillance (NNIS) System Report, data summary from January 1992 through June 2004, issued October 2004. Am J Infect Control 2004;32(8):470–85.
24. Schleifer KH, Kilpper-Balz R, Kraus J, et al. Relatedness and classification of *Streptococcus mutans* and "mutans-like" streptococci. J Dent Res 1984;63(8): 1047–50.
25. Turina M, Cheadle WG. Clinical challenges and unmet needs in the management of complicated skin and skin structure, and soft tissue infections. Surg Infect (Larchmt) 2005;6(Suppl 2):23–36.
26. Anaya DA, McMahon K, Nathens AB, et al. Predictors of mortality and limb loss in necrotizing soft tissue infections. Arch Surg 2005;140(2):151–7.
27. Sharma S. Toxic shock syndrome. 2006. Available at: http://www.emedicine.com/med/topic2292.htm. Accessed October 20, 2008.
28. Fischetti VA, Novick RP, Ferretti JJ, et al. Gram-positive pathogens. Washington, DC: ASM Press ; 2000.
29. Marothi YA, Agnihotri H, Dubey D. Enterococcal resistance—an overview. Indian J Med Microbiol 2005;23(4):214–9.
30. Leclercq R, Derlot E, Duval J, et al. Plasmid-mediated resistance to vancomycin and teicoplanin in *Enterococcus faecium*. N Engl J Med 1988;319(3):157–61.
31. Uttley AH, Collins CH, Naidoo J, et al. Vancomycin-resistant enterococci. Lancet 1988;1(8575–6):57–8.
32. Murray BE. Vancomycin-resistant enterococcal infections. N Engl J Med 2000; 342(10):710–21.
33. Karlowsky JA, Jones ME, Draghi DC, et al. Prevalence and antimicrobial susceptibilities of bacteria isolated from blood cultures of hospitalized patients in the United States in 2002. Ann Clin Microbiol Antimicrob 2004;3:7–15.
34. Franklin GA, Moore KB, Snyder JW, et al. Emergence of resistant microbes in critical care units is transient, despite an unrestricted formulary and multiple antibiotic trials. Surg Infect (Larchmt) 2002;3(2):135–44.
35. Perichon B, Courvalin P. Heterologous expression of the enterococcal vanA operon in methicillin-resistant *Staphylococcus aureus*. Antimicrob Agents Chemother 2004;48(11):4281–5.
36. Whitener CJ, Park SY, Browne FA, et al. Vancomycin-resistant *Staphylococcus aureus* in the absence of vancomycin exposure. Clin Infect Dis 2004;38(8): 1049–55.
37. Rice LB. Antimicrobial resistance in gram-positive bacteria. Am J Infect Control 2006;34(5 Suppl 1):S11–9.
38. Tunger A, Aydemir S, Uluer S, et al. In vitro activity of linezolid and quinupristin/dalfopristin against gram-positive cocci. Indian J Med Res 2004;120(6):546–52.
39. Sunenshine RH, McDonald LC. *Clostridium difficile*-associated disease: new challenges from an established pathogen. Cleve Clin J Med 2006;73(2):187–97.

40. Barbut F, Petit JC. Epidemiology of *Clostridium difficile*-associated infections. Clin Microbiol Infect 2001;7(8):405–10.
41. Bignardi GE. Risk factors for *Clostridium difficile* infection. J Hosp Infect 1998; 40(1):1–15.
42. Dial S, Alrasadi K, Manoukian C, et al. Risk of *Clostridium difficile* diarrhea among hospital inpatients prescribed proton pump inhibitors: cohort and case-control studies. CMAJ 2004;171(1):33–8.
43. Dial S, Delaney JA, Barkun AN, et al. Use of gastric acid-suppressive agents and the risk of community-acquired *Clostridium difficile*-associated disease. JAMA 2005;294(23):2989–95.
44. Pepin J, Saheb N, Coulombe MA, et al. Emergence of fluoroquinolones as the predominant risk factor for *Clostridium difficile*-associated diarrhea: a cohort study during an epidemic in Quebec. Clin Infect Dis 2005;41(9):1254–60.
45. Cone JB, Wetzel W. Toxic megacolon secondary to pseudomembranous colitis. Dis Colon Rectum 1982;25(5):478–82.
46. George WL, Rolfe RD, Finegold SM. Treatment and prevention of antimicrobial agent-induced colitis and diarrhae. Gastroenterology 1980;79(2):366–72.
47. Kelly CP, Pothoulakis C, LaMont JT. *Clostridium difficile* colitis. N Engl J Med 1994;330(4):257–62.
48. Johnson JR, Kuskowski MA, Menard M, et al. Similarity between human and chicken *Escherichia coli* isolates in relation to ciprofloxacin resistance status. J Infect Dis 2006;194(1):71–8.
49. Salyers AA, Gupta A, Wang Y. Human intestinal bacteria as reservoirs for antibiotic resistance genes. Trends Microbiol 2004;12(9):412–6.
50. Paterson DL, Bonomo RA. Extended-spectrum beta-lactamases: a clinical update. Clin Microbiol Rev 2005;18(4):657–86.
51. Cosgrove SE. The relationship between antimicrobial resistance and patient outcomes: mortality, length of hospital stay, and health care costs. Clin Infect Dis 2006;42(Suppl 2):S82–9.
52. Stone PW, Gupta A, Loughrey M, et al. Attributable costs and length of stay of an extended-spectrum beta-lactamase-producing *Klebsiella pneumoniae* outbreak in a neonatal intensive care unit. Infect Control Hosp Epidemiol 2003;24(8):601–6.
53. Kwok A, Lam T, Katelaris P, et al. *Helicobacter pylori* eradication therapy: indications, efficacy and safety. Expert Opin Drug Saf 2008;7(3):271–81.
54. Weir DM, Stewart J. Immunology. 8th edition. Edinburgh, UK: Churchill Livingstone; 1997.
55. Rahal JJ. Novel antibiotic combinations against infections with almost completely resistant *Pseudomonas aeruginosa* and *Acinetobacter species*. Clin Infect Dis 2006;43(Suppl 2):S95–9.
56. Onderdonk AB, Kasper DL, Cisneros RL, et al. The capsular polysaccharide of *Bacteroides fragilis* as a virulence factor: comparison of the pathogenic potential of encapsulated and unencapsulated strains. J Infect Dis 1977;136(1):82–9.
57. Mims C, Dockrell H, Goering R, et al. Medical microbiology. 3rd edition. Mosby; 2004.

The Stressed Host Response to Infection: The Disruptive Signals and Rhythms of Systemic Inflammation

Stephen F. Lowry, MD, FACS, FRCS(Edin) (Hon)

KEYWORDS

- Inflammation • Sepsis • Systems biology • Surgery
- Infection • Heart rate variability

Recent surveys document an increasing incidence of community-acquired and noso-comial infections in the United States, with a significant proportion of these infections occurring in an increasingly aged population with underlying health problems.[1,2] Among surgical patients, the stresses of operation or injury also increase the risks for infection and solid organ dysfunction across all population demographics.[3] The present incidence of acquired infection approximating 2% to 3% is likely to continue to increase among nontrauma surgical patients.[4]

THE STRESSED CLINICAL PHENOTYPE

The manifestation of systemic inflammatory response syndrome (SIRS) criteria is the common clinical phenotype of stressed surgical patients. Concerns have repeatedly been expressed that SIRS lacks sufficient specificity and prognostic value since the time the concept was originally proposed as a mechanistically based risk stratification system.[5,6] The SIRS concept does retain value within surgical populations in which morbidity and mortality risks are correlated to the expression and duration of SIRS.[3,7–9]

In essence, the SIRS phenotype reflects the presence of consequential systemic inflammation and suggests increasing risk for complications and an adverse outcome if the criteria are manifested over an extended period. The initial inflammatory stimulus for SIRS may arise from any number of etiologies, including "sterile" stresses, such as pancreatitis, or cross-sectional tissue injury resulting from involuntary injury or surgical

This work was supported by grant GM-34695 from the National Institutes of Health.
Department of Surgery, University of Medicine and Dentistry of New Jersey-Robert Wood Johnson Medical School, 125 Paterson Street, Suite 7300, New Brunswick, NJ 08901, USA
E-mail address: lowrysf@umdnj.edu

interventions. These injuries incite autonomic nervous and neuroendocrine signals that induce limited SIRS criteria, such as leukocytosis[10,11] and increased heart rate, but the simultaneous presence of three or more SIRS criteria is infrequent without overt activation of the innate immune system. It remains to be determined whether this activation can arise solely from sterile signals, such as injured tissues or, in many cases, really signifies activation by means of undetected endogenous or exogenous pathogen ligands.[12]

Evolution did not anticipate the successes of current surgical care or exogenous resuscitation or organ system support and antimicrobial therapies. Many mechanisms of the host response to localized and systemic inflammation have been defined at the molecular level, and recent summaries of these insights relevant to surgical patients have been published.[13–16] We are also increasingly aware of important endogenous variables unique to the individual host. These include, among others, the problems of confounding conditions or treatments and ageing influences, in addition to less overt influences arising from genetic variation. Each of these components contributes to variability in the expressed phenotype of individual patients. In this review, some insights from molecular investigations of inflammatory processes are discussed in the context of host-specific factors and clinical management practices in surgical patients with an acquired infection. The discussion briefly outlines conserved innate immune and neuroendocrine system responses that may transiently restore destabilizing insults.

Acute stressful conditions often precede the secondary insult of pathogen invasion in surgical patients. As a consequence, the so-called "two-hit" model of inflammatory insult has become the commonly accepted paradigm for stressful injury. We are cognizant that the second hit may be sterile or pathogen induced in nature. Although the secondary insult in the context of SIRS is generally perceived to occur 1 or more days after the initial insult, some have suggested that a demonstrable secondary host response may be elicited within a matter of hours after the initial traumatic event.[9] Most prevailing models of secondary insult disregard the role of unknown variables in considering how intrinsic regulatory signals, as well as pathogen virulence, interact during ongoing stress. The discussions in this article address the question as to how an existing non–pathogen-induced stress receives signals from endogenous (patient specific) and exogenous (treatment or pathogen) influences that modify the phenotypes and outcomes of an acquired infection.

LOCAL INFLAMMATORY SIGNALS

In mounting a defense against invasion by foreign organisms, the innate immune responses may well destroy injured and normal tissues and delay processes of wound repair and resolution of inflammation. To facilitate this immune activation, escalation, and resolution, Nathan[17,18] has described a "go-no go" binary information flow between immune cells and injured tissues as a necessary command and control system. The reader is referred to his outstanding discussions for greater detail.[17,18] Tissue molecular signals directing the resolution of localized inflammation are also programmed at an early juncture,[19] although the regulation of these processes during systemic inflammatory conditions is unclear. Contemporary injury science is seeking to define how host recognition systems distinguish and differentially respond to the states of sterile and nonsterile insult.

The immune response to tissue damage must propagate this information within the injury site against a background of systemic inflammatory responses that have potential to disrupt this controlled information exchange and cellular reprogramming.[20]

A significant injury focus is not isolated from systemic endogenous signals that modulate tissue blood flow, cellular metabolism, and what are early containment-enforcing anti-inflammatory signals. The host receives input signals regarding the status of the injury site(s) by means of a combination of soluble and "hard-wired" information channels. This bidirectional information exchange is conveyed by several classes of soluble mediators and by direct neural tissue sensing of mediators at local sites.[21–24]

THE RESPONSE TO THE INITIAL INSULT
Manifestations of the Initial Insult

There may be little evidence of a systemic response in subjects with mild or modest injury.[3] An insult of sufficient magnitude to induce several SIRS criteria induces systemic responses that encompass many features of a proinflammatory state, including activation of the coagulation and complement cascades, in addition to leukocyte and endothelial cell activation. Munford and Pughin[23] have discussed the temporal dynamics of this initial proinflammatory systemic response that evolves in short order to become anti-inflammatory in nature.

The Neuroendocrine Response

Activation of the hypothalamic-pituitary-adrenal axis (HPA) is the classic neuroendocrine response to stressors, including sterile tissue injury, hypoperfusion, or pathogen invasion.[25,26] In a previously healthy host, the initial injury-induced HPA activation elicits a hypermetabolic response and serves to maintain hemodynamic stability acutely, facilitate reprogramming of acute-phase proteins, and exert anti-inflammatory activity. Importantly, HPA activation also promotes an early systemic net anti-inflammatory signal as reflected in reduced levels of several proinflammatory mediators or priming of immune cells for production of anti-inflammatory molecules, such as interleukin (IL)-10.[11] The duration of these HPA-induced anti-inflammatory signals seems to be limited, however, and they probably dissipate within a few hours to days after the initial insult.[10,11]

Neuroendocrine system activation also includes several recently identified peptides that may act in parallel to HPA-derived signals and serve as bridging signals to adaptive immune generation.[27] These anti-inflammatory peptides act, in part, by way of the cyclic adenosine monophosphate (cAMP)-protein kinase A (PKA) signaling pathway and are inducible by infectious ligands. The durability of signaling by means of these neuropeptides in the context of ongoing severe inflammation is largely unknown, but they may serve as an alternative anti-inflammatory mechanism as the influence of other HPA-derived signals wanes.

SIGNALS FOR INNATE IMMUNE SYSTEM ACTIVATION

As noted previously, the innate immune system is initially activated at the local tissue injury site. Resident cells initiate this response and amplify signals for further recruitment of neutrophils and macrophages. These cells express cell surface pattern recognition receptors (PRRs) that detect invariant conserved molecular patterns and foreign nucleic acid structures, allowing the detection of a wide range of microbial pathogens. There are several PRR families that have been identified[28] as signal transducers for threatening exogenous (extra- and intracellular pathogen) molecules and endogenous (nonviable or injured tissue) products. The well-described Toll-like receptors serving these functions also interact with more recently defined intracellular signaling molecules, such as nucleotide oligomerization domain (NOD)-like receptors (NLRs) and a multiprotein cellular complex (inflammasome) that activates cellular caspases.[29]

These later mechanisms lend potential breadth and intensity to the innate inflammatory repertoire, although, again, the activity of NLRs and the inflammasome pathways have not been well described during conditions of sustained stress.[30,31]

During conditions of sterile injury, the cognate ligands for PRRs include diverse products of disrupted cells, including, among others, heat shock proteins, mitochondrial peptides bearing the N-formyl group hyaluronic acid, and the transcription factor HMGB1.[17,18,30,31] The Toll-family receptors are increasingly implicated as receptors for these ligands.[29,32]

In many cases, the early systemic responses to sterile injury are indistinguishable from those arising from infection and many of the same cellular activation events are observed.[33] This is not surprising, given that signals derived from tissue injury and infection converge on the same receptors. Hence, a major consideration is how the immune system recognizes such non–pathogen-induced signals[29] and provides informational cues that constrain the more damaging inflammatory responses invoked by microbial invasion.[17]

Rhythms After the First Hit

Homeostasis exhibits rhythmic physiologic and biochemical activities. The temporal predictability of this endogenous control is presumed to confer acute adaptive advantages[34] that likely extend to modulating systemic illnesses and solid organ function[35] over extended periods.

Circadian entrainment

The molecular regulatory components of the circadian clock[36] generate synchronization that coordinates phase relations among numerous internal rhythms.[37] Indeed, many gene products of the core circadian clock are embedded in regulatory networks necessary for normal cell function.[38] During health, circadian rhythms entrained by light and dark and food intake cycles are readily detectable as neuroendocrine secretory and autonomic activities, including heart rate and blood pressure.

As discussed elsewhere in this article, these entrainment cues are frequently altered in stressed hospitalized patients, and the consequences of this loss of environmental cues have yet to be fully defined in the context of stress.[39] Recent data document that inflammation-inducing ligands, including endotoxin[40] and tumor necrosis factor-α (TNFα),[41] suppress the expression of clock regulatory genes in the suprachiasmic nucleus and in peripheral tissues. This linkage of innate immune system activation to circadian rhythm control has yet to be explored in the setting of persistent systemic inflammation.

Autonomic rhythms

Autonomic function also exhibits circadian rhythmicity as assessed by measures of heart rate variability (HRV).[42] This daily fluctuation in frequency and power spectra has implications for sympathetic and parasympathetic balance and the acute regulation of systemic inflammatory activity. Autonomic imbalance, reflected by sympathetic activity excess (or parasympathetic attenuation), is associated with increased morbidity in patients who have severe sepsis.[43] A reduction in parasympathetic activity may be associated with diminished capacity to exert vagal cholinergic control over proinflammatory mediator activity.[44] Reductions in implied vagal nerve activity have now been noted during inflammatory conditions associated with endotoxinemic conditions in humans[45] and in experimental conditions of sterile systemic inflammation.[46] Hence, continued attenuation of vagal activity during SIRS may impede this alternative mechanism for controlling inflammatory balance.

Endocrine rhythms

The secretion of endocrine hormones is also subject to circadian rhythms and to intermittent stimuli, such as feeding and emotion.[47] As detailed elsewhere, a characteristically enhanced endocrine hormone profile is elicited during the early-phase response to injury or infection.[18,26,48,49] These hormone signals promote acute-phase metabolic and immunologic programming of target tissues.

Pathogens of the Initial Insult

Comprehensive discussions of the spectrum of initial pathogens complicating surgical illnesses are provided elsewhere in this issue. The reader is also referred to recent overviews of pathogen recognition mechanisms and discussion of virulence acquisition[28,29,50] and to discussions of plausible genetic determinants of pathogen recognition and immune responsiveness.[51–53] Most such reports do not, however, discuss these factors in the context of an existing non–pathogen-induced host response.

Modifiers of the Initial Injury Response

A healthy person subjected to an acute insult relies on stereotypic responses to recognize, contain, and resolve local sites of injury or pathogen invasion. The concept of a prototypical "healthy" host response must, however, be modified by patient-specific (endogenous) factors, some of which are discussed elsewhere in this article **(Fig. 1)**. It can be conjectured that initial host responses are more influenced by these

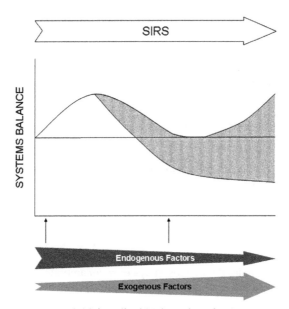

Fig.1. The host response to an initial sterile "hit" (stress), such as trauma or surgery, includes activation of inflammation-responsive systems (eg, innate immune system) modified primarily by the magnitude of insult and patient-specific (endogenous) factors. As the systemic inflammatory response arising from an initial stress continues, patient management and pathogen virulence (exogenous factors) assume a more prominent influence on the balance of systems activity. Responses lower than the basal level generally reflect reduced end-organ responsiveness (tolerance) and reduced signal input variance (adaptability). The interactions between endogenous and exogenous factors lead to uncertainty (gray area) over time about systems activity and overall responsiveness to secondary insults, such as infection.

endogenous host-specific factors than during later phases of SIRS, when therapies or interventions, iatrogenic misadventure, and diminished host adaptability become more consequential.

Age

More than 50% of patients receiving intensive care are older than 65 years of age.[1] Advancing age is clearly associated with increased morbidity and mortality. The relation between age-related immune competence and confounding illness is, however, more complex than commonly appreciated.[54,55] Epidemiologic data attest to the concept of "immuno-ageing," wherein proinflammatory innate immune responsiveness is reasonably well preserved among many older subjects.[56] The ageing population exhibits increased cytokine markers of low-grade inflammation (eg, IL-6), and this is associated with increased risk for development of infection[57] and other stressful events.[58] Elderly subjects challenged with lipopolysaccharide (LPS) also exhibit a more prolonged febrile response and hypotension,[56,59,60] in addition to prolonged and enhanced cytokine responses during pneumococcal pneumonia.[61]

Although some theories of ageing suggest that innate immune response capacity is sustained, at least in part, by the accumulated influences of noxious challenges, such as oxidative stress,[62] there may be other interacting factors that promote proinflammatory competence during ageing. For instance, the diminution of autonomic variability, particularly of vagal activity, that accompanies advancing age[42] may promote enhanced TNFα activity during initial stress. By contrast, physical conditioning enhances parasympathetic system signaling and provides a survival advantage to physically fit elderly patients during acute inflammatory stress by attenuating cytokine excesses.

The process of immunosenescence, or age-related defects in the human immune system, affects principally the adaptive immune response.[55,56] There is a gradual loss of T-cell repertoire from naive CD8 T cells and reduced response to neoantigens in elderly subjects. Concomitantly, there is a gradual shift from a type 1 cytokine response (eg, IL-2, interferon-γ [IFNγ], TNFα) toward a type 2 response (eg, IL-4, IL-6, IL-10, IL-15) that further impairs cell-mediated immunity.

Gender

It is widely assumed that gender influences the initial inflammatory response and risk profile resulting from injury. A discussion of the possible mechanisms underlying this canon is extensively presented elsewhere.[63,64] Nevertheless, recent single-institution reports,[65] multi-institutional prospective studies,[66,67] and report compilations[68] question the validity of the assumed female gender benefit among trauma patients. There are also conflicting reports regarding gender-based responses to lesser inflammatory challenges, such as to endotoxin.[69,70] Suffice it to say that, at present, there are no consistent gender-specific differences in systemic inflammatory responses reported among humans subjected to an initial sterile or pathogen-induced stress.

Confounding Illness and Treatment

There has been surprisingly little prospective correlation of acute inflammatory responses among noncardiac surgical patients that has carefully assessed the influence of confounding illnesses. Indeed, the precise classification of relevant confounding illness remains in flux.[54] Pittet and colleagues[71] noted several preexisting conditions that influenced the outcome of bacteremia in surgical patients, including, among others, recent surgery, antibiotic therapy, and previous cardiogenic shock or resuscitation. However dated this observation may be, the importance of such conditions suggests that a recent systemic inflammatory condition may predispose to infection and adversely influence outcome.

Genetic Factors

Inheritance contributes to the risk for premature life-threatening infection.[72] Although the mechanisms for this increased risk are not defined, there are identifiable low- and high-inflammatory cytokine response patterns among random subjects[73] and a strong genetic linkage for stimulated cytokine production among monozygotic twins.[74] Genome manipulations in animals clearly suggest that genetic variation within key cell signaling or response pathways may alter local and systemic innate and adaptive immune responses.[75] Genetic variation within homologous loci among humans is also likely to influence the host capacity to recognize and resolve tissue inflammation or respond to pathogen invasion. Genetic variation may also contribute to the expressed magnitude and duration of the SIRS phenotype, as suggested, for example, by variable cholinesterase activities and the resultant response to endotoxin.[76]

Initial Interventions

Resuscitation

It is recognized that fluid resuscitation modifies host inflammatory responses to infectious[77,78] or noninfectious insults.[79–81] Variations in fluid resuscitation regimens also result in varying inflammatory responses among older patients.[82] It is presently unknown if these initial resuscitation-modified inflammatory changes influence later immune, endocrine, and autonomic capacities during later phases of the SIRS condition. Substantial information regarding some of these issues may be forthcoming when detailed analyses of large multi-institutional studies are reported.[83]

Antimicrobial therapy

As discussed elsewhere in this issue, there is little doubt that inappropriate use of antimicrobial therapies increases the risk for overall infection and the emergence of resistant organisms. The use of prophylactic agents in patients with initial sterile stress has received limited study as to systemic inflammatory responses. It is clear, however, that inadequate antimicrobial therapy independently increases outcome risk among patients who have SIRS and develop nosocomial infection.[84] This adverse effect is likely enhanced among surgical patients who have complex illness.[51,85]

RESPONSES TO SUBSEQUENT INSULTS

The components of host response from an initial insult are more clearly defined than are those resulting from secondary events (see **Fig. 1**). The various clinical phenotypes and outcome trajectories resulting from prolonged stress in conjunction with infection have been debated for years. Several prominent overviews of this complex topic have been published.[86–89]

Although a de novo infectious challenge, in and of itself, yields variation in early host responses,[90] the later phases of SIRS promote an even broader palate of functional system(s) phenotypes as intervention-related influences interact with endogenous determinants. There may be conflicting signals being transmitted in parallel and, in some cases, isolation of tissues from the normal feedback controls of the uncomplicated state.[91] Persistent proinflammatory activity is manifest, for example, by continued coagulation system activation,[92] even as other markers of proinflammatory activity may be waning.[90] Simultaneously, variations in the competence of innate and adaptive immune defenses become evident within some tissue sites.[20,93–95] The mechanisms underlying this evolved condition of innate immune "tolerance" and diminished capacity for neoantigen responses are more thoroughly discussed elsewhere.[21,96] An important feature of SIRS is a persistent acute-phase response that experimental studies suggest may modify immune competence and solid organ function.[97–99] In the context of ongoing inflammation, altered innate immune competence may occur by means of gene-silencing programs or other mechanisms.[20,29,100]

Altered Rhythms During the Secondary Insult

Not infrequently, a prolonged stress state manifests diminishing amplitude, frequency, and efficiency of autonomic and neuroendocrine signaling.[91,101] For example, there have been several reports documenting diminished time domain measures of HRV among critically ill infected and injured patients[43,102–105] that correlate to increased solid organ dysfunction and mortality risk. Reduced host adaptability, as reflected in such measures of total power, may serve as a surrogate marker of organ systems' "connectedness" and of overall host capacity to respond effectively to inflammatory stressors.[101,106]

Disturbances in short-term variability and longer term circadian rhythmicity of neuroendocrine hormone secretion are also observed during prolonged inflammatory illness.[48,49] Attenuated hormone rhythmicity and signal amplitude are known to associate with ischemic events[47] and may likewise contribute to disordered metabolic and immune functions.[39,48,49] An intriguing association of reduced cardiac rate variability to adrenal cortical tolerance (or relative insufficiency) has been noted in some injured patients.[107]

Pathogens of the Second Hit

The SIRS state promotes loss of adaptive immune surveillance that likely enhances virulence factor acquisition in some bacterial species.[21,50,108] Although de novo infection may elicit distinctive gene expression patterns within immune cells,[109,110] immune cell expression signatures during acquired infections seem to converge during ongoing inflammation.[111–113] These observations suggest that a diminished immune system repertoire (variability) reflects another aspect of altered host adaptability.

MODIFIERS OF THE SECONDARY INSULT
Age

Age-related diminutions of immune and endocrine functions[114] and autonomic signal attenuation may all contribute to adverse outcomes among elderly patients. There is currently limited insight across the age spectrum as to how prominently these endogenous factors contribute to loss of adaptability during prolonged stress.

Genetic Factors

Most genetic association studies within seriously ill patients have been reported from mixed populations of community-acquired and nosocomial infections. The caveats for deriving definitive conclusions from existing clinical gene association studies have been discussed.[51,53] Nevertheless, there have been some single-institution prospective studies of highly stressed at-risk surgical populations, such as those with trauma and burns, that are highly suggestive of genetic contribution to nosocomial infectious risk. For example, functional single-nucleotide polymorphisms of proinflammatory cytokines[51,115–117] and pathogen recognition receptors[116,118] repeatedly associate with enhanced infection risk in stressed patients. Interestingly, these polymorphisms do not overtly modulate human responses[119] during health but only seem to enhance risk and alter responses in the context of ongoing stress.

THE INFLUENCES OF CURRENT TREATMENT PRACTICES

Little is known about how currently "acceptable" treatment practices (exogenous factors) might alter host adaptability. Several such strategies have been adopted after prospective demonstrations of improved outcomes that also exhibited some diminution of inflammatory markers. Interestingly, most of these adopted support modalities are designed to reduce signal input variance to the stressed host. Several current management practices are briefly discussed to speculate as to how invariant clinical management practices might alter the phenotypes and systemic responses of stressed patients.

Mechanical Ventilation

Current management of respiratory failure generally conforms to protective strategies that impose constraints to variations in volume, pressure, or oxygenation parameters.[120–123] These approaches seem to promote the resolution of initial pulmonary inflammation and related organ system dysfunction.[123] How these management practices influence inflammatory responses to a later tissue injury or infection challenge remains a matter of some conjecture.

Glucose Control

The clinical management concept of rigid glucose level control (reduced variability) has been rapidly adopted by the intensivist community.[124] There is now some reconsideration of this rigorous protocol,[125] and the issue of how varying ranges of glucose and insulin control may modulate inflammatory responses remains open to question.[126,127]

Route and Composition of Feeding

The use of parenteral nutrition has greatly diminished as a management practice among stressed patients.[128] Several inflammatory mediator responses may be potentiated during continuous parenteral feeding.[129–131] Some data suggest that these enhanced responses may be related to the composition of parenteral feeding regimens.[132] Importantly, continuous enteral or parenteral feeding may dampen cellular and systemic regulatory signals exerted by autonomic and circadian rhythms.[133] Hence, alternative management strategies designed to enhance variability of nutrient provision might further leverage any benefits of nutritional support.

REFERENCES

1. Angus DC, Linde-Zwirble WT, Lidicker J, et al. Epidemiology of severe sepsis in the United States: analysis of incidence, outcome, and associated costs of care. Crit Care Med 2001;29:1303–10.
2. Martin GS, Mannino DM, Eaton S, et al. The epidemiology of sepsis in the United States from 1979 through 2000. N Engl J Med 2003;348:1546–54.
3. Osborn TM, Tracy JK, Dunne JR, et al. Epidemiology of sepsis in patients with traumatic injury. Crit Care Med 2004;32:2234–40.
4. Vogel TR, Dombrovskiy VK, Lowry S. Postoperative sepsis: are we improving outcomes? Surg Infections 2008; in press.
5. Bone RC. Toward an epidemiology and natural history of SIRS (systemic inflammatory response syndrome). JAMA 1992;268:3452–5.
6. Bone RC, Balk RA, Cerra FB, et al. Definitions for sepsis and organ failure and guidelines for the use of innovative therapies in sepsis. The ACCP/SCCM

Consensus Conference Committee. American College of Chest Physicians/ Society of Critical Care Medicine. Chest 1992;101:1644–55.

7. Napolitano LM, Ferrer T, McCarter RJ Jr, et al. Systemic inflammatory response syndrome score at admission independently predicts mortality and length of stay in trauma patients. J Trauma 2000;49:647–52.

8. Talmor M, Hydo L, Barie PS. Relationship of systemic inflammatory response syndrome to organ dysfunction, length of stay, and mortality in critical surgical illness: effect of intensive care unit resuscitation. Arch Surg 1999;134:81–7.

9. Tschoeke SK, Hellmuth M, Hostmann A, et al. The early second hit in trauma management augments the proinflammatory immune response to multiple injuries. J Trauma 2007;62:1396–403.

10. Barber AE, Coyle SM, Marano MA, et al. Glucocorticoid therapy alters hormonal and cytokine responses to endotoxin in man. J Immunol 1993;150:1999–2006.

11. van der Poll T, Coyle SM, Barbosa K, et al. Epinephrine inhibits tumor necrosis factor-alpha and potentiates interleukin 10 production during human endotoxemia. J Clin Invest 1996;97:713–9.

12. Carcillo JA. Searching for the etiology of systemic inflammatory response syndrome: is SIRS occult endotoxemia? Intensive Care Med 2006;32:181–4.

13. Giannoudis PV. Current concepts of the inflammatory response after major trauma: an update. Injury 2003;34:397–404.

14. Keel M, Trentz O. Pathophysiology of polytrauma. Injury 2005;36:691–709.

15. Robertson CM, Coopersmith CM. The systemic inflammatory response syndrome. Microbes Infect 2006;8:1382–9.

16. Smith JW, Gamelli RL, Jones SB, et al. Immunologic responses to critical injury and sepsis. J Intensive Care Med 2006;21:160–72.

17. Nathan C. Points of control in inflammation. Nature 2002;420:846–52.

18. Nathan C. Neutrophils and immunity: challenges and opportunities. Nat Rev Immunol 2006;6:173–82.

19. Serhan CN, Savill J. Resolution of inflammation: the beginning programs the end. Nat Immunol 2005;6:1191–7.

20. Cavaillon JM, Adrie C, Fitting C, et al. Reprogramming of circulatory cells in sepsis and SIRS. J Endotoxin Res 2005;11:311–20.

21. Angele MK, Faist E. Clinical review: immunodepression in the surgical patient and increased susceptibility to infection. Crit Care 2002;6:298–305.

22. Molina PE. Neurobiology of the stress response: contribution of the sympathetic nervous system to the neuroimmune axis in traumatic injury. Shock 2005;24:3–10.

23. Munford RS, Pugin J. Normal responses to injury prevent systemic inflammation and can be immunosuppressive. Am J Respir Crit Care Med 2001;163:316–21.

24. Tracey KJ. The inflammatory reflex. Nature 2002;420:853–9.

25. Chrousos GP. The hypothalamic-pituitary-adrenal axis and immune-mediated inflammation. N Engl J Med 1995;332:1351–62.

26. Lowry SF. Host metabolic response to injury. In: Gallin J, Fauci A, editors, Advances in host defense mechanisms, vol 6. New York: Raven Press; 1986. p. 169–90.

27. Gonzalez-Rey E, Chorny A, Delgado M. Regulation of immune tolerance by anti-inflammatory neuropeptides. Nat Rev Immunol 2007;7:52–63.

28. Akira S, Uematsu S, Takeuchi O. Pathogen recognition and innate immunity. Cell 2006;124:783–801.

29. Barton GM. A calculated response: control of inflammation by the innate immune system. J Clin Invest 2008;118:413–20.

30. Petrilli V, Papin S, Tschopp J. The inflammasome. Curr Biol 2005;15:R581.
31. Zedler S, Faist E. The impact of endogenous triggers on trauma-associated inflammation. Curr Opin Crit Care 2006;12:595–601.
32. Mollen KP, Anand RJ, Tsung A, et al. Emerging paradigm: toll-like receptor 4—sentinel for the detection of tissue damage. Shock 2006;26:430–7.
33. Chen CJ, Kono H, Golenbock D, et al. Identification of a key pathway required for the sterile inflammatory response triggered by dying cells. Nat Med 2007;13:851–6.
34. Fuller PM, Lu J, Saper CB. Differential rescue of light- and food-entrainable circadian rhythms. Science 2008;320:1074–7.
35. Martino TA, Oudit GY, Herzenberg AM, et al. Circadian rhythm disorganization produces profound cardiovascular and renal disease in hamsters. Am J Physiol Regul Integr Comp Physiol 2008;294:R1675–83.
36. Reppert SM, Weaver DR. Coordination of circadian timing in mammals. Nature 2002;418:935–41.
37. Turek FW. Staying off the dance floor: when no rhythm is better than bad rhythm. Am J Physiol Regul Integr Comp Physiol 2008;294:R1672–4.
38. Kohsaka A, Bass J. A sense of time: how molecular clocks organize metabolism. Trends Endocrinol Metab 2007;18:4–11.
39. Carlson DE, Chiu WC. The absence of circadian cues during recovery from sepsis modifies pituitary-adrenocortical function and impairs survival. Shock 2008;29:127–32.
40. Okada K, Yano M, Doki Y, et al. Injection of LPS causes transient suppression of biological clock genes in rats. J Surg Res 2008;145:5–12.
41. Cavadini G, Petrzilka S, Kohler P, et al. TNF-alpha suppresses the expression of clock genes by interfering with E-box-mediated transcription. Proc Natl Acad Sci U S A 2007;104:12843–8.
42. Bonnemeier H, Richardt G, Potratz J, et al. Circadian profile of cardiac autonomic nervous modulation in healthy subjects: differing effects of aging and gender on heart rate variability. J Cardiovasc Electrophysiol 2003;14:791–9.
43. Annane D, Trabold F, Sharshar T, et al. Inappropriate sympathetic activation at onset of septic shock: a spectral analysis approach. Am J Respir Crit Care Med 1999;160:458–65.
44. Tracey KJ. Physiology and immunology of the cholinergic antiinflammatory pathway. J Clin Invest 2007;117:289–96.
45. Alvarez SM, Katsamanis Karavidas M, Coyle SM, et al. Low-dose steroid alters in vivo endotoxin-induced systemic inflammation but does not influence autonomic dysfunction. J Endotoxin Res 2007;13:358–68.
46. van Westerloo DJ, Giebelen IA, Florquin S, et al. The vagus nerve and nicotinic receptors modulate experimental pancreatitis severity in mice. Gastroenterology 2006;130:1822–30.
47. Steptoe A, Wardle J, Marmot M. Positive affect and health-related neuroendocrine, cardiovascular, and inflammatory processes. Proc Natl Acad Sci U S A 2005;102:6508–12.
48. Van den Berghe G, de Zegher F, Bouillon R. Clinical review 95: acute and prolonged critical illness as different neuroendocrine paradigms. J Clin Endocrinol Metab 1998;83:1827–34.
49. Van den Berghe GH. The neuroendocrine stress response and modern intensive care: the concept revisited. Bur 1999;25:7–16.
50. van der Poll T, Opal SM. Host-pathogen interactions in sepsis. Lancet Infect Dis 2008;8:32–43.

51. Imahara SD, O'Keefe GE. Genetic determinants of the inflammatory response. Curr Opin Crit Care 2004;10:318–24.

52. Moine P, Abraham E. Immunomodulation and sepsis: impact of the pathogen. Shock 2004;22:297–308.

53. Villar J, Maca-Meyer N, Perez-Mendez L, et al. Bench-to-bedside review: understanding genetic predisposition to sepsis. Crit Care 2004;8:180–9.

54. Dhainaut JF, Claessens YE, Janes J, et al. Underlying disorders and their impact on the host response to infection. Clin Infect Dis 2005;41(Suppl 7)):S481–9.

55. Gruver AL, Hudson LL, Sempowski GD. Immunosenescence of ageing. J Pathol 2007;211:144–56.

56. Opal SM, Girard TD, Ely EW. The immunopathogenesis of sepsis in elderly patients. Clin Infect Dis 2005;41(Suppl 7):S504–12.

57. Yende S, Tuomanen EI, Wunderink R, et al. Preinfection systemic inflammatory markers and risk of hospitalization due to pneumonia. Am J Respir Crit Care Med 2005;172:1440–6.

58. Cesari M, Penninx BW, Newman AB, et al. Inflammatory markers and onset of cardiovascular events: results from the health ABC study. Circulation 2003; 108:2317–22.

59. Krabbe KS, Bruunsgaard H, Hansen CM, et al. Ageing is associated with a prolonged fever response in human endotoxemia. Clin Diagn Lab Immunol 2001;8: 333–8.

60. Krabbe KS, Bruunsgaard H, Qvist J, et al. Hypotension during endotoxemia in aged humans. Eur J Anaesthesiol 2001;18:572–5.

61. Bruunsgaard H, Skinhoj P, Qvist J, et al. Elderly humans show prolonged in vivo inflammatory activity during pneumococcal infections. J Infect Dis 1999;180: 551–4.

62. Butcher SK, Lord JM. Stress responses and innate immunity: aging as a contributory factor. Aging Cell 2004;3:151–60.

63. Choudhry MA, Bland KI, Chaudry IH. Gender and susceptibility to sepsis following trauma. Endocr Metab Immune Disord Drug Targets 2006;6:127–35.

64. Choudhry MA, Bland KI, Chaudry IH. Trauma and immune response—effect of gender differences. Injury 2007;38:1382–91.

65. Magnotti LJ, Fischer PE, Zarzaur BL, et al. Impact of gender on outcomes after blunt injury: a definitive analysis of more than 36,000 trauma patients. J Am Coll Surg 2008;206:984–91.

66. Sperry JL, Nathens AB, Frankel HL, et al. Characterization of the gender dimorphism after injury and hemorrhagic shock: are hormonal differences responsible? Crit Care Med 2008;36:1838–45.

67. Sperry JL, Friese RS, Frankel HL, et al. Male gender is associated with excessive IL-6 expression following severe injury. J Trauma 2008;64:572–8.

68. Proctor KG. Gender differences in trauma theory vs. practice: comments on "Mechanism of estrogen-mediated intestinal protection following trauma-hemorrhage: p38 MAPK-dependent upregulation of HO-1" by Hsu JT, et al. Am J Physiol Regul Integr Comp Physiol 2008;294:R1822–4.

69. Coyle SM, Calvano SE, Lowry SF. Gender influences in vivo human responses to endotoxin. Shock 2006;26:538–43.

70. van Eijk LT, Dorresteijn MJ, Smits P, et al. Gender differences in the innate immune response and vascular reactivity following the administration of endotoxin to human volunteers. Crit Care Med 2007;35:1464–9.

71. Pittet D, Thievent B, Wenzel RP, et al. Importance of pre-existing co-morbidities for prognosis of septicemia in critically ill patients. Intensive Care Med 1993;19:265–72.
72. Sorensen TI, Nielsen GG, Andersen PK, et al. Genetic and environmental influences on premature death in adult adoptees. N Engl J Med 1988;318:727–32.
73. Wurfel MM, Park WY, Radella F, et al. Identification of high and low responders to lipopolysaccharide in normal subjects: an unbiased approach to identify modulators of innate immunity. J Immunol 2005;175:2570–8.
74. de Craen AJ, Posthuma D, Remarque EJ, et al. Heritability estimates of innate immunity: an extended twin study. Genes Immun 2005;6:167–70.
75. De Maio A, Torres MB, Reeves RH. Genetic determinants influencing the response to injury, inflammation, and sepsis. Shock 2005;23:11–7.
76. Ofek K, Krabbe KS, Evron T, et al. Cholinergic status modulations in human volunteers under acute inflammation. J Mol Med 2007;85:1239–51.
77. Rivers E, Nguyen B, Havstad S, et al. Early goal-directed therapy in the treatment of severe sepsis and septic shock. N Engl J Med 2001;345:1368–77.
78. Rivers EP, Ahrens T. Improving outcomes for severe sepsis and septic shock: tools for early identification of at-risk patients and treatment protocol implementation. Amsterdam, The Netherlands: Elsevier Inc; 2008.
79. Lang K, Boldt J, Suttner S, et al. Colloids versus crystalloids and tissue oxygen tension in patients undergoing major abdominal surgery. Anesth Analg 2001;93:405–9.
80. Lang K, Suttner S, Boldt J, et al. Volume replacement with HES 130/0.4 may reduce the inflammatory response in patients undergoing major abdominal surgery. Can J Anaesth 2003;50:1009–16.
81. McKinley BA, Valdivia A, Moore FA. Goal-oriented shock resuscitation for major torso trauma: what are we learning? Curr Opin Crit Care 2003;9:292–9.
82. Boldt J, Ducke M, Kumle B, et al. Influence of different volume replacement strategies on inflammation and endothelial activation in the elderly undergoing major abdominal surgery. Intensive Care Med 2004;30:416–22.
83. Moore FA, McKinley BA, Moore EE, et al. Inflammation and the host response to injury, a large-scale collaborative project: patient-oriented research core—standard operating procedures for clinical care. III. Guidelines for shock resuscitation. J Trauma 2006;61:82–9.
84. Harbarth S, Garbino J, Pugin J, et al. Inappropriate initial antimicrobial therapy and its effect on survival in a clinical trial of immunomodulating therapy for severe sepsis. Am J Med 2003;115:529–35.
85. Imahara SD, Nathens AB. Antimicrobial strategies in surgical critical care. Curr Opin Crit Care 2003;9:286–91.
86. Annane D, Bellissant E, Cavaillon JM. Septic shock. Lancet 2005;365:63–78.
87. Bone RC. Immunologic dissonance: a continuing evolution in our understanding of the systemic inflammatory response syndrome (SIRS) and the multiple organ dysfunction syndrome (MODS). Ann Intern Med 1996;125:680–7.
88. Hotchkiss RS, Karl IE. The pathophysiology and treatment of sepsis. N Engl J Med 2003;348:138–50.
89. Singer M, De Santis V, Vitale D, et al. Multiorgan failure is an adaptive, endocrine-mediated, metabolic response to overwhelming systemic inflammation. Lancet 2004;364:545–8.

90. Kellum JA, Kong L, Fink MP, et al. Understanding the inflammatory cytokine response in pneumonia and sepsis: results of the genetic and inflammatory markers of sepsis (GenIMS) study. Arch Intern Med 2007;167:1655–63.

91. Buchman TG. Nonlinear dynamics, complex systems, and the pathobiology of critical illness. Curr Opin Crit Care 2004;10:378–82.

92. Rangel-Frausto MS, Pittet D, Costigan M, et al. The natural history of the systemic inflammatory response syndrome (SIRS). A prospective study. JAMA 1995;273:117–23.

93. Cavaillon JM, Annane D. Compartmentalization of the inflammatory response in sepsis and SIRS. J Endotoxin Res 2006;12:151–70.

94. Munoz C, Carlet J, Fitting C, et al. Dysregulation of in vitro cytokine production by monocytes during sepsis. J Clin Invest 1991;88:1747–54.

95. Rogy MA, Oldenburg HS, Coyle S, et al. Correlation between acute physiology and chronic health evaluation (APACHE) III score and immunological parameters in critically ill patients with sepsis. Br J Surg 1996;83:396–400.

96. Cavaillon JM, Adrie C, Fitting C, et al. Endotoxin tolerance: is there a clinical relevance? J Endotoxin Res 2003;9:101–7.

97. Lagoa CE, Bartels J, Baratt A, et al. The role of initial trauma in the host's response to injury and hemorrhage: insights from a correlation of mathematical simulations and hepatic transcriptomic analysis. Shock 2006;26:592–600.

98. Renckens R, Roelofs JJ, Knapp S, et al. The acute-phase response and serum amyloid A inhibit the inflammatory response to Acinetobacter baumannii Pneumonia. J Infect Dis 2006;193:187–95.

99. Renckens R, van Westerloo DJ, Roelofs JJ, et al. Acute phase response impairs host defense against Pseudomonas aeruginosa pneumonia in mice. Crit Care Med 2008;36:580–7.

100. McCall CE, Yoza BK. Gene silencing in severe systemic inflammation. Am J Respir Crit Care Med 2007;175:763–7.

101. Lowry SF, Calvano SE. Challenges for modeling and interpreting the complex biology of severe injury and inflammation. J Leukoc Biol 2008;83:553–7.

102. Morris JA Jr, Norris PR, Ozdas A, et al. Reduced heart rate variability: an indicator of cardiac uncoupling and diminished physiologic reserve in 1,425 trauma patients. J Trauma 2006;60:1165–73.

103. Norris PR, Morris JA Jr, Ozdas A, et al. Heart rate variability predicts trauma patient outcome as early as 12 h: implications for military and civilian triage. J Surg Res 2005;129:122–8.

104. Norris PR, Ozdas A, Cao H, et al. Cardiac uncoupling and heart rate variability stratify ICU patients by mortality: a study of 2088 trauma patients. Ann Surg 2006;243:804–12.

105. Winchell RJ, Hoyt DB. Analysis of heart-rate variability: a noninvasive predictor of death and poor outcome in patients with severe head injury. J Trauma 1997; 43:927–33.

106. Godin PJ, Buchman TG. Uncoupling of biological oscillators: a complementary hypothesis concerning the pathogenesis of multiple organ dysfunction syndrome. Crit Care Med 1996;24:1107–16.

107. Morris JA Jr, Norris PR, Waitman LR, et al. Adrenal insufficiency, heart rate variability, and complex biologic systems: a study of 1,871 critically ill trauma patients. J Am Coll Surg 2007;204:885–92.

108. Wu L, Estrada O, Zaborina O, et al. Recognition of host immune activation by Pseudomonas aeruginosa. Science 2005;309:774–7.

109. Jenner RG, Young RA. Insights into host responses against pathogens from transcriptional profiling. Nat Rev Microbiol 2005;3:281–94.
110. Nau GJ, Richmond JF, Schlesinger A, et al. Human macrophage activation programs induced by bacterial pathogens. Proc Natl Acad Sci U S A 2002;99: 1503–8.
111. Johnson SB, Lissauer M, Bochicchio GV, et al. Gene expression profiles differentiate between sterile SIRS and early sepsis. Ann Surg 2007;245:611–21.
112. Ramilo O, Allman W, Chung W, et al. Gene expression patterns in blood leukocytes discriminate patients with acute infections. Blood 2007;109:2066–77.
113. Tang BM, McLean AS, Dawes IW, et al. Gene-expression profiling of gram-positive and gram-negative sepsis in critically ill patients. Crit Care Med 2008;36:1125–8.
114. Chahal HS, Drake WM. The endocrine system and ageing. J Pathol 2007;211: 173–80.
115. Cobb JP, Mindrinos MN, Miller-Graziano C, et al. Application of genome-wide expression analysis to human health and disease. Proc Natl Acad Sci U S A 2005;102:4801–6.
116. Barber RC, Aragaki CC, Rivera-Chavez FA, et al. TLR4 and TNF-alpha polymorphisms are associated with an increased risk for severe sepsis following burn injury. J Med Genet 2004;41:808–13.
117. Menges T, Konig IR, Hossain H, et al. Sepsis syndrome and death in trauma patients are associated with variation in the gene encoding tumor necrosis factor. Crit Care Med 2008;36:1456–62, e1–6.
118. Agnese DM, Calvano JE, Hahm SJ, et al. Human toll-like receptor 4 mutations but not CD14 polymorphisms are associated with an increased risk of gram-negative infections. J Infect Dis 2002;186:1522–5.
119. Calvano JE, Bowers DJ, Coyle SM, et al. Response to systemic endotoxemia among humans bearing polymorphisms of the Toll-like receptor 4 (hTLR4). Clin Immunol 2006;121:186–90.
120. Ventilation with lower tidal volumes as compared with traditional tidal volumes for acute lung injury and the acute respiratory distress syndrome. The Acute Respiratory Distress Syndrome Network. N Engl J Med 2000;342:1301–8.
121. Forel JM, Roch A, Marin V, et al. Neuromuscular blocking agents decrease inflammatory response in patients presenting with acute respiratory distress syndrome. Crit Care Med 2006;34:2749–57.
122. Parsons PE, Eisner MD, Thompson BT, et al. Lower tidal volume ventilation and plasma cytokine markers of inflammation in patients with acute lung injury. Crit Care Med 2005;33:1–6.
123. Ranieri VM, Suter PM, Tortorella C, et al. Effect of mechanical ventilation on inflammatory mediators in patients with acute respiratory distress syndrome: a randomized controlled trial. JAMA 1999;282:54–61.
124. Van den Berghe G, Wilmer A, Hermans G, et al. Intensive insulin therapy in the medical ICU. N Engl J Med 2006;354:449–61.
125. Angus DC, Abraham E. Intensive insulin therapy in critical illness. Am J Respir Crit Care Med 2005;172:1358–9.
126. Stegenga ME, van der Crabben SN, Blumer RM, et al. Hyperglycemia enhances coagulation and reduces neutrophil degranulation, whereas hyperinsulinemia inhibits fibrinolysis during human endotoxemia. Blood 2008;112:82–9.
127. Vanhorebeek I, Langouche L, Van den Berghe G. Glycemic and nonglycemic effects of insulin: how do they contribute to a better outcome of critical illness? Curr Opin Crit Care 2005;11:304–11.

128. Rhee P, Hadjizacharia P, Trankiem C, et al. What happened to total parenteral nutrition? The disappearance of its use in a trauma intensive care unit. J Trauma 2007;63:1215–22.

129. Fong YM, Marano MA, Barber A, et al. Total parenteral nutrition and bowel rest modify the metabolic response to endotoxin in humans. Ann Surg 1989;210: 449–56.

130. Lowry SF. The route of feeding influences injury responses. J Trauma 1990;30: S10–5.

131. van der Poll T, Levi M, Braxton CC, et al. Parenteral nutrition facilitates activation of coagulation but not of fibrinolysis during human endotoxemia. J Infect Dis 1998;177:793–5.

132. van der Poll T, Coyle SM, Levi M, et al. Fat emulsion infusion potentiates coagulation activation during human endotoxemia. Thromb Haemost 1996;75:83–6.

133. Lowry SF. A new model of nutrition influenced inflammatory risk. J Am Coll Surg 2007;205:S65–8.

Antimicrobial Agents for Surgical Infections

Nilam P. Patel, PharmD, BCPS[a], Mark A. Malangoni, MD, FACS[b,c],*

KEYWORDS

- Antibiotics • Antifungals • Infections
- Antimicrobial prophylaxis

The discovery of antibiotics is one of the major advances in the treatment of infectious diseases. Millions of lives have been saved, and death caused by many infections has plummeted with their use. Despite this advance, microorganisms remain ubiquitous in nature and infections continue to occur because of contamination and the invariable susceptibility of humans to disease.

As bacteria and fungi have become exposed to antibiotics, they have developed resistance to these drugs in a number of unique ways. This response has been countered by the development and production of newer agents that are less susceptible to bacterial resistance; however, bacteria in particular continue to create new ways to protect themselves from annihilation. This is particularly true among staphylococci and many gram-negative organisms. In addition, many of the more effective drugs are encumbered by adverse reactions that can limit their use and effectiveness (**Table 1**).

Antibiotics are typically used in three distinct situations: (1) empiric therapy, (2) definitive therapy, and (3) prophylaxis. Empiric treatment is used for the initial treatment of an infection, often without specific identification of the responsible pathogen or pathogens. In this situation, it is important to choose therapy based on the suspected organisms responsible for the infection. This can be influenced by the disease under consideration, the susceptibility of the patient, and the environment in which the disease has occurred. In general, broad-spectrum therapy is initiated in these situations. It is critical to perform cultures and to de-escalate therapy based on the antimicrobial sensitivity in 24 to 72 hours, when results are generally available.

If the responsible pathogens have been identified, definitive therapy is used. Patient susceptibility remains an important consideration, because some patients may not be able to tolerate the development of antimicrobial resistance while being treated. The goal of definitive therapy is to provide optimal chance for cure by using a narrow-spectrum, cost-effective, and safe agent. Because many infections in surgical patients are

[a] Critical Care, Department of Pharmacy, 2500 MetroHealth Medical Center, Cleveland, OH 44109–1998, USA
[b] Case Western University School of Medicine, Cleveland, OH, USA
[c] Department of Surgery, H-914, 2500 MetroHealth Medical Center, Cleveland, OH 44109–1998, USA
* Corresponding author.
E-mail address: mmalangoni@metrohealth.org (M.A. Malangoni).

Surg Clin N Am 89 (2009) 327–347
doi:10.1016/j.suc.2008.09.005
0039-6109/08/$ – see front matter
surgical.theclinics.com

Table 1
Common antimicrobial agents used in the management of surgical infections

Drug	Common Indications	Spectrum of Activity	Dose	Mode of Elimination	Notable Adverse Drug Reactions	Comments
Penicillins						
Penicillin G	Infections caused by clostridia and streptococci	Very limited	1–4 million units IV q 4–6 h	Renal	Allergic reactions, diarrhea, nausea	—
Penicillinase-resistant						
Dicloxacillin	Infections caused by *Staphylococcus aureus*, methicillin-sensitive	MSSA	250–500 mg po q 6 h	Fecal, renal	Allergic reactions, diarrhea, nausea	—
Nafcillin	Infections caused by *S aureus*, methicillin-sensitive	MSSA	0.5–2 g IV q 4–6 h	Hepatic	Allergic reactions, diarrhea, nausea	Modification of dose may be necessary for patients with both renal and hepatic dysfunction; platelet dysfunction with higher doses
Oxacillin	Infections caused by *S aureus*, methicillin-sensitive	MSSA	0.5–2 g IV q 4–6 h	Hepatic	Allergic reactions, diarrhea, nausea	No dosage adjustment needed unless CrCl <10 mL/min
Aminopenicillins						
Ampicillin	UTI, bacteremia	Includes *Enterococcus faecalis*	0.5–1 g po q 6 h; 1–2 g IV q 4–6 h	Renal	Allergic reactions, diarrhea, nausea	—
Amoxicillin	UTI	Includes *E faecalis*	250–500 mg po q 8 h	Renal	Allergic reactions, rash, diarrhea, nausea	—
Penicillin β-lactamase inhibitor						
Amoxicillin-clavulanate	SSTI	MSSA, PSP, PCN S, pneumococcus, anaerobes	500 mg q 8 h or 875 mg q 12 h po	Renal	Allergic reactions, diarrhea, nausea, cholestatic jaundice	Sometimes used off-label for oral switch with IAI

Drug	Indications	Spectrum	Dose	Elimination	Adverse effects	Comments
Ampicillin-sulbactam	SSTI, IAI, sinusitis	MSSA, PSP, PCN S pneumococcus, anaerobes	1.5–3 g IV q 6 h	Renal	Allergic reactions, diarrhea, nausea	Limited use because of high incidence of resistant gram-negatives
Piperacillin-tazobactam	IAI, SSTI, HAP	Very broad spectrum including *Pseudomonas aeruginosa*, Enterobacteraciae, MSSA, anaerobes, *E faecalis*.	3.375 g IV q 6 h	Renal	Allergic reactions, diarrhea, nausea	—
Ticarcillin-clavulanate	IAI, SSTI, HAP, UTI	Very broad spectrum including *Stenotrophomonas maltophilia*; less active against *P aeruginosa* than piperacillin-tazobactam	3.1 g IV q 6–8 h	Renal	Allergic reactions, diarrhea, nausea	Do not mix with aminoglycosides because of potential inactivation
Cephalosporins						
First generation						
Cefazolin	UTI, SSTI, early HAP, AP	Primarily gram-positive	1–2 g IV q 6 h	Renal	Allergic reactions, diarrhea	Limited activity against gram-negatives
Second generation						
Cefotetan	AP, UTI	Some gram-negatives with anaerobic coverage including *Bacteroides fragilis*	1–2 g IV q 8 h	Renal	Allergic reactions, hypoprothrombinemia, GI disturbances	—
Cefoxitin	IAI, UTI, AP	Some gram-negatives with anaerobic coverage including *B fragilis*	2 g IV q 6 h	Renal	Allergic reactions, GI disturbances	Increasing resistance to gram-negatives

(continued on next page)

Table 1
(*continued*)

Drug	Common Indications	Spectrum of Activity	Dose	Mode of Elimination	Notable Adverse Drug Reactions	Comments
Third generation						
Cefotaxime	IAI, SSTI, HAP	Gram-positive including *S pneumoniae*; gram-negatives	2 g IV q 8 h	Renal	Allergic reactions, GI disturbances	No pseudomonal coverage
Ceftazidime	HAP, SSTI	Gram-negatives including *P aeruginosa*	1–2 g IV q 8 h	Renal	Allergic reactions, GI disturbances	Induces extended-spectrum lactamase, no gram-positive coverage
Ceftizoxime	SSTI, HAP	Gram-positives and gram-negatives	1–3 g IV q 6–8 h	Renal	Allergic reactions, GI disturbances	
Ceftriaxone	IAI, SSTI, HAP	Good activity against *S. pneumoniae* and *Haemophilus influenzae*	1–2 g IV q 12–24 h	Fecal, renal	Allergic reactions, GI disturbances	No dosing adjustment needed in renal insufficiency; use higher dose and shorter dosing interval when treating meningitis
Fourth generation						
Cefepime	IAI, SSTI, HAP, UTI	MSSA, broad gram-negative activity including *P aeruginosa*	1–2 g IV q 12 h	Renal	Allergic reactions, GI disturbances	—
Carbapenems						
Doripenem	IAI, HAP	Broad spectrum of activity including *P aeruginosa*	500 mg IV q 8 h	Renal	—	—

Drug	Indications	Spectrum	Dosing	Elimination	Adverse effects	Comments
Ertapenem	IAI, SSTI, AP	Gram-positive and gram-negatives; anaerobes	1 g IV q 24 h	Renal	Allergic reactions, diarrhea, thrombocytopenia, abnormal LFTs	Useful for prophylaxis in colorectal operations; not active against *P aeruginosa*, enterococcus, Acinetobacter or *H influenzae*
Imipenem-cilastatin	IAI, SSTI, HAP	Broad spectrum of activity includes *A calcoaceticus-baumanni* complex	0.5-1 g IV q 6 h	Renal	Fever, rash, nausea, vomiting, diarrhea, seizures	Avoid in chronic renal failure; useful for acute sinusitis in hospitalized patients
Meropenem	IAI, SSTI	Broad spectrum of activity includes *A calcoaceticus-baumanni* complex	1-2 g IV q 8 h	Renal	Nausea, vomiting, diarrhea, rash	Useful to treat meningitis after craniotomy or ventriculostomy; useful for acute sinusitis in hospitalized patients. Higher doses should be used to treat meningitis.
Monobactams						
Aztreonam	IAI, SSTI, HAP	No activity against gram-positives or anaerobes	1-2 g IV q 6-8 h	Renal	Rash, diarrhea, nausea, vomiting, elevated transaminases	Useful for patients with non-IgE β-lactam allergy
Aminoglycosides						
Amikacin	Bone, RTI, and septicemia, other infections caused by susceptible gram-negative organisms	Gram-negatives including *P aeruginosa*	Serious gram-negative infections: 7.5-10 mg/kg/dose IV q 8-12 h ODA: 15-20 mg/kg/d	Renal	Nephrotoxicity and ototoxicity with trough levels >8	Use higher end of dosing range for patients who have increased volume of distribution (trauma, burns); goal peak serum level for life-threatening infections is 25-35mcg/ml; trough levels <8mcg/ml; must adjust dose in renal insufficiency

(continued on next page)

Table 1
(continued)

Drug	Common Indications	Spectrum of Activity	Dose	Mode of Elimination	Notable Adverse Drug Reactions	Comments
Gentamicin	Bone, RTI, UTI, IAI (in combination), septicemia	Gram-negatives including P aeruginosa, may be used synergistically to treat susceptible S aureus	Synergy: 1 mg/kg/dose IV q 8–12 h Serious gram-negative infections: 2–3 mg/kg/dose q 8–12 h ODA: 5–7 mg/kg/d	Renal	Nephrotoxicity and ototoxicity with trough levels >2	Use higher end of dosing range for patients who have increased volume of distribution (trauma, burns); goal peak serum level for life threatening infections 8–10 µg/mL; trough levels <2 µg/mL; when used for synergy goal peak levels: 3–4 µg/mL and trough <1 µg/mL; must adjust dose in renal insufficiency
Tobramycin	Infections caused by susceptible gram-negative organisms	Gram-negatives including P. aeruginosa, may be used synergistically to treat susceptible S aureus	Synergy: 1 mg/kg/dose IV q 8–12 h Serious gram-negative infections: 2–3 mg/kg/dose q 8–12 h ODA: 5–7 mg/kg/d	Renal	Nephrotoxicity and ototoxicity with trough levels >2	
Quinolones						
Ciprofloxacin	UTI; pyelonephritis; LRTI; SSTI; bone and joint, IAI (in combination with metronidazole); infectious diarrhea; febrile neutropenia; HAP; CA-MRSA	Enterobacteriaceae, P aeruginosa, Serratia, H influenzae, M catarrhalis, Neisseria gonorrhoeae, atypicals (Chlamydia, Mycoplasma, Legionella)	400 mg IV q 8–12 h 500–750 mg po q 12 h	Renal	Mental status changes with higher doses; seizures, QT prolongation (higher incidence with moxifloxacin than with other quinolones); tendon rupture; arthropathy; interstitial nephritis; increase transaminases	Best activity in class versus P aeruginosa; unreliable activity against enterococci, staphylococci, and streptococci; must adjust dose when CrCl <30 mL/min
Levofloxacin	CAP, LRTI, URTI, UTI, acute sinusitis, SSTI, pyelonephritis, prostatitis	Enterobacteriaceae, H influenzae, M catarrhalis, N gonorrhoeae, atypicals, S pneumoniae, ± MSSA	500–750 mg IV or po q 24 h	Renal		Has some activity against P aeruginosa; adjust dose when CrCl <50 mL/min

Moxifloxacin	CAP, URTI, SSTI, IAI	Enterobacteriaceae, H influenzae, M catarrhalis, N gonorrhoeae, atypicals, S pneumoniae, MSSA, + anaerobes	400 mg IV or po q 24 h	Primarily fecal		No P aeruginosa activity, little urinary activity; no adjustment needed in renal failure; avoid use in patients with severe cirrhosis
Macrolides, lincosamides						
Azithromycin	Acute pharyngitis, URTI, LRTI, SSTI, CAP, acute sinusitis	Some gram-positive activity, less than erythromycin; atypicals (Legionella, Chlamydia, Mycoplasma), H influenzae; best activity against Legionella	RTI, SSTI: 500 mg on day 1 followed by 250 mg/day days 2–5; CAP: 500 mg q 24 h	Hepatic	GI disturbances; elevated transaminases; QTc prolongation (rare)	Also covers N meningitis, N gonorrhoeae; substrate of CYP 3A4 but minimal drug interactions
Clarithromycin	Acute pharyngitis, URTI, LRTI, SSTI, CAP, acute sinusitis	Similar spectrum to azithromycin; however, less activity against gram-negatives, such as H influenzae and M catarrhalis	250–500 mg q 12 h or extended release 1 g q 24 h	Hepatic	Hepatoxicity, metallic taste	Substrate and inhibitor of CYP450 3A4
Erythromycin	URTI, SSTI	Highly active against group A β-hemolytic streptococci, PCN-sensitive S aureus	Base: 250–500 mg po q 6–12 h 500 m–1 g IV q 6 h (max 4 g/24 h)	Hepatic	Transient hearing loss with large doses IV, GI disturbances, QTc prolongation	Substrate and inibitor of CYP450 3A4 system, many drug interactions

(continued on next page)

Table 1
(continued)

Drug	Common Indications	Spectrum of Activity	Dose	Mode of Elimination	Notable Adverse Drug Reactions	Comments
Clindamycin	Sinusitis, necrotizing SSTI, alternative to β-lactams for surgical prophylaxis	Staphylococci sp Streptococci sp, anaerobes: CA-MRSA	150–450 mg po q 6–8 h 300–900 mg IV q 6–8 h	Hepatic	Diarrhea, elevated LFTs; *Clostridium difficile* enterocolitis	Useful alternative for patients with penicillin allergy; no activity against enterococci, MRSE, or MRSA
Ketolides						
Telithromycin	CAP, URTI, sinusitis	*S pneumoniae, H influenzae, M catarrhalis,* atypicals	800 mg po q d	Hepatic	QTc prolongation, hepatic failure, myasthenia gravis exacerbations	Use cautiously with other agents that prolong QTc interval; is substrate for and inhibits CYP450 3A4; monitor for potential drug interactions
Tetracyclines/glycylcyclines[8,23,24]						
Doxycycline	UTI	Rickettsia, atypicals (*Legionella, Chlamydia, Mycoplasma*), Spirochetes, non-TB mycobacteria. Doxycycline has good activity against *S pneumoniae* (not penicillin resistant). Minocycline has very good activity against *S aureus* and coagulase-negative staphylococci; CA-MRSA	100 mg IV or po q 12 h	Hepatic; substrate of CYP3A4 system	Photosensitivity; hepatotoxicity; esophageal ulceration (minimized with adequate fluid intake with capsule or tablet)	Calcium, magnesium, and aluminum containing products decrease intestinal absorption considerably. Fatal nephrotoxicity seen when administered with methoxyflurane anesthetics. Anticonvulsants decrease tetracycline levels; potentiation of warfarin effects; increased digoxin levels seen when given with doxycycline
Minocycline	Anthrax, rickettsial diseases, acute intestinal amebiasis		200 mg IV or po initial dose followed by 100 mg q 12 h	Renal		

Drug	Indication	Spectrum	Dose	Elimination	Adverse effects	Comments
Tigecycline	SSTI, IAI	MSSA, MRSA, GISA, MRSE, S pyogenes, S agalactiae, S pneumoniae, VRE, gram-negative aerobes, some anaerobic activity	100 mg IV × 1 followed by 50 mg IV q 12 h		Nausea and vomiting	No activity against P aeruginosa. Not ideal for blood stream infections because plasma levels drop soon after completion of infusion. Excellent tissue penetration. Reduce dose in severe hepatic insufficiency
Polymyxins[6,8,25]						
Colistin/ colistimethate/ polymyxin E	Infection caused by susceptible gram-negative bacteria, particularly multiple drug resistant organisms	Active against most multiple drug resistant gram-negative aerobes including P aeruginosa; no activity against Proteus sp, Providencia, Burkholderia, and Serratia sp	2.5–5 mg/kg/d in 2–4 divided doses; max daily dose is 300 mg	Renal; dose must be significantly adjusted in renal insufficiency	Neurotoxicity, nephrotoxicity	Available for inhaled use; use adjusted body weight for dosing in obesity
Polymyxin B			15,000–25,000 units/kg/d q 12 h			Significantly higher fluid volume associated with each dose when compared with colistimethate
Agents for drug-resistant gram-positive infections[8,24,26–28]						
Daptomycin	SSTI, bacteremia, right-sided endocarditis	Gram-positive aerobes including E faecalis (vancomycin-susceptible strains only), E faecium (including VRE), MSSA, MRSA, MSSE, MRSE, S agalactiae, S pyogenes	SSTI: 4 mg/kg IV q 24 h Bacteremia or right-sided endocarditis: 6 mg/kg IV q 24 h	Renal	Elevations in creatine phosphokinase; monitor creatine phosphokinases weekly; elevation in LFTs	Poor efficacy for treatment of pneumonia, rapidly inactivated. Discontinue any 3-hydroxy-3-methylglutaryl coenzyme A reductase inhibitors on initiation of daptomycin because of increased risk of rhabdomyolysis. Administer q 48 h when CrCl <30 mL/min

(continued on next page)

Table 1 (continued)

Drug	Common Indications	Spectrum of Activity	Dose	Mode of Elimination	Notable Adverse Drug Reactions	Comments
Linezolid	SSTI, CAP	*E faecium, E faecalis* (vancomycin resistant) MSSA, MRSA, MSSA, MSSE	600 mg IV or po q 12 h	Hepatic	Thrombocytopenia; myelosuppression (generally seen with use >2 weeks); lactic acidosis; increased LFTs; optic neuropathy	Monitor complete blood count weekly. Linezolid is a monoamine oxidase inhibitor. Use with a selective serotonin reuptake inhibitor may precipitate serotonin syndrome, discontinue selective serotonin reuptake inhibitors before initiating linezolid and monitor for signs and symptoms of serotonin syndrome. No dosage adjustment necessary in renal or hepatic failure
Quinupristin/ dalfopristin	*E faecium* (vancomycin-resistant) bacteremia, SSTI	MRSA, MSSA, streptococci sp	7.5 mg/kg IV q 8 h	Hepatic	Myalgias, arthralgias, hyperbilirubinemia	Significantly inhibits CYP3A4 system; many drug interactions
Vancomycin	Treatment of infections caused by staphylococcal and streptococcal sp; used orally for staphylococcal entercolitis and *C difficile* colitis	*Enterococcus* sp (not VRE), MSSA, MRSA, *Streptococcus* sp	10–15 mg/kg/dose q 8–12 h *C difficile* colitis: 125–250 mg po q 6 h	Renal	Ototoxicity with high levels (>80 µg/mL), interstitial nephritis, nephrotoxicity	Trough levels should be monitored and targeted for efficacy. Levels of 5–15 µg/mL are acceptable for most infections. Levels of 15–20 µg/mL may be needed for such infections as meningitis, endocarditis, pneumonia secondary to MRSA, and osteomyelitis. Adjust dose in renal insufficiency

Miscellaneous agents[8,29-32]

Chloramphenicol	Serious infections caused by susceptible strains of bacteria	Good gram-negative, gram-positive, and anaerobic activity; no activity against *P aeruginosa*	50–100 mg/kg/d IV q 6 h; maximum daily dose 4 g/day	Hepatic	Serious and fatal blood dyscrasias; monitor complete blood count while on therapy; gray baby syndrome; GI disturbances	Therapeutic levels: 15–20 µg/mL Toxic levels: >40 µg/mL Avoid use in severe hepatic impairment
Nitazoxanide	Treatment of diarrhea caused by *Cryptosporidium parvum* or *Giardia lambia*; alternative for *C difficile* colitis	Active against a broad range of parasites, *Bacteroides sp, C difficile*, gram-positive aerobes	500 mg po q 12 h	Hepatic to active metabolite	Diarrhea, nausea, increase in LFTs	—
Metronidazole	IAI, *C difficile* colitis	Gram-negative anaerobes: *Bacteroides sp, Fusobacterium sp.* Gram-positive anaerobes: *Clostridium sp*; activity against other gram-positive anaerobes is variable	500 mg IV or po q 6–8 h	Hepatic	Disulfiram reaction when administered with alcohol, GI disturbances, confusion.	Reduce dose in severe hepatic impairment. Decrease interval to q 12 h when CrCl <10 mL/min
Rifampin	Adjunctive therapy for treatment of gram-positive bacteremia; CA-MRSA	Aerobic and anaerobic gram-positive and enteropathogenic gram-negatives	300–600 mg po q 12–24 h	Hepatic	Hepatotoxicity, red/orange body fluids, central nervous system toxicity	Do not use alone because of rapid development of resistance. Potent inducer of CYP450 system. Many drug interactions

(continued on next page)

Table 1
(continued)

Drug	Common Indications	Spectrum of Activity	Dose	Mode of Elimination	Notable Adverse Drug Reactions	Comments
Rifaximin	Alternative therapy for relapsing or refractory C. difficile colitis	Aerobic and anaerobic gram-positive and enteropathogenic gram-negatives	200 mg po q 8 h or 400 mg q 12 h	Unchanged in feces	GI disturbances	Not absorbed po
Sulfamethoxazole-trimethoprim	CA- MRSA, SSTI, treatment of choice for S maltophilia, first line agent for UTI	MSSA, MRSA, Escherichia coli, S maltophilia, Pneumocystis carinii	UTI: 800/160 mg po q 12 h; S maltophilia or P carinii pneumonia: 15–20 mg/kg/d IV or po in 3–4 divided doses CA-MRSA: 2 DS tablets (800/160) q 12 h or up to 10 mg/kg/d in divided doses	Renal	Rash, SJS, TEN, crystalluria, hyperkalemia with higher doses	Dosing interval must be adjusted in renal failure
Amphotericin[8,33–35]						
Amphotericin B Liposomal amphotericin Lipid complex amphotericin Amphotericin B cholestryl complex	Candidemia, aspergillosis, crypococcal meningitis	Candida sp, Aspergillus sp, histoplasmosis, Cryptococcus	0.25–1 mg/kg/d IV 3–6 mg/kg/d IV based on indication 5 mg/kg/d IV 3–4 mg/kg/d IV	Renal	Nephrotoxicity (less with lipid products); infusion-related reactions (rigors, chills, hypotension, itching, electrolyte abnormalities)	Lipid products are generally better tolerated than nonlipid amphotericin

Echinocandins[8,36,37]

	Indications	Spectrum	Dosing	Elimination	Adverse Effects	Comments
Anidulafungin	Esophageal candidiasis, candidemia, invasive candidiasis	*Aspergillus* sp, *Candida* sp. Variable against *C parapsilosis*. No activity against *Cryptococcus neoformans* or *Fusarium*.	Esophageal candidiasis: 100 mg followed by 50 mg q d. All other indications: 200 mg followed by 100 mg q d	Spontaneous degradation	Hepatotoxicity	Limited drug interactions, well tolerated
Micafungin	Only indicated for esophageal candidiasis and prophylaxis against *Candida* after stem cell transplant		Esophageal candidiasis: 150 mg q d. Prophylaxis: 50 mg q d	Hepatic		
Caspofungin	Treatment of invasive *Aspergillus* and candidal infections, candidemia, empiric therapy for suspected fungal infections in febrile neutropenia		70 mg IV followed by 50 mg q d			

Azoles[8,38,39]

	Indications	Spectrum	Dosing	Elimination	Adverse Effects	Comments
Fluconazole	Candidiasis	*C albicans*	400–1600 mg followed by 200–800 mg q 24 h IV or po	Renal	Hepatotoxicity	Use with caution in patients with hepatic failure. May need to use higher doses for nonalbicans sp
Itraconazole	Blastomycosis, histoplasmosis, aspergillosis	*C albicans*, *Aspergillus* sp, *Cryptococcus*	200 mg q 12 h IV or po × 4 doses followed by 200 mg IV q d	Hepatic	Hepatotoxicity, QTc prolongation, negative inotropic effects with IV administration	Variable activity against nonalbicans should not be used in patients with CrCl <30 mL/min because of accumulation of the vehicle. Potent inhibitor of CYP450 system

(continued on next page)

Table 1
(continued)

Drug	Common Indications	Spectrum of Activity	Dose	Mode of Elimination	Notable Adverse Drug Reactions	Comments
Voriconazole	Invasive aspergillosis	C albicans, C krusei, C tropicalis, C glabrata, C parapsilosis, Aspergillus sp	6 mg/kg IV q 12 h × 2 doses followed by 4 mg/kg q 12 h 200 mg po q 12 h	Hepatic	Visual disturbances, hepatotoxicity, rash	Do not use when CrCl <50 mL/min because of accumulation of IV vehicle. PO dose is 100 mg q 12 when patients weight <40 kg.
Miscellaneous antifungals						
Flucytosine	Used in combination with other agents in management of candidiasis, crytococcosis	Candida and Cryptococcus	50–150 mg/kg/d po q 6 h	Renal	Cardiotoxicity, myelosuppression, hepatotoxicity	Dose must be adjusted in renal failure. Do not use alone because resistance develops quickly in vivo

Abbreviations: AP, antimicrobial prophylaxis; CA-MRSA, community-acquired MRSA; CAP, community-acquired pneumonia; CrCl, creatinine clearance; GI, gastrointestinal; GISA, glycopeptide intermediate *S aureus*; HAP, hospital-acquired infection; IAI, intra-abdominal infection; LFT, liver function tests; LRTI, lower respiratory tract infection; MRSA, methicillin-resistant *S aureus*; MRSE, methicillin resistant *S epidermidis*; MSSA, methicillin-sensitive *S aureus*; ODA, once-daily administration; PCN, penicillin; PRP, penicillin-resistant pneumococcus; PSP, penicillin-sensitive pneumococcus; RTI, respiratory tract infection; SJS, Stevens-Johnson syndrome; SSTI, skin and soft tissue infection; TEN, toxic epidermal necrolysis; URTI, upper respiratory tract infection; UTI, urinary tract infection; VRE, vancomycin-resistant enterococcus.

polymicrobial, definitive therapy may involve using a broader-spectrum agent or multiple antimicrobial agents administered concurrently. In other cases, definitive therapy may require two drugs given in combination for synergy to achieve bactericidal activity against the microorganism or to prevent resistance from developing.

Another important use of antimicrobials in surgical patients is for prophylaxis, particularly in the perioperative period. This is the most common reason for prescribing parenteral antibiotics in the health care environment. Recommendations for the use of prophylactic antibiotics are based on the risk of surgical site infection, the susceptibility of the patient, and the exposure of the incision to contamination and environmental effects.

In each of these circumstances, it is important to select the proper agent, dose, and dosing interval. It may be necessary to repeat the perioperative dose depending on the length of operation.

The duration of treatment can vary based on the disease being treated, the intensity of the infection, and host susceptibility. In general, there is little Class I information about the duration of treatment for most infections. When these data are available, they should be followed. In the absence of discrete information, it is best to treat the patient until the acute signs of infection (fever, leukocytosis, tachycardia, and tachypnea) have resolved. Some organisms, such as *Staphylococcus aureus*, have a tendency to disseminate through the bloodstream or may be more difficult to eradicate, requiring a longer duration of treatment.

Although age is usually not a determinant in the selection of antimicrobial agents, the loss of renal function that can accompany advanced age can be a concern. Even though the initial serum creatinine may be in the normal range, creatinine clearance is often reduced in elderly patients. Patients with pre-existing renal insufficiency or diminished renal function cannot tolerate treatment with potentially nephrotoxic drugs, such as gentamicin or amphotericin B. Adjustment for hepatic dysfunction is more difficult to predict for drugs that rely on liver metabolism or excretion. Because of this, the dose of these agents is usually done on an empiric basis and serum drug levels should be monitored when possible in this situation.

The availability of many effective oral antimicrobials has allowed one to minimize the duration of parenteral treatment in many circumstances. As an infection comes under control with intravenous treatment, it is often possible to "switch" to oral therapy, given that there is an appropriate drug with appropriate gastrointestinal absorption available, and the patient has had a return in gastrointestinal function. The switch allows for continuation of treatment at a lower cost, is more convenient for the patient, and can result in earlier discharge from the hospital. If the same antimicrobial being given parenterally does not have an oral form, there is often another agent available within the same drug class that can substitute. At times, it is necessary actually to switch to another class of drug that is effective according to the sensitivity report.

PENICILLINS

The discovery and mass production of penicillin stands as a landmark in the history of antibiotics. These agents are bactericidal, have a low toxicity, and are widely distributed throughout the body. With time, there has been increasing antimicrobial resistance to the older agents and newer penicillins have a much greater spectrum of activity, particularly against gram-negatives. The β-lactam structure of penicillin has served as the basis for synthetic penicillins and cephalosporins. Newer agents are products of manipulation of the β-lactam ring that have led to a broader spectrum of activity and increased resistance to enzymatic degradation by β-lactamases and penicillin-binding proteins. The combination of β-lactamase inhibitors with some of the newer agents has further increased their efficacy. These agents are generally active without the need for metabolization. About 3% to 10% of the population is allergic to penicillins, which is a major limitation to their use.[1]

CEPHALOSPORINS

The cephalosporins are a large group of β-lactam–based antibiotics that have multiple indications for usage and possess many of the same essential characteristics as penicillins. Cephalosporins are classified by generations. In general, there is increasing gram-negative activity and decreasing gram-positive activity as one progresses from first- to third-generational drugs. Certain agents possess unique activity profiles. Cefotetan and cefoxitin, two second-generation cephalosporins also referred to as "cephamycins," have a unique pharmacologic structure that confers effectiveness against *Bacteroides fragilis*. Cefepime, currently the only fourth-generation cephalosporin, is highly active against both gram-positive and gram-negative bacteria, including *Pseudomonas*.[2]

Cephalosporins have a very favorable efficacy-to-toxicity profile. Like penicillins, they are susceptible to β-lactamases and penicillin-binding protein inactivation. Besides having multiple indications for use in different disease states, cephalosporins are the mainstay for perioperative antimicrobial prophylaxis. The allergic cross-reactivity with penicillin allergy is less than 5% and only 1% to 2% of patients without a penicillin allergy are allergic to cephalosporins. These drugs should be avoided if the patient has a Type I IgE-mediated penicillin allergy (anaphylaxis, angioedema).

CARBAPENEMS

This class of drugs is also based on a β-lactam ring but has a structure that is more resistant to bacteria than many penicillins and cephalosporins. Carbapenems have a very broad spectrum of activity including anaerobic bacteria. Imipenem has been combined with cilastatin to avoid inactivation and accumulation of a potentially toxic metabolite. Patients with central nervous system lesions, a history of seizures, or renal failure should be given imipenem-cilastatin with caution, because drug-related seizure activity has been seen in these patients. The allergic cross-reactivity of carbapenems with penicillins is similar to cephalosporins. These drugs should be avoided if the patient has a Type I IgE-mediated penicillin allergy (anaphylaxis, angioedema).[3]

MONOBACTAMS

Aztreonam is currently the only monobactam available. It has excellent activity against gram-negative bacteria, but no activity against gram-positives or anaerobes. This drug is also susceptible to β-lactamases. There is minimal cross-reactivity in patients with penicillin allergy. Because this drug has no major nephrotoxicity or ototoxicity, it is useful to treat patients with renal insufficiency.[4]

AMINOGLYCOSIDES

Aminoglycosides were introduced into practice in the 1970s. Surprisingly, even with antimicrobial resistance on the rise, aminoglycosides continue to be effective against most gram-negative organisms with little development of resistance. In addition to their activity against gram-negative organisms, gentamicin and tobramycin have also demonstrated synergistic activity against *Enterococcus* and *Staphylococcus* sp when combined with vancomycin, cefazolin, or nafcillin. In this case, lower serum levels and hence a lower dose are needed than for the treatment of infections caused by gram-negative organisms.[5,6]

There are some issues that may make aminoglycosides less than ideal to use. Generally speaking, aminoglycosides have poor tissue penetration. In addition, the risk of nephrotoxicity requires monitoring of serum aminoglycoside levels, which also adds expense to their use. The risk of nephrotoxicity is greater with more frequent dosing and when other nephrotoxic agents are given concurrently. Appropriate monitoring of serum levels, dosage adjustment for age, renal function, and weight can decrease the risk of nephrotoxicity. Once-daily administration (ODA), or so-called "high-dose" aminoglycoside therapy, has also been demonstrated to decrease the incidence of nephrotoxicity. ODA involves administering a single large dose of aminoglycosides (≥ 5 mg/kg gentamicin or ≥ 15 mg/kg of amikacin) every 24, 36, or 48 hours. ODA maximizes the peak/minimum inhibitory concentration (MIC) ratio while allowing time for adequate clearance of drug. ODA should not be used in patients with ascites, burns of greater than 20% of total body surface area, pregnancy, chronic renal failure, as perioperative prophylaxis, or in patients greater than 70 years of age. It can be extremely difficult to achieve appropriate peak levels in patients who have an increased volume of distribution. In addition, fluctuating renal function increases the risk of drug accumulation. Because there is always a significant period of time where plasma levels are negligible, ODA should always be used in conjunction with another antimicrobial agent when treating serious infections caused by gram-negative organisms, ideally an extended-spectrum β-lactam or a carbapenem.

MACROLIDES

Most macrolide use in surgical patients is for the management of skin and soft tissue infections and respiratory tract infections. When determining which macrolide to use, there are some important considerations. Clarithromycin is available only in oral form. Both azithromycin and erythromycin are available intravenously. Erythromycin is poorly tolerated and has many drug interactions and, as a result, has fallen out of favor for the management of most infections. Aztihromycin has virtually no major drug interactions, is well tolerated, and has a broad spectrum of activity.[7,8]

QUINOLONES

Ciprofloxacin, levofloxacin, and moxifloxacin are the main quinolones used in surgical practice. Both ciprofloxacin and levofloxacin have a role in the management of hospital-acquired infections including pneumonia caused by *Pseudomonas*. It is imperative, however, that they be used in conjunction with another antibiotic (eg, piperacillin-tazobactam) when treating *Pseudomonas aeruginosa* infections because of a higher incidence of treatment failure when used alone. Both levofloxacin and moxifloxacin are effective in the management of community-acquired pneumonia. Moxifloxacin has broader anaerobic activity, which makes it useful in the treatment of skin and soft tissue infections and intra-abdominal infections.[8–11]

ANTIFUNGALS

Amphotericin B has been the mainstay of antifungal treatment. Unfortunately, it is associated with major toxic side effects, particularly nephrotoxicity, that often limit its usefulness. The development of lipid formulations that are less toxic has allowed for effective treatment of fungal infections resistant to other agents. Azoles are effective against many fungi but lack the broad spectrum of activity of amphotericin B preparations. Some non-albicans *Candida* species are resistant to fluconazole or can become resistant while on therapy. The echinocandins are newer agents that do not have the same problems with toxicity as amphotericin B and have similar antifungal activity. There has been much made of the efficacy of these newer agents, yet their superiority to fluconazole has been questioned, particularly in view of their greater cost.[12,13]

PHARMACOKINETIC AND PHARMACODYNAMIC CONSIDERATIONS IN THE SURGICAL PATIENT

Surgical patients experience many pharmacokinetic and pharmacodynamic changes that may affect the success of therapy. When choosing an empiric antibiotic, it is just as important to select the correct dose and interval as it is to pick the right drug. Dosing antibiotics according to pharmacokinetic and pharmacodynamic principles can decrease the incidence of both treatment failure and the development of resistance.[14–18]

All antibiotics can be classified as either concentration-dependent or time-dependent. Concentration-dependent antibiotics refer to those where higher concentrations result in more rapid and complete killing. Higher peak/MIC and area under the curve/MIC correlate best with efficacy. Concentration-dependent antimicrobials include the quinolones, metronidazole, amphotericin, and aminoglycosides.

Time-dependent antibiotics are characterized by saturation of killing that occurs at low multiples of MIC (4–8 × MIC) and the extent of killing depends on time of exposure. In this circumstance, efficacy correlates with time greater than MIC. Time-dependent antimicrobials include the β-lactams, clindamycin, macrolides, azoles, and vancomycin.

Postantibiotic effect refers to the persistent suppression of bacterial regrowth following exposure to an antibiotic. It is measured in time (hours). A long postantibiotic effect prevents bacterial regrowth when antibiotic levels fall below the MIC. Most antibiotics exhibit a postantibiotic effect for gram-positive organisms but the duration is short. Aminoglycosides, quinolones, tetracyclines, macrolides, chloramphenicol, and rifampin exhibit a prolonged postantibiotic effect for gram-negative organisms.

When choosing the proper antimicrobial dose, one must consider the patient's volume of distribution. Trauma and burn patients often receive massive quantities of fluid during resuscitation, which can lead to an increase in volume of distribution for many hydrophilic agents, such as the aminoglycosides and β-lactams. It is not unusual for these patients to require higher than normal doses to achieve normal therapeutic levels. Gentamicin and tobramycin doses as high as 5 to 7 mg/kg/dose and amikacin at 10 to 15 mg/kg/dose may be necessary to reach goal peak serum levels. Conversely, these same patients may experience a decrease in renal or hepatic clearance of antimicrobials because of hypoperfusion. When this occurs, the dosing interval should be lengthened. The dosing interval also should be lengthened in patients with acute renal insufficiency and those needing renal replacement therapy. Typically, the dose of antibiotics cleared through renal excretion needs to be adjusted when creatinine clearance is less than 50 mL/min. When dosing drugs for patients who are on continuous renal replacement therapy, it is safe to assume the creatinine clearance is less than 30 mL/min while requiring continuous renal replacement therapy. In the event that a patient is converted to traditional hemodialysis, dosing should be readjusted to a creatinine clearance of less than 10 mL/min.

Burn patients with more than 20% to 30% total body surface area burns experience an increased drug clearance. These patients should be monitored closely and dosing intervals may need to be shortened for adequate treatment. For example, it is not unusual to adjust the interval of vancomycin dosing to every 6 to 8 hours rather than the usual every 12 hours to maintain therapeutic trough levels in this group of patients.

Another challenge is adequately dosing obese patients. There are conflicting reports regarding the appropriate method to dose obese patients. Although some recommend higher than normal doses, others suggest that no dose adjustment is needed. Interestingly, kidneys harvested from obese donors have been demonstrated to have a significantly higher glomerular planar surface area compared with nonobese donors. This may potentially lead to increased clearance of drugs and the need for a more frequent dosing interval. Some authorities have recommended increasing the dose of cephalosporins administered for perioperative antimicrobial prophylaxis to all patients who weigh more than 80 kg.

CONSIDERATIONS IN MANAGEMENT OF MULTIDRUG-RESISTANT ORGANISMS

Resistance to commonly used agents is increasing and remains a constant threat. Knowing the variety of available options is crucial when selecting empiric treatment. The approach to choosing empiric antimicrobial therapy should be based on the organisms anticipated to be responsible for the disease being treated.[19–22]

If a resistant gram-positive organism is suspected, such as methicillin-resistant *S aureus* (MRSA) or vancomycin-resistant enterococcus, vancomycin (MRSA only), linezolid, quinupristin-dalfopristin, daptomycin, or tigecycline are options for treatment. Because of the greater cost of linezolid therapy, vancomycin remains the first-line agent to treat MRSA infections. Linezolid should be considered for patients who are not clinically improving while receiving vancomycin. Daptomycin should not be used for treatment of pneumonia because it is rapidly inactivated by surfactant. Tigecycline is useful in the management of multiple drug resistant (MDR) infections; however, it should be avoided if treating sepsis or a bacteremia. This is because of rapid tissue distribution following infusion causing plasma levels to drop, which could lead to potential treatment failure.

Patients with community-acquired MRSA have a different resistance profile than those with nosocomial MRSA. Community-acquired MRSA is usually responsive to trimethoprim-sulfamethoxazole, clindamycin, and linezolid, all of which can be given orally.

The management of infections secondary to MDR organisms, such as *Acinetobacter calcoaceticus* or *Acinetobacter baumanii*, *P aeruginosa*, *Escherichia coli*, *Klebsiella pneumoniae*, and *Stenotrophomonas maltophilia*, is complicated because of enzymatic degradation. Of particular concern are organisms that produce extended-spectrum β-lactamase and AmpC β-lactamase. Unfortunately, simple and reliable testing methods to detect these organisms have not been established. Extended-spectrum β-lactamase–mediated resistance should be considered, however, if an organism is demonstrated to be resistant to ceftazidime on the sensitivity panel. If an organism is resistant to both ceftazidime and cefoxitin, AmpC-mediated resistance should be suspected. In either scenario, the sensitivity panel may show that the organisms are sensitive to the extended-spectrum β-lactams, such as piperacillin-tazobactam. It is imperative that these drugs not be used in this situation because resistance can develop in vivo leading to treatment failure. Meropenem or imipenem remain the agents of choice for the treatment of extended-spectrum β-lactamase– and AmpC β-lactamase–producing organisms.

The induction of carbapenemases has led to exploration and reintroduction of older, more toxic agents, such as polymyxin B and colistimethate. These agents remain highly effective against gram-negatives, including MDR organisms. They have been used successfully as monotherapy and in combination with other antimicrobials to treat MDR pseudomonal and acinetobacter infections. Sulfamethoxazole-trimethoprim is the agent of choice to treat *S maltophilia* infections, whereas tigecycline, ticarcillin-clavulanate, and the fluoroquinolones are alternative agents. Tigecycline has also been used in the management of MDR *A baumanii* infection. As previously mentioned, this drug should be avoided if bacteremia is suspected.

REFERENCES

1. Wright AJ. The penicillins. Mayo Clin Proc 1999;74:290–307.
2. Marshall WF, Blair JE. The cephalosporins. Mayo Clin Proc 1999;74:187–95.
3. Hellinger WC, Brewer NS. Carbapenems and monobactams: imipenem, meropenem, and aztreonam. Mayo Clin Proc 1999;74:420–34.
4. Terrell CL. Antifungal agents. Part II. The azoles. Mayo Clin Proc 1999;74:78–100.
5. Drusano GL, Ambrose PG, Bhavnani SM, et al. Back to the future: using aminoglycosides again and how to dose them optimally. Clin Infect Dis 2007;45:753–60.
6. Kaye D. Current use for old antibacterial agents: polymyxins, rifampin, and aminoglycosides. Infect Dis Clin North Am 2004;18:669–89.
7. Alvarez-Elcoro S, Enzler MJ. The macrolides: erythromycin, clarithromycin, and azithromycin. Mayo Clin Proc 1999;74:613–34.
8. Lacy CF, Armstrong LL, Goldman MP, et al. Lexicomp's drug information handbook. 15th edition. Hudson(OH): Lexicomp; 2007.
9. Owens RC, Ambrose PG. Antimicrobial safety: focus on fluoroquinolones. Clin Infect Dis 2005;41:S144–57.
10. Stein GE. The methoxyfluoroquinolones: gatifloxacin and moxifloxacin. Infect Med 2000;17:564–70.
11. O'Donnell JA, Gelone ST. The newer fluoroquinolones. Infect Dis Clin North Am 2004;18:691–716.
12. Patel R. Antifungal agents. Part I. Amphotericin B preparations and flucytosine. Mayo Clin Proc 1998;73:1205–25.
13. Sobel JD, Revankar SJ. Echinocandins: first-choice or first-line therapy for invasive candidiasis? N Engl J Med 2007;356:2525–6.
14. Smilack JD. The tetracyclines. Mayo Clin Proc 1999;74:727–9.
15. Drew RH. Emerging options for treatment of invasive, multidrug-resistant *Staphylococcus aureus* infections. Pharmacotherapy 2007;27:227–49.
16. Michalopoulos A, Falagas ME. Colistin and polymyxin B in critical care. Crit Care Clin 2008;24:377–91.
17. Mohr JF, Murray BE. Vancomycin is not obsolete for the treatment of infection caused by methicillin-resistant *Staphylococcus aureus*. Clin Infect Dis 2007;44:1536–42.
18. Tedesco KL, Rybak MJ. Daptomycin. Pharmacotherapy 2004;24:41–57.
19. Narita M, Tsuji BT, Yu VL. Linezolid-associated peripheral and optic neuropathy, lactic, and serotonin syndrome. Pharmacotherapy 2007;27:1189–97.
20. Kasten MJ. Clindamycin, metronidazole, and chloramphenicol. Mayo Clin Proc 1999;74:825–33.
21. Fox LM, Saravolatz LD. Nitazoxanide: a new thiazolide antiparasitic agent. Clin Infect Dis 2005;40:1173–80.
22. Adachi JA, DuPont HL. Rifaximin: a novel nonabsorbed rifamycin for gastrointestinal disorders. Clin Infect Dis 2006;42:541–7.
23. Falagas ME, Valkimadi PE, Huang YT, et al. Therapeutic options for *Stenotrophomonas maltophilia* infections beyond co-trimoxazole: a systematic review. J Antimicrob Chemother. 2008 Jul 28 [Epub ahead of print].

24. Wong-Beringer A, Krienglauykiat J. Systemic antifungal therapy: new options, new challenges. Pharmacotherapy 2003;23:1441–62.
25. Ashley ESD, Lew R, Lewis JS, et al. Pharmacology of systemic antifungal agents. Clin Infect Dis 2006;43:S28–39.
26. Chen SCA, Sorrell TC. Antifungal agents. Med J Aust 2007;187:404–9.
27. Cappelletty D, Eiselstein-McKitrick K. The echinocandins. Pharmacotherapy 2007;27:369–88.
28. Morris M, Villmann M. Echinocandins in the management of invasive fungal infections, part 1. Am J Health Syst Pharm 2006;63:1693–703.
29. Sabo JA, Abdel-Rahman SM. Voriconazole: a new triazole antifungal. Ann Pharmacother 2000;34:1032–43.
30. DeBeule K, Van Gestel J. Pharmacology of itraconazole. Drugs 2001;61(Suppl): 27–37.
31. Bergman SJ, Speil C, Short M, et al. Pharmacokinetic and pharmacodynamic aspects of antibiotic use in high risk populations. Infect Dis Clin North Am 2007;21: 821–46.
32. Estes L. Review of pharmcokinetics and pharmacodynamics of antimicrobial agents. Mayo Clin Proc 1998;73:1114–22.
33. Bonate PL. Pathophysiology and pharmacokinetics following burn injury. Clin Pharmacokinet 1990;18:118–30.
34. Pai MP, Bearden DT. Antimicrobial dosing considerations in obese adult patients. Pharmacotherapy 2007;27:1081–91.
35. Pea F, Viale P, Furlanut M. Antimicrobial therapy in critically ill patients. Clin Pharmacokinet 2005;44:1009–34.
36. Jacoby GA, Munoz-Price LS. The new β-lacatamases. N Engl J Med 2005;352: 380–91.
37. Nathisuwan S, Burgess DS, Lewis JS. Extended-spectrum β-lacatamases: epidemiology, detection, and treatment. Pharmacotherapy 2001;21:920–8.
38. Giamarellou K, Kanellakopoulou K. Current therapies for Pseudomonas aeruginosa. Crit Care Clin 2008;24:261–78.
39. Reid GE, Grim SA, Aldeza CA, et al. Rapid development of Acinetobacter baumannii resistance to tigecycline. Pharmacotherapy 2007;27:1198–201.

Adjunctive Measures for Treating Surgical Infections and Sepsis

Matthew C. Byrnes, MD[a,b,*], Greg J. Beilman, MD[a]

KEYWORDS

- Sepsis bundles • Adjunctive therapy • Activated protein C
- Vasopressors • Glycemic control

Sepsis results in significant mortality, morbidity, and hospital expenditures. Sepsis has been defined as infection associated with the systemic inflammatory response syndrome. Sepsis is considered "severe" when end organ dysfunction is caused by the sepsis syndrome. Severe sepsis has a mortality of 20% to 50%, with a resulting cost of $50,000 per patient.[1–4] With 751,000 cases annually, severe sepsis is the 10th most common cause of death in the United States.

The focal point of the management of sepsis and its resultant sequelae remains early diagnosis, prompt institution of antimicrobial therapy, appropriate resuscitation, and adequate source control. Nonetheless, many patients who are treated according to these principles still succumb to this disease. Accordingly, numerous adjunctive treatments have been studied and implemented over the past several decades. Unfortunately, the history of sepsis treatment has been fraught with more failures than successes.[5] To date, there have been no interventions that have been demonstrated to be efficacious by multiple large, well-designed, multicenter, randomized clinical trials.[6] Several therapies, such as intravenous immunoglobulin and corticosteroids, have fallen out of favor. Other therapies, such as vasopressin administration for septic shock have undulated in their popularity among critical care physicians. More recent research into therapies or care models including tight blood glucose management, early goal-directed therapy, drotrecogin alfa (activated), protocolization of care, and intensivist management have demonstrated positive results. Further research is being conducted to verify the success of these initial trials. This article summarizes the available adjunctive treatments for severe sepsis. Interventions with evidence supporting benefit in populations of patients with sequelae of sepsis are listed in **Box 1**.

[a] Department of Trauma, Division of Surgical Critical Care, University of Minnesota, MMC 11, 420 Delaware Street SE, Minneapolis, MN 55455, USA
[b] Department of Trauma, North Memorial Medical Center, 3300 Oakdale Avenue, Robbinsdale, MN 55422, USA
* Corresponding author. Division of Surgical Critical Care, University of Minnesota, MMC 11, 420 Delaware Street SE, Minneapolis, MN 55455.
E-mail address: byrne147@umn.edu (M.C. Byrnes).

Surg Clin N Am 89 (2009) 349–363
doi:10.1016/j.suc.2008.09.001
0039-6109/08/$ – see front matter © 2009 Elsevier Inc. All rights reserved.

surgical.theclinics.com

> **Box 1**
> **Adjunctive Therapies Demonstrating Evidence of Benefit in ICU Patients**
>
> Low tidal volume ventilation in acute lung injury/ARDS
>
> Recombinant human activated Protein C
>
> "Tight" glucose control
>
> Early appropriate antibiotic administration
>
> Intensivist management
>
> Early goal-directed therapy
>
> Sepsis "bundles"

ACTIVATED PROTEIN C

Activated Protein C is an endogenous peptide that is activated by thrombin coupled with thromobomodulin.[7] This acts as a natural anticoagulant via inhibition of factors Va and VIIIa. It also possesses anti-inflammatory activity via inhibition of tumor necrosis factor (TNF)-α, interleukin (IL)-1, and IL-6.[8] Activated protein C levels have been demonstrated to be inappropriately reduced among patients with severe sepsis.[9–12] Further, patients with reduced levels of activated protein C have been shown to have increased risk of death. Sepsis is associated with marked inflammation and microvascular coagulation,[11,12] which could potentially be attenuated by normalization of protein C levels. Accordingly, it was hypothesized that administration of activated protein C would reduce the risk of death in severe sepsis. Results of preclinical and phase 2 trials bolstered this hypothesis.[13]

The Recombinant Human Activated Protein C Worldwide Evaluation of Severe Sepsis (PROWESS) trial was the first large-scale phase 3 trial to demonstrate efficacy for a therapeutic agent in reducing the risk of death in sepsis.[8] This study was conducted from 1998 to 2000 in 164 centers in 11 countries. There were 1728 patients randomized in a 1:1 double-blinded fashion to receive an infusion of recombinant human activated protein C (drotrecogin alfa [activated], trade name Xigris) or placebo. Other components of sepsis management were left to the discretion of the treating physician. Inclusion criteria included sepsis and organ dysfunction within 24 hours of randomization. There were a variety of exclusion criteria, including platelet count lower than 30,000 and chronic renal failure (refer to package insert for full details). The primary end point was all-cause mortality at 28 days. The trial was terminated after the second planned interim analysis demonstrated efficacy of the study medication versus placebo. Patient characteristics were similar between placebo and treatment groups. One quarter of patients underwent a surgical procedure. The average APACHE II score was 25 in each group. The risk of death at 28 days was significantly lower among the patients in the drotrecogin alfa group (30.8% versus 24.7%, $P = .005$, **Fig. 1**). This difference in survival was noted within a few days of administration of the study medications. The incidence of severe hemorrhagic complications was higher in the drotrecogin alfa (activated) group, but this did not reach statistical significance (3.5% versus 2%, $P = .06$). A subsequent analysis reported that the mortality benefit was most pronounced among patients with an APACHE score of 25 or higher.[14] The results of the PROWESS trial were corroborated by a single arm, phase 3B trial.[15] The American arm of the Extended Evaluation of Recombinant Human Activated Protein C United States (ENHANCE) trial enrolled 273 adult patients treated with drotrecogin alfa (activated). There were with similar inclusion and exclusion criteria as the PROWESS trial. There was no placebo arm. The 28-day mortality was 26.4%,

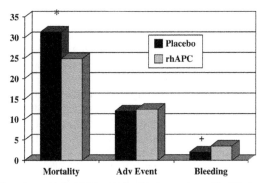

Fig. 1. Outcomes of patients in the PROWESS trial. (*Data from* Ely EW, Laterre PF, Angus DC, et al. Drotrecogin alfa (activated) administration across clinically important subgroups of patients with severe sepsis. Crit Care Med 2003;31(1):12–9.) * $P = .005$, + $P = .06$.

which was similar to the intervention group and lower than the placebo group in the PROWESS trial. Four percent of patients suffered serious bleeding complications.

Drotrecogin alfa (activated) was approved for use by the Food and Drug Administration (FDA) in the United States in 2001. The largest treatment effect was seen among patients with more severe sequelae of sepsis (higher APACHE II scores, multiple organ dysfunctions, or septic shock). Accordingly, the pharmaceutical company was charged with performing an additional trial among septic patients with a lower risk of death.[16] The Administration of Drotrecogin Alfa (Activated) in Early Stages of Severe Sepsis (ADDRESS) trial was developed to evaluate patients with less severe sepsis (APACHE 2 score <25 or single organ failure). Although the trial had planned to enroll 12,000 patients, it was terminated before full enrollment secondary to futility. The study enrolled 2613 patients. The 28-day mortality rate was similar between the groups (17% versus 18.5%, $P = .34$). The risk of serious bleeding was higher with the study group (2.4% versus 1.2%, $P = .02$).

The REsearching severe Sepsis and Organ dysfunction in children: gLobal perspective (RESOLVE) trial was conducted to evaluate the efficacy of drotrecogin alfa (activated) in pediatric patients.[17] Trial design was similar to previous studies. There was no difference in 28-day mortality between the groups (17.5% versus 17.2%, $P = .93$).

On the basis of these trials, drotrecogin alfa (activated) is licensed in the United States for patients with sepsis, APACHE 2 score 25 or higher, and age 18 or older. The efficacy of the medication has only been demonstrated when treating patients within 24 to 48 hours of the first organ failure. It is administered as a 96-hour infusion with a dose of 24 μg/kg/h. It should be stopped 1 to 2 hours before any procedure and can be restarted 1 hour after minor or percutaneous procedures and 12 hours after major procedures if hemostasis has been established. Use of this drug in patients with significant risk of bleeding (eg, severe thrombocytopenia, recent neurosurgery, or cerebrovascular event) is contraindicated.

The FDA was initially ambivalent regarding the decision to approve drotrecogin alfa (activated).[18] There were concerns about a change in trial design in the middle of patient enrollment. The European agency approved drotrecogin alfa (activated) with the stipulation that such approval would be reviewed annually. A statement was published suggesting that an additional phase 3 trial was needed to confirm safety and efficacy of the medication.[19] This generated significant controversy.[20,21] While the medication remains approved for use, a second phase 3 trial in the appropriate patient group (adult sepsis patients with high risk of death) is planned, which is expected to yield results by 2011.

CORTICOSTEROIDS

The use of corticosteroids in the management of septic shock has been debated for many years. High doses of corticosteroids were used 2 decades ago with unfavorable results.[22,23] High-dose corticosteroids gave way to lower, "physiologic" doses, which have generated significant controversy in the past few years.

There are multiple reasons for suspecting that corticosteroids would be beneficial in septic shock. Corticosteroids have potent anti-inflammatory effects, via a multitude of mechanisms.[24] As such, it was felt that corticosteroids could mitigate the hyper-inflammatory response of sepsis. Further, multiple authors have described a state of "relative adrenal insufficiency" in sepsis.[25] This condition is characterized by a decreased response of the adrenal glands to ACTH. Finally, vascular responsiveness to catecholamines is dependent upon adequate levels of cortisol.[26] Administration of low-dose hydrocortisone has been demonstrated to improve mean arterial pressure in vasopressor-dependent patients.

With this background, Annane and colleagues[27] conducted a randomized, double-blinded trial comparing low-dose hydrocortisone (50 mg every 6 hours) and fludrocor-tisones (50 µg every day) with placebo. Inclusion criteria consisted of severe sepsis with hypotension for at least 1 hour despite adequate fluid resuscitation and vasopres-sors. Patients were also given a corticotropin stimulation test to evaluate for "relative adrenal insufficiency." Resolution of the need for vasopressors was more common among patients treated with steroids (57% versus 40%, $P = .001$). Additionally, among patients with relative adrenal insufficiency, mortality was reduced by treating patients with steroids (63% versus 53%, $P = .02$).

Although the use of low-dose hydrocortisone became standard of care, there were concerns about its efficacy. The degree of shock among patients evaluated by Annane and colleagues was especially severe. It was unclear if these results applied to less severe septic shock. As a result, the Corticosteroid Therapy of Septic Shock (CORTICUS) trial was conducted. Inclusion criteria included sepsis with hypotension requiring use of vasopressors.[28] However, this trial enrolled patients with a much less severe shock state. Although patients enrolled in this study had to meet the criteria for septic shock, they did not have to have refractory hypotension despite use of maximum doses of va-sopressors. Mortality was similar between the corticosteroid-treated group and the placebo group (34.3% versus 31.5%, $P = .51$). The corticosteroid group demonstrated more rapid reversal of shock but developed more episodes of superinfection.

As a result of the CORTICUS trial, an international sepsis guideline has removed corticotropin stimulation tests from the standard sepsis management algorithm.[29] Hydrocortisone is now recommended only in patients with septic shock poorly responsive to vasopressor therapy. Some authors, however, have disagreed with these conclusions drawn from the CORTICUS trial.[30]

A final group worth consideration includes patients who were previously on long-term corticosteroid therapy. These patients have been excluded from most trials. Accordingly, it may be reasonable to provide "stress dose" corticosteroids to these patients during their acute stress event. Also, a corticosteroid taper is recommended upon completion of all doses of corticosteroids to avoid an increase in proinflamma-tory mediators after abrupt discontinuation of corticosteroid therapy.[31]

VASOPRESSOR/INOTROPIC MEDICATIONS

Vasopressor or inotropic medications are a standard temporizing component in the management of septic shock. They do not alter the septic response; rather, the goal of vasopressor administration is to maintain an adequate perfusion pressure until the hypotensive response to sepsis abates. Although it is generally agreed that hypotension should be avoided, the optimum vasopressor and blood pressure targets are controversial. For the purposes of this discussion, these two classes of agents will be considered together.

Choice of Agent

There are several medications available for clinical use. Norepinephrine (Levophed) is the most commonly used vasopressor. It has effects on both alpha and beta adrenergic receptors, resulting in both increased inotropy and peripheral vasoconstriction. Epinephrine has activity similar to norepinephrine, with more beta-adrenergic effects. Dopamine has effects on dopaminergic receptors at low doses, beta-adrenergic effects at moderate doses, and alpha-adrenergic effects at higher doses. Phenylephrine (Neosynephrine) has mostly alpha agonist activity. Accordingly, it induces peripheral vasoconstriction without increasing cardiac contractility. This increases afterload, which may decrease cardiac output. Dobutamine, in contrast, has primarily beta adrenergic activity, producing increased inotropy and peripheral vasodilation. Vasopressin induces peripheral vasoconstriction via V receptors. Dopamine has historically been considered the vasopressor of choice.[32] The Surviving Sepsis guidelines recommended dopamine or norepinephrine as first line agents.[29]

Sakr and colleagues[33] evaluated patients in septic shock in an observational prospective fashion. About one third of these patients received dopamine, while the remainder never received dopamine. Mortality was significantly higher among patients treated with dopamine (42.9% versus 35.7%, $P = .02$). Dopamine was also an independent risk factor for mortality in multivariate analysis. Another prospective, observational study reported lower mortality when norepinephrine was used to improve mean arterial pressure in septic shock (62% versus 82%, $P<.001$).[32]

Excessive vasoconstriction has been a concern with use of vasopressors; however, DeBacker and colleagues[34] reported that splanchnic blood flow was similar with use of norepinephrine or dopamine, but was reduced with epinephrine. Additionally, mesenteric perfusion has been reported to be preserved among patients with septic shock treated with norepinephrine compared with severe sepsis without shock.[35]

Vasopressin has been extensively studied over the past decade. There is a relative vasopressin deficiency among patients in septic shock.[36] Further, the use of vasopressin has been demonstrated to reduce the doses of catecholamines required to maintain adequate arterial pressures.[37] Vasopressin was prospectively evaluated in a randomized, double-blinded fashion.[38] Patients in septic shock were randomized to receive a titratable infusion of norepinephrine or vasopressin in addition to their current regimen of vasopressors. Patients with less severe septic shock (<15 µg/min norepinephrine) had improved mortality with vasopressin infusions (35.7% versus 26.5%, $P = .05$). Mortality was not reduced by infusion of vasopressin among patients with more severe septic shock.

In summary, norepinephrine and dopamine remain the primary initial vasopressors in the treatment of septic shock. Vasopressin should be considered an important adjunct vasopressor. Epinephrine may be considered as a second line agent. Phenylephrine has a minimal role in the treatment of septic shock.

Goals

The goal of vasopressor therapy is to maintain an adequate perfusion pressure to supply end-organ vascular beds. Animal studies have indicated that there is loss of autoregulation with mean arterial pressures lower than 60 mm Hg.[39] A general goal of titrating vasopressors to a mean arterial pressure of 65 mm Hg has been recommended; however, this must be adjusted for individual patients who have higher or lower blood pressures at baseline. In patients receiving vasopressor therapy, it is key to maintain adequate preload through volume resuscitation to prevent splanchnic vasoconstriction.

INTENSIVE GLUCOSE MANAGEMENT

Critical illness is often associated with hyperglycemia.[40] Various stress mechanisms, such as secretion of glucagon, catecholamines, and cortisol work to enhance blood glucose levels. This is adaptive in the short run in that it provides glucose to the brain during times of stress. Hyperglycemia, however, may be deleterious to long-term outcomes. Hyperglycemia impairs neutrophil function, which may increase infectious risks. Additionally, patients suffering from myocardial infarction have been demonstrated to have increased mortality if their blood glucose levels were elevated.[41]

With this background, Van Den Berghe and colleagues[42] performed a randomized trial comparing critically ill patients managed with intensive insulin therapy to patients managed with a standard regimen. The blood glucose target for the intensive therapy arm was 80 to 110 mg/dL. The target for the standard therapy arm was 180 to 200 mg/dL. Patients treated with intensive insulin therapy had a significantly reduced mortality (8% versus 4.6%, $P<.04$). These patients also had a reduced rate of renal failure and critical illness polyneuropathy. Several limitations of this trial should be noted. The study group, in a surgical ICU, contained a high proportion of cardiovascular surgery patients, and very few patients had infections at the time of study entry. They also received a high glucose load in the first 24 hours postoperatively, as aggressive nutrition was begun in the immediate postoperative time period.

A similar study was conducted among patients admitted to a medical ICU.[43] Again, patients were randomized to intensive insulin therapy or standard therapy. The results of this study, however, failed to demonstrate a mortality benefit of intensive insulin therapy in the intent-to-treat group (**Fig. 2**), although there was survival benefit in patients remaining in the ICU longer than 3 days.

Only one randomized trial has been conducted that has focused solely on patients with severe sepsis.[44] Patients with severe sepsis were randomized to receive therapy as described in the previous trials. This trial, however, was terminated early secondary to

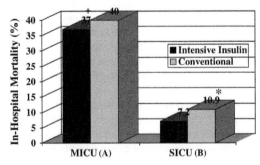

Fig. 2. Effects of intensive insulin therapy on patients in an medical intensive care unit (MICU) (*A, data from* Van den Berghe G, Wilmer A, Hermans G, et al. Intensive insulin therapy in the medical ICU. N Engl J Med 2006;354(5):449–61) and an surgical intensive care unit (SICU) (*B, data from* van den Berghe G, Wouters P, Weekers F, et al. Intensive insulin therapy in the critically ill patients. N Engl J Med 2001;345(19):1359–67.) * $P = .01$, + $P =$ not significant.

safety concerns. Mortality was not reduced among patients treated with intensive insulin therapy, but the risk of severe hypoglycemia (serum glucose <40 mg/dL) was significantly higher among patients treated with intensive insulin therapy (17% versus 4.1%, P<.0001). Since hypoglycemia can be associated with deleterious outcomes, such as stroke and death, the investigators felt obligated to terminate the trial. There is currently a large ongoing trial (NICE-SUGAR, The Normoglycaemia in Intensive Care Evaluation [NICE] and Survival Using Glucose Algorithm Regulation [SUGAR] Study), randomizing patients to two different blood glucose targets, which has enrolled over 6000 patients in 35 international ICUs. Results are expected within the next 1 to 2 years.

In summary, intensive insulin therapy has received significant attention over the past decade. While one large single center trial demonstrated improved outcomes with this regimen, subsequent trials have failed to replicate those results. Current international recommendations have been made to maintain blood glucose levels lower than 150 mg/dL.[29] Maintenance of blood glucose between 80 and 110 mg/dL may carry a significant risk of hypoglycemia.

FLUID RESUSCITATION

Although vasopressors remain a cornerstone for maintenance of adequate blood pressure in septic shock, they should only be administered in conjunction with efforts at restoring effective intravascular volume. The most effective fluid to achieve this goal is quite controversial.

There are three broad categories of intravenous fluids: crystalloid, albumin, and nonalbumin colloid. Crystalloid fluids consist of balanced salt solutions. Lactated Ringer's solution and normal saline are the most commonly used crystalloid solutions, although sterile water with sodium bicarbonate can occasionally be used. Large volumes of normal saline can induce a metabolic acidosis due to the chloride load (154 mEq/L) in this fluid. Lactated Ringer's contains potassium (though only 4 meq/L), which may be problematic in hyperkalemic patients. The theoretic advantage of albumin is the ability to provide smaller volumes of fluid to resuscitate the intravascular space. As a result of the large oncotic pressure, a significant percentage of the volume administered with albumin solutions remains intravascular.[45] In comparison, only 25% of an isotonic crystalloid solution remains intravascular.[46] These differences may potentially allow for more rapid resuscitation with albumin with less resultant edema. Albumin, however, is more expensive than crystalloid and can potentiate pulmonary edema in patients with "leaky" capillaries.

Numerous studies have been conducted to evaluate crystalloid versus colloid. In a meta-analysis, the Cochrane collaboration reported that albumin increases the risk of mortality in injured patients.[47] A subsequent meta-analysis disputed these results.[48] The most important trial to date was published in 2004. Nearly 7000 patients were randomized to receive 4% albumin or saline for resuscitation fluids.[49] There were no significant differences in outcomes between the groups. There was a trend toward reduced mortality among septic patients resuscitated with albumin (30.7% versus 35.3%, P = .09).

Nonalbumin colloid solutions generally contain a large molecular weight starch that does not filter through capillary junctions. As a result, these solutions possess significant oncotic pressure. They have been developed as less expensive and potentially more effective versions of albumin. A recent randomized trial evaluated septic patients who were resuscitated with lactated Ringer's solution or 10% pentastarch.[44] Patients receiving pentastarch had higher rates of renal failure and had a trend toward increased mortality.

In summary, albumin and isotonic crystalloid solutions are both effective volume expanders in septic shock. To date there is no compelling evidence in support of one solution over the other. Nonalbumin colloids carry additional risks that are not posed by albumin or crystalloid.

OTHER PHARMACEUTICAL AGENTS

Many pharmaceutical agents have been developed with the goal of altering the septic response. Nearly all, with the exception of drotrecogin alfa (activated) have failed.[5] Trials have been performed on compounds that block endotoxin, found in all gram-negative bacteria. Other trials have evaluated blockade of TNF-α.[50] The use of the naturally occurring IL-1 receptor antagonist has also been studied.[51] All of these trials have either failed to demonstrate a benefit, or have actually resulted in increased mortality.

Intravenous immunoglobulins (IVIG) have been studied since the 1980s for the treatment of severe sepsis. Meta-analyses have suggested that administration of IVIG is beneficial in severe sepsis, with the IgA and IgM preparations being the most beneficial.[52,53] It should be noted that the trials used for the meta-analyses were of variable quality. A recent large, randomized trial failed to demonstrate a benefit to administration of intravenous IgG to patients with severe sepsis.[54] As a result, this medication is not currently recommended for severe sepsis.

OTHER ADJUNCTIVE THERAPIES OF SEPSIS

There are several other adjunctive therapies to the management of sepsis. These include low tidal volume ventilation, stress ulcer prophylaxis, and deep vein thrombosis prophylaxis.

The acute respiratory distress syndrome network (ARDSnet) trial evaluated patients ventilated with low tidal volumes (5–7 mL/kg) versus patients with higher tidal volumes (12 mL/kg).[55] There was a mortality benefit associated with low tidal volumes in patients with ARDS or acute lung injury. Although this trial did not focus on septic patients, this recommendation has been extended to septic patients with acute lung injury.

Patients with severe sepsis are at increased risk of stress ulceration secondary to reduced gastric perfusion. Respiratory failure is also an independent risk factor for stress ulceration.[56] The recommended agents are H2 blockers or proton pump inhibitors. The benefit of these medications must be balanced against the potential for increasing colonization of the stomach with pathogenic bacteria, which can increase the risk for ventilator-associated pneumonia.[57]

Critically ill patients are at significant risk for deep vein thrombosis. This can be a fatal complication if untreated or undiagnosed. Prophylaxis against deep vein thrombosis should be provided with either unfractionated heparin (dosed three times per day rather than twice daily) or low molecular weight heparin. Low molecular weight heparin has been recommended in the highest risk patients. Since drotrecogin alfa (activated) has antithrombotic activity, there is a theoretic risk of increased bleeding among patients receiving both heparin and drotrecogin alfa. In a prospective study, however, there was actually an increased mortality among patients treated with drotrecogin alfa (activated) and placebo compared with drotrecogin alfa (activated) and heparin. Further, coadministration of prophylactic heparin and drotrecogin alfa did not appear to increase bleeding risks.[58] Accordingly, chemical deep vein thrombosis prophylaxis should not be withheld from patients simply because they are receiving an infusion of drotrecogin alfa (activated).

EARLY GOAL-DIRECTED THERAPY

The philosophy of early goal-directed therapy ties together two important concepts in the treatment of sepsis: prompt intervention and titration of therapies to specific end points. The first concept has been well demonstrated in a number of arenas. For instance, antibiotic therapy is much more efficacious when delivered early in sepsis than in a delayed fashion.[59] As sepsis progresses, global hypoxia may develop in the setting of prolonged perfusion defects.[60] As cell death begins to occur as a result of inadequate tissue oxygen delivery, the sepsis syndrome may become resistant to later resuscitation. Thus, prompt resuscitation has been associated with improved outcomes and it is now recommended as a standard of care.

The concept of titrating therapy to specific end points has a history of mixed results. There are a variety of markers that can be used to assess tissue perfusion. Markers of global perfusion include lactic acid serum concentrations, base deficit, and central venous oxygen saturation. Central venous oxygen (CVO_2) saturation correlates with global oxygen delivery and uptake. As oxygen use becomes delivery dependent, CVO_2 saturation begins to fall. At levels of less than 70%, oxygen use is felt to be delivery dependent and efforts aimed at improving delivery may be warranted. Hemodynamic markers of resuscitation include cardiac index, central venous pressure, pulmonary artery wedge pressure, and oxygen delivery. Clinical indicators of perfusion include urinary output, capillary refill, and mental status. Any of these markers can provide a goal or an end point for resuscitation. However, increasing oxygen delivery to the tissues to supranormal levels, in an effort to treat tissue hypoxia, failed to improve outcomes.[61] Other efforts aimed at directing therapy to specific goals have similarly failed.[62]

In contrast, in 2001, Rivers and colleagues[63] reported successful results of early goal-directed therapy. In this single-center study, 263 patients were randomized to receive early goal-directed therapy (EGDT) or standard care in the emergency room. The protocol for EGDT was as follows:

- Oximetric central venous catheters were placed to measure central venous pressure (CVP) and central venous hemoglobin oxygen saturation (C_vO_2).
- 500-mL aliquots of isotonic crystalloid were given by bolus infusion to achieve a central venous pressure greater than 8 mm Hg.
- Mean arterial pressure was maintained at 65 mm Hg or higher with vasopressors.
- If the C_vO_2 saturation was still less than 70%, blood was transfused to a hematocrit of 30.
- If the C_vO_2 saturation was still less than 70%, dobutamine was started.

Mortality was significantly lower among patients randomized to EGDT (48.2% versus 33.3%, $P = .01$). These patients also received more fluid in the first 6 hours (5 versus 3.5 L) but then received less fluid in hours 7 to 72 (10.6 versus 8.6 L). This approach may ultimately have been successful because of its emphasis on early resuscitation of the septic patient rather than the specific components of the protocol. Nonetheless, aspects of this approach have become standard for the initial resuscitation of patients with septic shock.

PROTOCOL-DIRECTED MANAGEMENT OF SEVERE SEPSIS

Although several adjunctive therapies for sepsis have been demonstrated to be effective, they have been incompletely implemented in practice. Reasons for inconsistent medical care of septic patients include lack of education as well as unintentional omission of accepted therapies. For instance, a physician may believe that prompt antibiotic administration is necessary, but fails to consider it in specific situations; alternatively, the physician may practice in a health care system that does not emphasize timely medication delivery.

The concept of a "bundle" has been developed to aid in the delivery of best practices. A bundle consists of several generally accepted, evidence-based practices that are implemented as a group. For instance, bundles may focus on ventilator management, sepsis resuscitation, or ongoing sepsis management. These bundles/protocols have been implemented in a number of hospitals with significant success.

Some sepsis bundles provide goals to be completed within 6 hours and 24 hours.[64] In one hospital, the 6-hour bundle was similar to the EGDT protocol. The 24-hour bundle included ongoing resuscitation and ventilator goals. It was found that noncompliance with the protocol increased risk of mortality by 100%.

Similar results were seen in a 1200-bed university hospital.[65] A standardized order set was developed for the management of septic shock. Patients managed in the emergency department before the initiation of the order set (n = 60) were compared with patients managed with the order set (n = 120). Mortality was markedly reduced among patients treated with the standardized order sets (48.3% versus 30.0%, n = 0.04). These patients also received a significantly higher volume of intravenous fluids and were more likely to receive appropriate antimicrobial therapy.

These results were also replicated internationally.[66] A national educational program on the treatment of sepsis was implemented in Spain. Fifty-nine intensive care units participated in the study. The educational program was multidisciplinary and was focused on health care professionals practicing in the emergency department, the ICU, and the wards. There were 10 hours of lectures dedicated to the program. As previously described, 6- and 24-hour bundles were developed. Patients treated before initiation of the educational program were compared with patients treated after the program was implemented. Mortality rates from sepsis were lower after initiation of the program (44% versus 39.7%, $P = .04$).

Finally, similar results were achieved in community-based hospitals.[67] A shock protocol was developed at a 180-bed community hospital. Time to intensivist arrival to the patient's bedside was reduced after the protocol was implemented. Mortality was also markedly reduced after implementation of the protocol (40.7% versus 28.2%, $P = .035$).

In summary, the implementation of protocol-based care has generally been associated with positive outcomes. To date, no study has reported worsened outcomes after implementation of a protocol to manage severe sepsis.

ROLE OF INTENSIVISTS

As intensive care units have matured into defined entities within hospitals, the role of critical care specialists has increased. The traditional model of surgical critical care consisted of surgeons or internists managing critically ill patients with the assistance of multiple consultants. This philosophy has shifted in recent years toward the development of consultative critical care services, in which an intensivist provides most of the minute-to-minute decision making with regard to management of a critically ill patient. While some intensive care units have shifted toward a "closed model," in which the intensivist is the sole attending physician for the patient, most units still operate as an "open" or "semi-open/collaborative" environment.

Although all surgeons should be familiar with the general approach to the septic patient, intensivists may be much more familiar with current best practices for the treatment of sepsis. Additionally, the intensivist is generally immediately available for patient management throughout the day. There are numerous problems with attempting to manage critically ill patients in the intensive care unit over the telephone while performing an operation. The maturation of intensivist consultative services provides bedside expertise during times in which the surgeon is unavailable. The surgeon, however, still should be familiar with sepsis research and protocols, so that patient care decisions can be made in a collaborative fashion.

The majority of studies that have evaluated the effect of intensivists on outcomes among critically ill patients have reported positive results. A meta-analysis of prospective observational studies[68] reported that 94% of the studies evaluated found a positive impact of high-intensity intensivist use (mandatory intensivist consultation) on outcome; the odds ratio for ICU mortality in patients treated by intensivists was 0.61. A recent study, however, questioned the results of these previous studies.[69] To date, none of these studies have focused exclusively on outcomes in septic patients.

SUMMARY

Sepsis syndromes associated with surgical infections represent a significant cause of morbidity and mortality around the world. Adjunctive therapies have been historically unsuccessful; however, more recent research is promising. Early diagnosis and resuscitation are key to optimizing outcomes. Additionally, adjunctive therapies, such as appropriate vasopressor management, use of drotrecogin alfa (activated) when warranted, control of hyperglycemia, and adherence to proven protocols can reduce mortality.

REFERENCES

1. Angus DC, Linde-Zwirble WT, Lidicker J, et al. Epidemiology of severe sepsis in the United States: analysis of incidence, outcome, and associated costs of care. Crit Care Med 2001;29(7):1303–10.
2. Martin GS, Mannino DM, Eaton S, et al. The epidemiology of sepsis in the United States from 1979 through 2000. N Engl J Med 2003;348(16):1546–54.
3. Chalfin DB, Holbein ME, Fein AM, et al. Cost-effectiveness of monoclonal antibodies to gram-negative endotoxin in the treatment of gram-negative sepsis in ICU patients. JAMA 1993;269(2):249–54.
4. Wheeler AP, Bernard GR. Treating patients with severe sepsis. N Engl J Med 1999;340(3):207–14.
5. Cohen J. Adjunctive therapy in sepsis: a critical analysis of the clinical trial programme. Br Med Bull 1999;55(1):212–25.
6. Werdan K. Mirror, mirror on the wall, which is the fairest meta-analysis of all? Crit Care Med 2007;35(12):2852–4.
7. Esmon CT. The protein C anticoagulant pathway. Arterioscler Thromb 1992;12(2):135–45.
8. Bernard GR, Vincent JL, Laterre PF, et al. Efficacy and safety of recombinant human activated protein C for severe sepsis. N Engl J Med 2001;344(10):699–709.
9. Fourrier F, Chopin C, Goudemand J, et al. Septic shock, multiple organ failure, and disseminated intravascular coagulation. Compared patterns of antithrombin III, protein C, and protein S deficiencies. Chest 1992;101(3):816–23.
10. Lorente JA, Garcia-Frade LJ, Landin L, et al. Time course of hemostatic abnormalities in sepsis and its relation to outcome. Chest 1993;103(5):1536–42.

11. Bone RC, Grodzin CJ, Balk RA. Sepsis: a new hypothesis for pathogenesis of the disease process. Chest 1997;112(1):235–43.
12. Esmon CT, Taylor FB Jr, Snow TR. Inflammation and coagulation: linked processes potentially regulated through a common pathway mediated by protein C. Thromb Haemost 1991;66(1):160–5.
13. Taylor FB Jr, Chang A, Esmon CT, et al. Protein C prevents the coagulopathic and lethal effects of Escherichia coli infusion in the baboon. J Clin Invest 1987;79(3):918–25.
14. Ely EW, Laterre PF, Angus DC, et al. Drotrecogin alfa (activated) administration across clinically important subgroups of patients with severe sepsis. Crit Care Med 2003;31(1):12–9.
15. Bernard GR, Margolis BD, Shanies HM, et al. Extended evaluation of recombinant human activated protein C United States Trial (ENHANCE US): a single-arm, phase 3B, multicenter study of drotrecogin alfa (activated) in severe sepsis. Chest 2004;125(6):2206–16.
16. Abraham E, Laterre PF, Garg R, et al. Drotrecogin alfa (activated) for adults with severe sepsis and a low risk of death. N Engl J Med 2005;353(13):1332–41.
17. Nadel S, Goldstein B, Williams MD, et al. Drotrecogin alfa (activated) in children with severe sepsis: a multicentre phase III randomised controlled trial. Lancet 2007;369(9564):836–43.
18. Kalil AC, Sun J. How many patients with severe sepsis are needed to confirm the efficacy of drotrecogin alfa activated? A Bayesian design. Intensive Care Med 2008;34:1804–11.
19. Warren HS, Suffredini AF, Eichacker PQ, et al. Risks and benefits of activated protein C treatment for severe sepsis. N Engl J Med 2002;347(13):1027–30.
20. Siegel JP. Assessing the use of activated protein C in the treatment of severe sepsis. N Engl J Med 2002;347(13):1030–4.
21. Ely EW, Bernard GR, Vincent JL. Activated protein C for severe sepsis. N Engl J Med 2002;347(13):1035–6.
22. Lefering R, Neugebauer EA. Steroid controversy in sepsis and septic shock: a meta-analysis. Crit Care Med 1995;23(7):1294–303.
23. Sprung CL, Caralis PV, Marcial EH, et al. The effects of high-dose corticosteroids in patients with septic shock. A prospective, controlled study. N Engl J Med 1984; 311(18):1137–43.
24. Meduri GU, Muthiah MP, Carratu P, et al. Nuclear factor-kappaB- and glucocorticoid receptor alpha-mediated mechanisms in the regulation of systemic and pulmonary inflammation during sepsis and acute respiratory distress syndrome. Evidence for inflammation-induced target tissue resistance to glucocorticoids. Neuroimmunomodulation 2005;12(6):321–38.
25. Rothwell PM, Udwadia ZF, Lawler PG. Cortisol response to corticotropin and survival in septic shock. Lancet 1991;337(8741):582–3.
26. Annane D, Bellissant E, Sebille V, et al. Impaired pressor sensitivity to noradrenaline in septic shock patients with and without impaired adrenal function reserve. Br J Clin Pharmacol 1998;46(6):589–97.
27. Annane D, Sebille V, Charpentier C, et al. Effect of treatment with low doses of hydrocortisone and fludrocortisone on mortality in patients with septic shock. JAMA 2002;288(7):862–71.
28. Sprung CL, Annane D, Keh D, et al. Hydrocortisone therapy for patients with septic shock. N Engl J Med 2008;358(2):111–24.
29. Dellinger RP, Levy MM, Carlet JM, et al. Surviving sepsis campaign: international guidelines for management of severe sepsis and septic shock: 2008. Crit Care Med 2008;36(1):296–327.

30. Marik PE, Pastores SM, Kavanagh BP. Corticosteroids for septic shock. N Engl J Med 2008;358(19):2069–70 [author reply 2070–1].
31. Keh D, Boehnke T, Weber-Cartens S, et al. Immunologic and hemodynamic effects of "low-dose" hydrocortisone in septic shock: a double-blind, randomized, placebo-controlled, crossover study. Am J Respir Crit Care Med 2003;167(4): 512–20.
32. Martin C, Viviand X, Leone M, et al. Effect of norepinephrine on the outcome of septic shock. Crit Care Med 2000;28(8):2758–65.
33. Sakr Y, Reinhart K, Vincent JL, et al. Does dopamine administration in shock influence outcome? Results of the Sepsis Occurrence in Acutely Ill Patients (SOAP) Study. Crit Care Med 2006;34(3):589–97.
34. De Backer D, Creteur J, Silva E, et al. Effects of dopamine, norepinephrine, and epinephrine on the splanchnic circulation in septic shock: which is best? Crit Care Med 2003;31(6):1659–67.
35. Meier-Hellmann A, Specht M, Hannemann L, et al. Splanchnic blood flow is greater in septic shock treated with norepinephrine than in severe sepsis. Intensive Care Med 1996;22(12):1354–9.
36. Landry DW, Levin HR, Gallant EM, et al. Vasopressin pressor hypersensitivity in vasodilatory septic shock. Crit Care Med 1997;25(8):1279–82.
37. Mutlu GM, Factor P. Role of vasopressin in the management of septic shock. Intensive Care Med 2004;30(7):1276–91.
38. Russell JA, Walley KR, Singer J, et al. Vasopressin versus norepinephrine infusion in patients with septic shock. N Engl J Med 2008;358(9):877–87.
39. Kirchheim HR, Ehmke H, Hackenthal E, et al. Autoregulation of renal blood flow, glomerular filtration rate and renin release in conscious dogs. Pflugers Arch 1987; 410(4–5):441–9.
40. McCowen KC, Malhotra A, Bistrian BR. Stress-induced hyperglycemia. Crit Care Clin 2001;17(1):107–24.
41. Malmberg K, Ryden L, Efendic S, et al. Randomized trial of insulin-glucose infusion followed by subcutaneous insulin treatment in diabetic patients with acute myocardial infarction (DIGAMI study): effects on mortality at 1 year. J Am Coll Cardiol 1995;26(1):57–65.
42. van den Berghe G, Wouters P, Weekers F, et al. Intensive insulin therapy in the critically ill patients. N Engl J Med 2001;345(19):1359–67.
43. Van den Berghe G, Wilmer A, Hermans G, et al. Intensive insulin therapy in the medical ICU. N Engl J Med 2006;354(5):449–61.
44. Brunkhorst FM, Engel C, Bloos F, et al. Intensive insulin therapy and pentastarch resuscitation in severe sepsis. N Engl J Med 2008;358(2):125–39.
45. Allison SP, Lobo DN. Debate: albumin administration should not be avoided. Crit Care 2000;4(3):147–50.
46. Devlin JW, Barletta JF. Albumin for fluid resuscitation: implications of the saline versus albumin fluid evaluation. Am J Health Syst Pharm 2005;62(6):637–42.
47. Human albumin administration in critically ill patients: systematic review of randomised controlled trials. Cochrane Injuries Group Albumin Reviewers. BMJ 1998; 317(7153):235–40.
48. Wilkes MM, Navickis RJ. Patient survival after human albumin administration. A meta-analysis of randomized, controlled trials. Ann Intern Med 2001;135(3):149–64.
49. Finfer S, Bellomo R, Boyce N, et al. A comparison of albumin and saline for fluid resuscitation in the intensive care unit. N Engl J Med 2004;350(22):2247–56.
50. Abraham E, Wunderink R, Silverman H, et al. Efficacy and safety of monoclonal antibody to human tumor necrosis factor alpha in patients with sepsis syndrome.

A randomized, controlled, double-blind, multicenter clinical trial. TNF-alpha MAb Sepsis Study Group. JAMA 1995;273(12):934–41.

51. Opal SM, Fisher CJ Jr, Dhainaut JF, et al. Confirmatory interleukin-1 receptor antagonist trial in severe sepsis: a phase III, randomized, double-blind, placebo-controlled, multicenter trial. The Interleukin-1 Receptor Antagonist Sepsis Investigator Group. Crit Care Med 1997;25(7):1115–24.

52. Kreymann KG, de Heer G, Nierhaus A, et al. Use of polyclonal immunoglobulins as adjunctive therapy for sepsis or septic shock. Crit Care Med 2007;35(12): 2677–85.

53. Laupland KB, Kirkpatrick AW, Delaney A. Polyclonal intravenous immunoglobulin for the treatment of severe sepsis and septic shock in critically ill adults: a systematic review and meta-analysis. Crit Care Med 2007;35(12):2686–92.

54. Werdan K, Pilz G, Bujdoso O, et al. Score-based immunoglobulin G therapy of patients with sepsis: the SBITS study. Crit Care Med 2007;35(12):2693–701.

55. Ventilation with lower tidal volumes as compared with traditional tidal volumes for acute lung injury and the acute respiratory distress syndrome. The acute respiratory distress syndrome network. N Engl J Med 2000;342(18):1301–8.

56. Cook DJ, Fuller HD, Guyatt GH, et al. Risk factors for gastrointestinal bleeding in critically ill patients. Canadian Critical Care Trials Group. N Engl J Med 1994; 330(6):377–81.

57. Kahn JM, Doctor JN, Rubenfeld GD. Stress ulcer prophylaxis in mechanically ventilated patients: integrating evidence and judgment using a decision analysis. Intensive Care Med 2006;32(8):1151–8.

58. Levi M, Levy M, Williams MD, et al. Prophylactic heparin in patients with severe sepsis treated with drotrecogin alfa (activated). Am J Respir Crit Care Med 2007;176(5):483–90.

59. Kollef MH, Sherman G, Ward S, et al. Inadequate antimicrobial treatment of infections: a risk factor for hospital mortality among critically ill patients. Chest 1999; 115(2):462–74.

60. Beal AL, Cerra FB. Multiple organ failure syndrome in the 1990s. Systemic inflammatory response and organ dysfunction. JAMA 1994;271(3):226–33.

61. Hayes MA, Timmins AC, Yau EH, et al. Elevation of systemic oxygen delivery in the treatment of critically ill patients. N Engl J Med 1994;330(24):1717–22.

62. Gattinoni L, Brazzi L, Pelosi P, et al. A trial of goal-oriented hemodynamic therapy in critically ill patients. SvO2 Collaborative Group. N Engl J Med 1995;333(16): 1025–32.

63. Rivers E, Nguyen B, Havstad S, et al. Early goal-directed therapy in the treatment of severe sepsis and septic shock. N Engl J Med 2001;345(19):1368–77.

64. Gao F, Melody T, Daniels DF, et al. The impact of compliance with 6-hour and 24-hour sepsis bundles on hospital mortality in patients with severe sepsis: a prospective observational study. Crit Care 2005;9(6):R764–70.

65. Micek ST, Roubinian N, Heuring T, et al. Before-after study of a standardized hospital order set for the management of septic shock. Crit Care Med 2006; 34(11):2707–13.

66. Ferrer R, Artigas A, Levy MM, et al. Improvement in process of care and outcome after a multicenter severe sepsis educational program in Spain. JAMA 2008; 299(19):2294–303.

67. Sebat F, Johnson D, Musthafa AA, et al. A multidisciplinary community hospital program for early and rapid resuscitation of shock in nontrauma patients. Chest 2005;127(5):1729–43.

68. Pronovost PJ, Angus DC, Dorman T, et al. Physician staffing patterns and clinical outcomes in critically ill patients: a systematic review. JAMA 2002;288(17): 2151–62.
69. Levy MM, Rapoport J, Lemeshow S, et al. Association between critical care physician management and patient mortality in the intensive care unit. Ann Intern Med 2008;148(11):801–9.

Prevention of Surgical Site Infection

John P. Kirby, MS, MD*, John E. Mazuski, MD, PhD

KEYWORDS

- Surgical site infection • Surgical wound infection
- Staphylococcus aureus
- Methicillin-resistant *Staphylococcus* aureus
- Antibiotic prophylaxis • Antimicrobial agents • Infection control

Surgical site infection (SSI) is an important postoperative complication. It is second only to urinary tract infection as the most common nosocomial infection in hospitalized patients. Based on extensive epidemiologic surveys, it has been estimated that SSI develops in at least 2% of hospitalized patients undergoing operative procedures, although this is a likely underestimate because of incomplete post-discharge data.[1] Other data indicate that SSI develops following 3% to 20% of certain procedures, and that the incidence is even higher in certain high-risk patients.[2]

There seems to be a perception among some surgeons that SSI is a relatively trivial infection. However, based on survey data, there were over 290,000 infections in hospitalized patients in 2002, and SSI was estimated to be directly responsible for 8205 deaths of surgical patients that year.[1] Thus, the mortality rate was 3% among patients who developed SSI. There is also significant morbidity associated with SSI; a large number of patients develop long-term disabilities as a result of poor wound healing and overt tissue destruction following these infections. Finally, the economic costs of SSI to both the patient and the health care delivery system are high.[3]

Because of their frequency and clinical significance, SSI rates are of interest to regulatory agencies and to the public at large. Public reporting of SSI rates by health care entities is increasingly required, and this mandate is being extended to individual surgeons. Further, a number of regulatory programs have been implemented that apply both financial incentives for following best practices in preventing SSI and financial penalties when such infections occur. It can be anticipated that such programs will expand in the future.

Department of Surgery, Washington University School of Medicine, Campus Box 8109, 660 S. Euclid Avenue, Saint Louis, MO 63110-1093, USA
* Corresponding author.
E-mail address: kirbyj@wustl.edu (J.P. Kirby).

Surg Clin N Am 89 (2009) 365–389
doi:10.1016/j.suc.2009.01.001
0039-6109/09/$ – see front matter © 2009 Elsevier Inc. All rights reserved.

DEFINITIONS

SSI is an infection that occurs somewhere in the operative field following a surgical intervention. The Centers for Disease Control and Prevention (CDC) considers SSI to include both incisional SSI and organ space SSI. Incisional SSI is subdivided into superficial and deep SSI, depending on whether the infection is limited to the skin and subcutaneous tissue only (superficial SSI) or extends into the deeper tissues, such as the fascial and muscular layers of the body wall (deep SSI). Organ/space SSI is an infection that occurs anywhere within the operative field other than where the body wall tissues were incised. Examples include intra-abdominal abscess developing after an abdominal operation, empyema developing after a thoracic operation, and osteomyelitis or joint infection developing after an orthopedic procedure.[4]

The National Healthcare Safety Network (NHSN) of the CDC has developed a series of criteria in an effort to objectively define SSI (**Box 1**). Although these criteria are relatively detailed, it is important to realize that the surgeon's judgment ultimately determines whether an SSI is present in equivocal cases. Thus, when there are erythematous changes around a wound or it is draining material that is not clearly purulent, it is important that the surgeon's opinion be clearly expressed as to whether or not an SSI is present.

RISK FACTORS FOR DEVELOPING SSI

The risk of developing SSI varies greatly according to the nature of the operative procedure and the specific clinical characteristics of the patient undergoing that procedure. Ultimately, it is necessary to consider a broad range of risk factors for developing preventative measures.

The CDC wound classification system[5–7] is widely used to capture some of the risk of infection related to the type of operative procedure. This classification scheme focuses primarily on the degree of contamination likely to be present during the operation (**Table 1**). Thus, during Class I (clean) procedures, only microorganisms from the skin and external environment are likely to be introduced into the wound. With Class II (clean-contaminated) procedures, there is additional exposure to microorganisms colonizing the epithelial surfaces and lumen of structures of the respiratory, digestive, genital, and urinary tracts, although contamination should be limited in scope. With Class III (contaminated), and Class IV (dirty-infected) procedures, there is progressively greater exposure of the wound to potential pathogenic microorganisms.

Although the CDC wound classification scheme allows some stratification of risk, it does not take into account other risks related to the operative procedure or patient characteristics. Two large epidemiologic surveys performed by the CDC in the 1970s and 1980s established the importance of these other factors in developing SSI. In 1985, the Study on the Efficacy of Nosocomial Infection Control identified an abdominal operation, an operation of longer duration (2 hours or more), and a patient having three or more discharge diagnoses as being risk factors for the development of SSI in addition to wound classification (contaminated or dirty-infected versus clean or clean-contaminated).[8] Subsequently, the National Nosocomial Infections Surveillance System (NNIS),[9] the predecessor of the current NHSN, simplified risk stratification to three factors: (1) CDC wound classification (contaminated or dirty-infected); (2) a longer duration operation, defined as one that exceeded the 75th percentile for a given procedure; and (3) the medical characteristics of the patient, as determined by an American Society of Anesthesiology (ASA) score of III, IV, or V (presence of a severe systemic disease that results in functional limitations, is life threatening, or is expected to preclude survival from the operation) at the time of the operation.

With the widespread introduction of laparoscopic techniques into the surgical arma-mentarium, this three-point risk index has been further modified.[10] A rule now calls for subtraction of one risk factor point when cholecystectomy or colon surgery is per-formed laparoscopically; however, for appendectomy and gastric surgery, subtraction of one point is done only if there are no other risk factors.

The impact of these risk factors can be seen in information provided by the NHSN about SSI rates for various operative procedures performed in 2006–2007.[11] Selected data from this publication are summarized in **Table 2**. Looking at these figures, it is apparent that even with risk adjustment, there are intrinsic disparities in SSI rates with different procedures. For instance, among patients with no risk factors who underwent breast or colonic operations, the rate of SSI was fivefold higher with colonic surgery than it was with breast surgery. Nonetheless, with each procedure, there is a major impact of additional risk factors; SSI rates double to quadruple as the number of risk factors increase. Thus, it is clear that the risk of SSI is related to factors other than just wound classification.

The primary use of these analyses is in monitoring trends in SSI rates and in allowing individual institutions to benchmark their data against national averages. However, these broad-based risk adjustments do not easily lead to targeted interventions for the prevention of SSI. For this, knowledge of more specific risk factors is needed. Multivariate analyses have identified large numbers of specific risk factors which place the patient at higher risk of developing a SSI: (1) patient characteristics, such as increased age or the presence of a remote infection at the time of the operation; (2) aspects of preoperative, intraoperative, and postoperative management, such as de-layed delivery of prophylactic antibiotics or flash sterilization of surgical instruments. One summary of risk factors, from the 1999 CDC guidelines on prevention of SSI, is reproduced in **Box 2**.[7] Although these risk factors are not necessarily independent of each other, they do provide potential targets for developing preventative measures.

MICROBIOLOGY

SSI is caused by microorganisms introduced into the surgical wound at the time of the operative procedure. Most of these microorganisms come from the patient's endog-enous flora, but occasionally the pathogenic organisms are acquired from an exoge-nous source, such as the air in the operating room, surgical equipment, implants or gloves, or even medications administered during the operative procedure.[7,12] When there is an unexplained local outbreak of SSI, investigations performed by infection control personnel may be useful in uncovering an exogenous source.

Large, cross-institutional surveys involving all surgical specialties have revealed that a small number of gram-positive cocci and gram-negative bacilli are responsible for most SSIs. The NNIS system categorized 17,671 isolates obtained from patients with SSI from 1986 to 1996.[13] Over one half of the isolates were gram-positive cocci; *Staphylococcus aureus* was the most commonly isolated organism, followed by coag-ulase-negative staphylococci, and *Enterococcus* spp. Approximately one third of the isolates were gram-negative bacilli, with *Escherichia coli*, *Pseudomonas aeruginosa*, and *Enterobacter* spp being the most frequently encountered gram-negative organ-isms. About 5% of the isolates were anaerobic bacteria. More recent surveys involving multiple[14] or single institutions[15,16] have corroborated these general findings, although the specific distribution of organisms differs somewhat, probably reflecting different types of surgical practices at individual institutions.

This general pattern masks significant variability in the microbiology of SSI accord-ing to the type of operative procedure.[7,12] For patients undergoing clean procedures,

Box 1

CDC criteria for defining an SSI

Superficial incisional SSI

Infection occurs within 30 days after the operative procedure

    and

involves only skin or subcutaneous tissue of the incision

    and

patient has at least one of the following:

    Purulent drainage from the superficial incision.

    Organisms isolated from an aseptically obtained culture of fluid or tissue from the superficial incision.

    At least one of the following signs or symptoms of infection: pain or tenderness; localized swelling, redness, or heat; and superficial incision is deliberately opened by surgeon and is culture-positive or not cultured. A culture-negative finding does not meet this criterion.

    Diagnosis of superficial incisional SSI by the surgeon or attending physician.

Deep incisional SSI

Infection occurs within 30 days after the operation if no implant is left in place or within 1 year if implant is in place and the infection appears to be related to the operative procedure

    and

involves deep soft tissues (eg, fascial and muscle layers) of the incision

    and

patient has at least one of the following:

    Purulent drainage from the deep incision but not from the organ/space component of the surgical site.

    A deep incision spontaneously dehisces or is deliberately opened by a surgeon and is culture-positive or not cultured when the patient has at least one of the following signs or symptoms: fever (>38°C) or localized pain or tenderness. A culture-negative finding does not meet this criterion.

    An abscess or other evidence of infection involving the deep incision is found on direct examination, during reoperation, or by histopathologic or radiologic examination.

    Diagnosis of a deep incisional SSI by a surgeon or attending physician.

Organ/Space SSI

Infection occurs within 30 days after the operation if no implant is left in place or within 1 year if implant is in place and the infection appears to be related to the operative procedure

    and

infection involves any part of the body (excluding the skin incision, fascia, or muscle layers) that is opened or manipulated during the operative procedure

    and

patient has at least one of the following:

    Purulent drainage from a drain that is placed through a stab wound into the organ/space.

Organisms isolated from an aseptically obtained culture of fluid or tissue in the organ/space.

An abscess or other evidence of infection involving the organ/space that is found on direct examination, during reoperation, or by histopathologic or radiologic examination.

Diagnosis of an organ/space SSI by a surgeon or attending physician.

Reprinted from Horan TC, Andrus M, Dudeck MA. CDC/NHSN surveillance definition of health care-associated infection and criteria for specific types of infections in the acute care setting. Am J Infect Control 2008;36:309–32; with permission.

staphylococci predominate as the cause of SSI, since these microorganisms are present on the skin at the site of most incisions. However, gram-negative and other enteric organisms colonize the skin at certain sites, including the axilla, perineum and groin; patients having incisions in those areas may have a SSI caused by gram-negative organisms. Thus, patients undergoing coronary artery bypass surgery are likely to have gram-positive organisms as the cause of a sternal wound infection, but are frequently found to have gram-negative organism as the cause of a leg wound infection.[17] With clean-contaminated or contaminated wounds, bacteria from the respiratory, gastrointestinal, genital, or urinary tracts contribute to the infection. For instance, gram-negative bacilli and anaerobic organisms are frequent causes of SSI

Table 1
Surgical wound classification

Class	Type	Description
I	Clean	An uninfected operative wound in which no inflammation is encountered and the respiratory, alimentary, genital, or uninfected urinary tract is not entered. In addition, clean wounds are primarily closed and, if necessary, drained with closed drainage. Operative incisional wounds that follow nonpenetrating (blunt) trauma should be included in this category if they meet the criteria
II	Clean-contaminated	An operative wound in which the respiratory, alimentary, genital, or urinary tracts are entered under controlled conditions and without unusual contamination. Specifically, operations involving the biliary tract, appendix, vagina, and oropharynx are included in this category, provided no evidence of infection or major break in technique is encountered
III	Contaminated	Open, fresh, accidental wounds. In addition, operations with major breaks in sterile technique (eg, open cardiac massage), or gross spillage from the gastrointestinal tract, and incisions in which acute, nonpurulent inflammation is encountered are included in this category
IV	Dirty-infected	Old traumatic wounds with retained devitalized tissue and those that involve existing clinical infection or perforated viscera. This definition suggests that the organisms causing postoperative infection were present in the operative field before the operation

Reprinted from Mangram AJ, Horan TC, Pearson ML, et al. Guideline for prevention of surgical site infection, 1999. Infect Control Hosp Epidemiol 1999;20:250–78.

Table 2 SSI rates (%) for selected procedures, according to risk index				
Procedure	Number of Risk Factors			
	0	1	2	3
Appendectomy	1.49		3.49	
Bile duct, liver, or pancreatic surgery	8.77		16.34	
Breast surgery	0.80	2.74	Not reported	
Colon surgery	4.18	6.07	8.01	10.86
Gastric surgery	1.84		4.86	
Herniorrhaphy (inpatient)	1.02	2.47	4.36	
Peripheral vascular bypass surgery	2.00	6.69		
Small bowel surgery	2.62	6.31		

Selective data reprinted from Edwards JR, Peterson KD, Andrus ML, et al. National Healthcare Safety Network (NHSN) Report, data summary for 2006 through 2007, issued November 2008. Am J Infect Control 2008;36:609–26.

following procedures involving the lower gastrointestinal tract.[7] Nonetheless, organisms derived from the skin may still contribute to these infections. In a recent trial of prophylactic antibiotics for subjects undergoing colorectal procedures, 11% of all isolates obtained from subjects with SSI were staphylococci, most of which were S aureus.[18] With Class IV (dirty-infected) wounds, it is generally assumed that pathogenic organisms already present in the operative field will be responsible for a subsequent SSI.[7] Finally, it should be noted that unique microbiological patterns may pertain to certain highly specialized procedures; for instance, enterococci are frequently found to be the pathogens causing SSI after liver transplantation.[19]

The most significant change in the microbiology of SSI has been the increased involvement of resistant microorganisms in these infections. The number of SSI caused by methicillin-resistant S aureus (MRSA) has increased dramatically.[20] Anderson and colleagues[14] found that MRSA was responsible for 17% of all severe SSIs developing in 1010 patients at 26 community hospitals in the Southeast, and accounted for 53% of the infections due to S aureus. Naylor and colleagues[21] documented MRSA in 40% of the severe postoperative SSIs developing in vascular surgery patients at 25 centers in Great Britain and Ireland. An increased occurrence of infections due to MRSA has also been recognized in studies of subjects undergoing cardiac, orthopedic, or plastic surgery procedures.[22–25] The emergence of the USA300 clone of MRSA, commonly referred to as community-acquired MRSA, may further impact the microbiology of SSI. This strain is recognized as being responsible for significant numbers of serious hospital-acquired staphylococcal infections;[26,27] a preliminary report also suggests its frequent involvement as a cause of SSI.[28]

The gram-negative bacilli isolated from patients with SSI also demonstrate increased resistance.[29,30] These resistant organisms likely result from prior exposure of the patient to the health care environment or broad spectrum antimicrobial therapy. The increasing resistance of gram-negative organisms causing SSI parallels their increasing resistance when they cause other nosocomial infections.[31]

Although infrequently identified in epidemiologic surveys, two infections, streptococcal gangrene due to Group A β-hemolytic streptococci and clostridial myonecrosis usually due to Clostridium perfringens, should be mentioned. These fulminant monomicrobial infections rarely develop following an operative procedure. The possibility of such an infection should be considered in a patient with clinical findings suggestive of

Box 2
Risk factors for SSI

Patient-related

Age

Nutritional status

Diabetes

Smoking

Obesity

Coexistent infections at a remote body site

Colonization with microorganisms

Altered immune response

Length of preoperative stay

Operation

Duration of surgical scrub

Skin antisepsis

Preoperative shaving

Preoperative skin preparation

Duration of operation

Antimicrobial prophylaxis

Operating room ventilation

Inadequate sterilization of instruments

Foreign material in the surgical site

Surgical drains

Surgical technique

    Poor hemostasis

    Failure to obliterate dead space

    Tissue trauma

Reprinted from Mangram AJ, Horan TC, Pearson ML, et al. Guideline for prevention of surgical site infection, 1999. Infect Control Hosp Epidemiol 1999;20:250–78.

severe sepsis or septic shock out of proportion to those expected in a patient with a typical postoperative SSI. Typically, soft-tissue infections due to these organisms manifest themselves early after an operative procedure, sometimes within the first 24 hours. Because of their rapidly progressive nature, early surgical management coupled with appropriate antimicrobial therapy is mandatory.[32]

PREVENTION OF SSI: GENERAL MEASURES

Interventions to prevent SSI are based on knowledge of the various risk factors that predispose a patient to develop such an infection and an understanding of the microbiology of SSI. In this section, general measures to prevent SSI will be discussed; subsequent sections will focus on some of the issues related to antimicrobial prophylaxis and other interventions that target specific pathogens. The interventions discussed in this and subsequent sections are summarized in **Table 3**.

Table 3
Selected interventions for prevention of SSI

Intervention	Evidence[a]	References
Preoperative		
Reduce hemoglobin A1c levels to <7% before operation	Class II data	Anderson et al[33]
Smoking cessation 30 d before operation	Class II data	Mangram et al,[7] Anderson et al[33]
Administer specialized nutritional supplements or enteral nutrition at severe nutritional risk for 7–14 d preoperatively; preoperative parenteral nutrition should not be routinely used, except selectively in patients with severe underlying malnutrition	Class I and Class II data with significant heterogeneity	Mangram et al,[7] Anderson et al,[33] Weimann et al,[40] Anonymous[42]
Adequately treat preoperative infections, such as urinary tract infections	Class II data	Mangram et al,[7] Anderson et al[33]
Decolonization of unselected patients with mupirocin is not currently recommended	Class I data	Mangram et al,[7] Anderson et al,[33] Kalmeijer et al,[83] Perl et al,[84] Konvalinka et al,[85] Suzuki et al,[92] Laupland and Conly[95]
Identification and decolonization of S aureus carriers may be a potentially useful intervention, but requires further investigation	Limited Class I data	Rao et al,[90] Hacek et al[91]
Preoperative showering with chlorhexidine is not currently recommended	Class I data	Mangram et al,[7] Anderson et al,[33] Webster and Osborne[45]
Perioperative preparations		
Remove hair only if it will interfere with the operation; hair removal by clipping immediately before the operation or with depilatories; no pre- or perioperative shaving of surgical site[b]	Class I data	Mangram et al,[7] Anderson et al,[33] Kjønniksen et al,[43] Bratzler and Hunt,[44] Springer[70]
Use an antiseptic surgical scrub or alcohol-based hand antiseptic for preoperative cleansing of the operative team members' hands and forearms	Class II data	Mangram et al,[7] Anderson et al[33]
Prepare the skin around the operative site with an appropriate antiseptic agent, including preparations based on alcohol, chlorhexidine, or iodine/iodophors	Class II data	Mangram et al,[7] Anderson et al,[33] Digison[46]

Administer prophylactic antibiotics for most clean-contaminated and contaminated procedures, and selected clean procedures; use antibiotics appropriate for the potential pathogens (Table 6)[b]	Strong Class I data	Mangram et al,[7] Bratzler and Hunt,[44] Anonymous,[67] Springer,[70] Classen et al[73]
Administer prophylactic antibiotics within 1 h before incision (2 h for vancomycin and fluoroquinolones)[b]	Strong Class II data	Mangram et al,[7] Bratzler and Hunt,[44] Anonymous,[67] Springer,[70] Classen et al[73]
Use higher dosages of prophylactic antibiotics for morbidly obese patients	Limited Class II data	Mangram et al,[7] Forse et al[38]
Use vancomycin as a prophylactic agent only when there is a significant risk of MRSA infection	Class I data	Mangram et al,[7] Anderson et al,[33] Anonymous,[67] Bolon et al,[96] Finkelstein et al[97]
Operating room environment		
Provide adequate ventilation, minimize operating room traffic, and clean instruments and surfaces with approved disinfectants	Class II and Class III data	Mangram et al,[7] Anderson et al[33]
Avoid flash sterilization	Class II data	Mangram et al,[7] Anderson et al[33]
Use laminar airflow for orthopedic implant procedures. A common practice of uncertain utility	Contradictory Class II data	Mangram et al,[7] Anderson et al,[33] Brandt et al[48]
Conduct of operation		
Carefully handle tissue, eradicate dead space, and adhere to standard principles of asepsis	Class III	Mangram et al,[7] Anderson et al[33]
Avoid use of surgical drains unless absolutely necessary	Limited Class I, Class II data	Mangram et al,[7] Barie[49]
Leave contaminated or dirty-infected wounds open, with the possible exception of wounds following operations for perforated appendicitis	Limited Class I, Class II data	Mangram et al,[7] Brasel et al,[50] Cohn et al[51]
Redose prophylactic antibiotics with short half-lives intraoperatively if operation is prolonged (for cefazolin if operation is >3 h) or if there is extensive blood loss	Limited Class I, Class II data	Mangram et al,[7] Scher,[74] Swoboda et al[75]

(continued on next page)

Table 3
(continued)

Intervention	Evidence[a]	References
Maintain intraoperative normothermia[c]	Class I; some contradictory Class II data	Mangram et al,[7] Anderson et al,[33] Bratzler and Hunt,[44] Sessler and Akca,[53] Kurz et al,[54] Barone et al,[55] Walz et al,[56] Springer[70]
Use 80% oxygen intraoperatively and immediately postoperatively. Not currently recommended, but a large clinical trial is evaluating the approach	Heterogeneous Class I data; meta-analysis supports use of this modality	Anderson et al,[33] Greif et al,[57] Pryor et al,[58] Belda et al,[59] Mayzler et al,[60] Meyhoff et al[62]
Postoperative management		
Discontinue prophylactic antibiotics within 24 h after the procedure (48 h for cardiac surgery and liver transplant procedures); preferably, discontinue prophylactic antibiotics after skin closure[b]	Class I; meta-analyses support single dose regimens for prophylaxis	Mangram et al,[7] Bratzler and Hunt,[44] Anonymous,[67] Springer,[70] Barie,[76] DiPiro et al,[77] McDonald et al[78]
Maintain serum glucose levels <200 mg/dL on postoperative days 1 and 2[d]	Class II data	Anderson et al,[33] Bratzler and Hunt,[44] Zerr et al,[63] Furnary et al,[64] Lazar et al,[65] Carr et al,[66] Springer[70]
Monitor wound for the development of SSI	Class III data	Mangram et al,[7] Anderson et al[33]
Infection control and surveillance		
Maintain an active surveillance system for monitoring incidence of SSI	Class II data	Mangram et al,[7] Anderson et al[33]
Provide feedback to practitioners regarding individual rates of SSI	Class II data	Mangram et al,[7] Anderson et al[33]

[a] Class I data from prospective, randomized, controlled trials or meta-analyses of such trials; Class II data from well-controlled prospective or retrospective studies with good study design; Class III data from uncontrolled studies, case series, or expert opinion. Evidence grades do not directly correspond to those provided in Mangram et al[7] and Anderson et al.[33]

[b] SCIP measure for cardiothoracic, vascular, colorectal surgical procedures, hip or knee arthroplasty, and hysterectomy.

[c] SCIP measure for colorectal procedures.

[d] SCIP measure for cardiac surgery procedures.

General measures to prevent SSI can be organized into those directed at the patient's preoperative risk factors and those that relate to perioperative management of the patient. With respect to the latter, considerations include the patient's and the operative team's preparations for surgery, the operating room environment, intraoperative techniques, and other aspects of the patient's intraoperative and postoperative cares.

As is typical with many medical therapies, there are varying degrees of scientific evidence supporting various interventions. Although some are supported by data from prospective randomized controlled trials or other high-quality studies, the evidence for many is based primarily on experience and expert opinion accumulated over the years, or even surgical dogma never subjected to rigorous evaluation. Practice guidelines summarizing recommendations and the evidence behind them for the prevention of SSI have been developed and updated by the CDC, most recently in 1999.[7] Since then, no comprehensive set of guidelines for the prevention of SSI have appeared, although a recent publication from the Society for Healthcare Epidemiology of America and the Infectious Diseases Society of America[33] summarizes the previous guidelines and provides some updates based on additional literature.[34–39]

The patient's pre-existing medical conditions are a major contributor to the risk of SSI. Significant numbers of patients undergoing operative procedures have one or more of the risk factors listed in **Box 2**. The preoperative history and physical examination will usually allow detection of these medical conditions. However, many of these risk factors are not readily amenable to intervention, even if a surgical procedure can be delayed. Age is obviously not a modifiable risk factor. Likewise, a prolonged preoperative hospital stay usually reflects the need for hospitalization of a seriously ill patient with a compromised physiologic state rather than an opportunity for intervention.[7] Treating obesity or restoring immune competence to a patient who is immunosuppressed is generally not feasible in the short term. Generally accepted measures for preventing SSI include (1) optimizing preoperative glucose levels and lowering hemoglobin A1C concentrations in patients with diabetes; (2) encouraging patients to stop smoking at least 30 days before a procedure; and (3) treating any concomitant infection preoperatively.[7,33] However, there are limited data indicating that these interventions successfully prevent SSI when applied to large populations. Small studies suggest that preoperative use of oral supplements or enteral nutrition for 7 to 14 days may reduce infectious complications such as SSI in patients at severe nutritional risk.[40] However, use of preoperative parenteral nutrition has been associated with an increased risk of infectious complications, unless targeted at severely malnourished patients.[41,42]

In contrast to interventions based on patients' preoperative medical conditions, there are somewhat more complete data regarding certain perioperative approaches for prevention of SSI. Preoperative hair removal by shaving, particularly when performed the night before the procedure, has been consistently found to increase SSI rates.[7,43] It is currently recommended that either hair not be removed or that it be removed by clipping immediately before the operation or by using non-caustic depilatories.[7,33,43] Appropriate hair removal is one of the measures currently monitored as part of the Surgical Care Improvement Project (SCIP),[44] an initiative developed by a partnership of nongovernmental and government organizations, including the American College of Surgeons, the CDC, and the Centers for Medicare and Medicaid Services (CMS).

Preoperative showering with antiseptic agents such as chlorhexidine has not been shown to have a beneficial impact on SSI rates.[7,33,45] However, appropriate skin preparation at the time of the operative procedure with an antiseptic agent is a well-established preventative measure. Acceptable antiseptic agents include alcohol, chlorhexidine, and iodine and iodophors, some of which now have been re-formulated to provide a longer duration of action.[7,33,46] Use of chlorhexidine as a skin preparation has been recommended for prevention of catheter-related blood-stream infections;[47] however, the available data have not conclusively shown that it, or any other surgical site preparation, is superior for the prevention of SSI.[7,46] Similarly, although preparation of surgical team members' hands and forearms is a firm recom-mendation, the data are inadequate to indicate that any specific antiseptic agent or method is preferable.

The operating room environment may be the source of contamination leading to SSI in a limited number of cases. Generally accepted environmental measures to prevent SSI include maintaining adequate ventilation, minimizing operating room traffic, avoid-ing flash sterilization of operating room equipment, and cleaning surfaces and equip-ment with approved disinfectants.[7,33] The use of laminar air flow in the operating room and respiratory isolation of the operating team have been suggested as additional measures to avoid infection, particularly during orthopedic implant procedures. However, high-quality data indicating that these interventions result in decreased infection rates are lacking,[7] and a recent investigation questions whether use of laminar air flow has any efficacy whatsoever.[48] Other aspects of the operating room environment, such as the types of surgical drapes or the attire of the surgical team, are of potential importance, but there is little information available indicating that any intervention related to these will directly impact the risk of SSI. Occasional outbreaks of SSI have been linked to the presence in the operating room of a team member with an active infection or colonization with a pathogenic organism; exclusion from the operating room is only recommended for individuals who have draining skin lesions or have been epidemiologically linked to patient infections.[7]

The conduct of the operation by the surgeon and surgical team is another potential, although largely unproven, arena in which the risk of SSI might be altered. Tradition-ally, surgeons are taught that gentle handling of tissues, thorough irrigation of contam-ination, complete removal of devitalized or necrotic tissues, and avoidance of dead space are all important in avoiding infection.[7,33] The use of drains has been associated with an increase rather than a decrease in the risk of SSI; in the absence of a clear indi-cation, use of drains is strongly discouraged.[49] Closure of a contaminated or dirty-in-fected wound remains a topic of debate. The universal rule that these wounds need to be left open has been challenged for some procedures. Using a decision analysis approach, Brasel and colleagues[50] found that many wounds could be safely closed following operations for perforated appendicitis. However, a prospective randomized trial comparing primary closure with initial open management of dirty-infected wounds revealed that routine primary closure led to significantly more infections; nonetheless, hospital lengths of stay and costs of care did not differ between the two groups.[51] Finally, there is little question that the use of minimally invasive approaches will decrease the risk of SSI; for instance, rates of SSI are significantly lower with laparo-scopic appendectomy compared with open appendectomy.[52]

With regard to management of the closed wound, various types of wound dress-ings, antibiotic ointments, and other adjuvants have been used. There are a number of new types of transparent, semipermeable, or antibacterial dressings available, some of which are marketed as being advantageous for the prevention of SSI. None-theless, there are almost no data indicating that any specific approach or method of postoperative wound management impacts SSI rates.

Several aspects of perioperative management, including avoidance of hypothermia, maintenance of high tissue oxygen concentrations, and treatment of hyperglycemia have been investigated in some detail with respect to prevention of SSI. A frequent intraoperative problem is the development of hypothermia.[53] A prospective trial of subjects undergoing colorectal operations found that subjects randomized to receive additional intraoperative warming to maintain normothermia (mean core temperature of 36.6°C) had a threefold reduction in SSI compared with subjects who did not receive supplemental warming (mean core temperature of 34.7°C).[54] These positive results have been called into question somewhat by subsequent nonrandomized studies, which did not replicate this benefit.[55,56] Nonetheless, maintenance of normothermia in patients undergoing colorectal procedures is one of the components currently monitored as part of the SCIP initiative.

More controversial is the use of increased inspired oxygen concentrations in the intraoperative and immediate postoperative periods. Four prospective randomized controlled trials compared use of 80% oxygen with 30% oxygen in subjects undergoing abdominal operations, primarily colorectal procedures.[57–60] Two of these trials found significant reductions in the rates of SSI with the use of higher oxygen concentrations.[57,59] One trial, which was underpowered, identified a trend toward fewer SSIs in subjects receiving 80% oxygen.[60] However, one trial found an increase rather than a decrease in the SSI rates of subjects randomized to receive higher oxygen concentrations.[58] A meta-analysis of these trials suggests the overall data favor use of higher oxygen concentrations;[61] but given the heterogeneity of the results, this is still considered an unresolved issue.[33] A large randomized clinical trial, currently underway in Denmark,[62] will hopefully allow this controversy to be definitively resolved.

Avoidance of significant hyperglycemia in the intraoperative and postoperative period appears important in preventing SSI, particularly in patients undergoing cardiac surgical procedures. The risk of developing deep SSI and mediastinitis was found to be significantly reduced in cardiac surgery patients when frequent monitoring of blood glucose concentrations, coupled with use of insulin infusions as needed to control glucose concentrations was performed intraoperatively and postoperatively. This reduced risk applied to both diabetic and non-diabetic patients.[63–66] Avoidance of serum glucose levels greater than 200 mg/dL at 6:00 AM on postoperative days 1 and 2 after cardiac surgery is one of the current performance measures of the SCIP initiative. Further, mediastinitis following coronary artery bypass surgery is a complication for which hospitals will receive no additional reimbursement from CMS, since it is considered a preventable infection.

With regard to other aspects of postoperative management, there are few interventions that have been recommended. Probably the most important detail is to monitor the surgical wound for the development of a SSI.[7,33] It is generally accepted that early management of an infected wound helps avoid a more major subsequent complication. Unfortunately, some surgical practitioners are reluctant to intervene when there is a suspected SSI, which allows the infection to progress.

In addition to the efforts of individual surgeons, an effective infection control program is important in reducing institution-wide rates of SSI. Components of a successful infection control program include adequate surveillance for SSI, which is becoming increasingly difficult as hospital lengths of stay decrease and more patients develop SSIs as outpatients, and feedback to individual surgical practitioners so that practices can be modified.[7,33]

PREVENTION OF SSI: ANTIMICROBIAL PROPHYLAXIS

Perioperative antimicrobial prophylaxis is widely used, and probably overused, for the prevention of SSI. In general, antimicrobial prophylaxis is recommended under two circumstances: (1) when the risk of infection is relatively high, as it is for many clean-contaminated or contaminated operations, such as colorectal procedures; or (2) when the subsequent development of SSI could have disastrous consequences, such as with procedures involving implantation of a prosthetic vascular graft or orthopedic hardware.[7,67] The use of antibiotic prophylaxis for certain clean procedures not meeting the second criteria, such as breast or hernia operations, remains controversial.[67,68] As noted in **Table 2**, infection rates increase substantially for these operations in the presence of a single NNIS risk factor, one of which is a higher ASA score, indicating the patient has significant underlying medical comorbidities. However, whether or not a decision to use antimicrobial prophylaxis can be based on that risk assessment is unknown, because no definitive large-scale trials of antimicrobial prophylaxis have been performed in which subjects were stratified according to medical risk factors.[69]

The general principles regarding antimicrobial prophylaxis include (1) selection of antimicrobial agents based on the likely pathogens responsible for a SSI with a particular operation; (2) administration of antibiotics shortly before the commencement of that operation such that serum and tissue levels are high at the time of incision and during the course of the operation; and (3) discontinuation of antimicrobial therapy at the end of the operation, or at most 24 to 48 hours after the procedure is completed.[37,67,69] Compliance with these principles (appropriate selection, timing, and duration of antimicrobial prophylaxis) are monitored as part of the SCIP initiative,[44,70] and are also included as measures in the Physician's Quality Reporting Initiative of CMS, which provides financial incentives to practitioners who follow best practices.

Extensive guidelines regarding agents for surgical prophylaxis were published by the American Society of Health-System Pharmacists guidelines in 1999. The CDC guidelines also provide some general information about the subject.[7] As part of the SCIP initiative, specific antimicrobial agents have been recommended for prophylaxis with certain operations: cardiothoracic, vascular or colorectal procedures, hip or knee arthroplasty, and hysterectomy.[44] These recommendations are periodically updated.[70] Prophylactic antibiotics for selected procedures are outlined in **Table 4**.

First and second generation cephalosporins are the preferred prophylactic agents for most surgical procedures.[7,44,67] For clean procedures, the primary consideration is activity against staphylococci, although for clean-contaminated procedures, particularly upper gastrointestinal or gynecologic procedures, coverage of gram-negative Enterobacteriacae is also a consideration. Both cefazolin and cefuroxime provide these antibacterial activities. Because of the large numbers of anaerobic bacteria in the lower gastrointestinal tract, anaerobic coverage is recommended for operations involving the distal small bowel, appendix, colon, and rectum. This can be provided by second generation cephalosporins with anti-anaerobic activity, such as cefoxitin or cefotetan, or by addition of an anti-anaerobic agent, such as clindamycin or metronidazole, to other first or second generation cephalosporins. For patients with significant β-lactam allergies, vancomycin or clindamycin is recommended for gram-positive coverage and aminoglycosides or fluoroquinolones are recommended when gram-negative activity is needed.[7,44,67]

Much of the data supporting use of first and second generation cepahlosporins for prophylaxis were derived from trials performed in the 1970s, 1980s, and early 1990s.[7,67] Other than aminoglycoside-based regimens, few other agents were extensively tested in those trials. In the recent past, there have been very few trials focusing on the use of antimicrobial agents for surgical prophylaxis. This means that current recommendations are derived from data generated before the widespread development of resistance among gram-positive and gram-negative bacteria and that there

Table 4
Prophylactic antimicrobial agents for selected surgical procedures

Procedure	Recommended Agents	Potential Alternatives	References
Cardiothoracic	Cefazolin or cefuroxime	Vancomycin,[a,b] clindamycin[b]	Mangram et al,[7] Weimann et al,[40] Anonymous,[67] Springer[70]
Vascular	Cefazolin or cefuroxime	Vancomycin,[a,b] clindamycin[b]	Mangram et al,[7] Weimann et al,[40] Anonymous,[67] Springer[70]
Gastroduodenal	Cefazolin	Cefoxitin, cefotetan, aminoglycoside[b,c] or fluoroquinolone[b,d] ± anti-anaerobe[e]	Mangram et al,[7] Anonymous[67]
Open biliary	Cefazolin	Cefoxitin, cefotetan, aminoglycoside[b,c] or fluoroquinolone[b,d] ± anti-anaerobe[e]	Mangram et al,[7] Anonymous[67]
Laparoscopic cholecystectomy	None	—	Anonymous[67]
Appendectomy, nonperforated	Cefoxitin, cefotetan, cefazolin + metronidazole	Ertapenem,[f] aminoglycoside[b,c] or fluoroquinolone[b,d] + anti-anaerobe[e]	Mangram et al,[7] Anonymous[67]
Colorectal	Cefoxitin, cefotetan, ampicillin/sulbactam, ertapenem, cefazolin + metronidazole	Aminoglycoside[b,c] or fluoroquinolone[b,d] + anti-anaerobe;[e] aztreonam[b] + clindamycin	Mangram et al,[7] Itani et al,[18] Weimann et al,[40] Anonymous,[67] Springer[70]
Hysterectomy	Cefazolin, cefuroxime, cefoxitin, cefotetan, ampicillin/sulbactam	Aminoglycoside[b,c] or fluoroquinolone[b,d] ± anti-anaerobe;[e] aztreonam[b] + clindamycin	Mangram et al,[7] Weimann et al,[40] Anonymous,[67] Springer[70]
Orthopedic implantation	Cefazolin, cefuroxime	Vancomycin,[a,b] clindamycin[b]	Mangram et al,[7] Weimann et al,[40] Anonymous,[67] Springer[70]
Head and neck	Cefazolin, clindamycin	—	Anonymous[67]

a In the absence of a β-lactam allergy, vancomycin use is only recommended for prophylaxis when there is a high incidence of infections due to resistant staphylococci.
b An alternative for patients with significant allergies to β-lactam agents.
c Gentamicin, tobramycin, netilmicin, or amikacin, although gentamicin is the aminoglycoside generally recommended for use for prophylaxis.
d Ciprofloxacin, levofloxacin, or moxifloxacin. Not approved by the FDA for use in surgical prophylaxis. Because of its anti-anaerobic spectrum of activity, moxifloxacin could potentially be used without an additional anti-anaerobic agent.
e Clindamycin or metronidazole.
f Approved by the FDA for use as a prophylactic agent only for colorectal procedures.

is little data available regarding the efficacy of newer antimicrobial agents for surgical prophylaxis.

Only two newer antibiotics have been approved by the United States Food and Drug Administration (FDA) for surgical prophylaxis over the past decade or so. Alatrofloxacin, a fluoroquinolone, was found comparable to cefotetan for prophylaxis with colorectal procedures;[71] however, this agent was subsequently withdrawn from the market. The other was ertapenem, which was evaluated against cefotetan in a prospective, randomized, controlled trial in subjects undergoing elective colorectal procedures. Overall, in the subset of evaluable subjects, 18% of those randomized to receive ertapenem developed a SSI compared with 31% of those who received cefotetan, a statistically significant difference. The difference was also significant in the modified intention-to-treat analysis.[18] Thus, ertapenem can be used for prophylaxis for colorectal procedures and probably other operations involving the lower gastrointestinal tract where anaerobic coverage is needed, and is now included in the SCIP recommendations as an acceptable agent for colorectal procedures.[70]

To achieve high concentrations in the tissues during an operative procedure, the timing of prophylactic antibiotics is critical. In experimental animal studies, infections were prevented only if antibiotics were administered immediately before or at the time a wound was made.[72] This observation was supported by data from a large prospective observational trial by Classen and colleagues.[73] In this study, subjects who received prophylactic antibiotics within a 2-hour period before the incision was made had the lowest incidence of SSI. Subjects who had antibiotics initiated more than 2 hours before the incision was made, and those whose antibiotics started more than 3 hours after the incision was made, had 6.7- and 5.8-fold increases in the risk of SSI, respectively. Even if antibiotics were started in the perioperative period, defined as 0 to 3 hours after the incision was made, the risk was still increased 2.4-fold, although this was not statistically significant. Thus, the general recommendation is that antibiotics should be administered within a 1-hour period before incision; however, a 2-hour time window is considered appropriate when vancomycin or fluoroquinolones are used, since these antibiotics need to be administered over a longer infusion time.[7,44,67]

Adequate serum and tissue concentrations may not be maintained over the course of the operation, particularly with longer procedures or use of antibiotics with shorter half-lives.[74] In addition, some patients may sustain rapid blood loss during a procedure, leading to inadequate concentrations of the prophylactic agent.[7,75] Antibiotic redosing is one solution to this problem. However, there are no firm guidelines with respect to this issue. Based on one study, it was recommended that cefazolin be redosed if the surgical procedure was longer than 3 hours.[7,67,74] With use of an agent with a longer half-life, such as ertapenem, redosing would not generally be necessary.[70]

Patients who are morbidly obese are another group of patients in whom achieving adequate antibiotic tissue levels can be challenging. One study noted low tissue levels of cefazolin when a 1-g dose was given preoperatively to morbidly obese subjects. This was overcome by using a higher 2-g dose. The use of the higher dose was associated with a decreased rate of SSI in these subjects.[38] Although no definitive recommendation can be made, the use of higher doses of prophylactic agents would seem appropriate for patients who are morbidly obese.[7]

When used for surgical prophylaxis, the duration of antibiotic therapy should be limited. With few exceptions, published guidelines recommend that antibiotics be discontinued within 24 hours of the operation.[7,44,67] A maximum 48-hour duration of prophylactic therapy has been permitted for patients undergoing cardiovascular and liver transplant procedures,[44,67] although there is significant controversy regarding the need for longer therapy in those patients.[44,69,76] Many authorities, in fact, question the utility of administering further antibiotics at all, once the incision is closed.[7,69,76] Reviews of the available data suggest that single-dose regimens are as effective as multiple-dose regimens for surgical prophylaxis.[77,78] Limiting the duration of antibiotic exposure should help curtail the development of resistant organisms and avoid other types of collateral damage, such as *Clostridium difficile*-associated disease.[7,39,67] Nonetheless, it is routinely found that the principle of early discontinuation of prophylactic antimicrobial therapy is frequently violated by surgical practitioners, and is the SCIP measure that seems most refractory to change.[39,44]

PREVENTION OF SSI: SPECIAL CONSIDERATIONS REGARDING STAPHYLOCOCCAL INFECTIONS

S aureus is responsible for more SSIs than any other microorganism. The incidence of SSI due to this organism appears to be increasing, as are the numbers of infections due to methicillin-resistant clones.[20] Thus, there is considerable interest in approaches that could help prevent the development of SSI due to *S aureus*, including those due to MRSA.

Many, if not most, infections due to *S aureus* develop in patients colonized with this organism. Colonization of normal individuals with *S aureus* is quite common, and is a recognized risk factor for SSI.[7] In epidemiologic surveys, approximately 25% to 30% of healthy individuals in the community were found to have their nares colonized with *S aureus*.[79–81] In these healthy populations, nasal colonization with MRSA was uncommon, with only 1.0% to 2.6% of individuals found to carry this resistant pathogen. However, in a nationwide prevalence study, the number of individuals colonized with MRSA doubled from 0.8% in 2001–2002 to 1.5% in 2003–2004.[81]

One potential approach to prevent SSI due to *S aureus* would be to preoperatively decolonize patients carrying this organism. Optimally, this approach would include preoperative screening of patients to detect those who were actually carriers of *S aureus*. This approach would be applicable both to patients colonized with methicillin-sensitive *S aureus* (MSSA) as well as those colonized with MRSA.

Preoperative decolonization of patients has been evaluated in a number of studies, although generally in unselected subjects rather than in confirmed carriers of *S aureus*. Topical mupirocin applied to the nares is the agent generally used for decolonization. Treatment with mupirocin eliminated nasal carriage of *S aureus* in 91% of colonized health care workers.[82] In trials of preoperative decolonization, mupirocin was effective in 85%, 83%, and 82% of subjects colonized with *S aureus*.[83–85]

Data from nonrandomized trials suggested that decolonization of unselected preoperative subjects with mupirocin was effective in reducing the incidence of SSI due to *S aureus*; in some, the overall rate of SSI was also reduced.[86–89] Recent studies of subjects undergoing orthopedic surgery, in which decolonization was applied only to subjects who were confirmed carriers of *S aureus,* also demonstrated improved outcomes with this approach.[90,91] However, four prospective randomized controlled trials failed to demonstrate any benefit with use of preoperative mupirocin in unselected preoperative subjects.[83–85,92] Recent meta-analyses of these randomized trials or of combined nonrandomized and randomized studies suggested that decolonization with mupirocin prevented SSI due to *S aureus*, but that an overall benefit in preventing SSI in general was less certain. The results appeared strongest for subjects undergoing cardiac or orthopedic procedures; the potential usefulness of this approach for patients undergoing general surgery was questionable.[93,94] Given the variable results, the efficacy of decolonization is still considered an open question.[33,95] Clearly, further research is warranted, which may be facilitated by the increased availability of rapid screening techniques allowing more facile detection of S aureus carriage.

With respect to decreasing the risk of SSI specifically due to MRSA, a widely employed approach is to use prophylactic antibiotics effective against MRSA. Generally, vancomycin is the antibiotic used for this purpose in the United States; however, other glycopeptide antibiotics, such as teicoplanin, may be used elsewhere. Guidelines provide relatively little guidance as to when to use vancomycin. The CDC guidelines indicate that routine use of vancomycin is not recommended, although it may be the agent of choice when there is a cluster of SSI due to MRSA or coagulase-negative staphylococci.[7] The ASHP guidelines suggest that vancomycin use should be restricted, although it is appropriate for surgical prophylaxis involving implantation of prosthetic materials at institutions where there is a high rate of infections due to MRSA or coagulase-negative staphylococci.[67] However, neither guideline states a threshold for the incidence of infections due to resistant staphylococci that should lead to routine use of vancomycin for prophylaxis.

In part, this is due to the relatively poor results seen with the use of glycopeptides for prophylaxis. A meta-analysis by Bolon, and colleagues[96] evaluated trials of subjects undergoing cardiac surgery randomized to receive prophylaxis with a glycopeptide or a β-lactam antibiotic. No benefits were seen with the use of glycopeptides; the trend was actually toward better results with use of β-lactam agents. In subgroup analyses, subjects who received glycopeptide prophylaxis were less likely to develop an infection due to a resistant gram-positive organism, but this advantage was more than offset by an overall increase in the numbers of gram-positive and total infections. A potential shortcoming of the meta-analysis is that the component studies took place before MRSA was widespread in the hospital setting; six of the seven studies were stated to occur in institutions where the prevalence of MRSA was low. Nonetheless, even in the institution where there was a high prevalence of MRSA, prophylaxis with vancomycin proved to be no better than prophylaxis with cefazolin.[97]

There are several reasons why vancomycin may not be the ideal prophylactic agent, even in settings where there is a high prevalence of methicillin-resistant staphylococci. Vancomycin requires a prolonged infusion time to avoid development of the red man syndrome related to histamine release;[98] this necessitates careful planning to ensure timely administration of the agent for prophylaxis. In addition, vancomycin distributes into tissues somewhat slowly; tissue concentrations may not be adequate to cover staphylococci in some patients.[99] Further, vancomycin has no activity against gram-negative organisms. Thus, if vancomycin is used as the sole agent for prophylaxis, coverage of common gram-negative bacillary pathogens will be lacking; however, administration of a second agent to provide gram-negative coverage further increases the complexity of the prophylactic regimen.[33] Finally, the therapeutic efficacy of vancomycin against staphylococci has been called into question recently.[100] Vancomycin is generally considered less effective than β-lactam agents when treating patients with infections due to MSSA, and there is some evidence that vancomycin is also less effective than other anti-MRSA agents for the treatment of infections due to MRSA. Additional research is urgently needed to determine optimal antibiotic prophylaxis in settings in which there is a high prevalence of MRSA, particularly since this high prevalence is increasingly becoming the rule rather than the exception.

MANAGEMENT OF SSI

SSI is suspected when there is erythema, drainage or fluctuance of the surgical incision, in the absence or presence of systemic signs of infection such as fever or leukocytosis.[32,101] Local signs of infection are usually apparent with superficial and deep SSI, although systemic signs are somewhat variable. In contrast, the presence of systemic signs of infection in the absence of local signs may indicate an organ/space infection or an infection originating from a source other than the surgical site.

The distinction between a superficial and a deep SSI may not be obvious on cursory examination; a necrotizing infection of the deeper tissues may progress if what was thought to be a superficial infection is neglected. Thus, the possibility of a necrotizing soft tissue infection should always be considered, especially when there is a particularly erythematous or painful wound, or patient appears more ill than would be expected with a relatively minor infection. The diagnosis of a necrotizing infection is best resolved by direct examination of the subcutaneous tissue and deeper layers.[32,101,102]

Treatment of SSI nearly always involves opening the incision and establishing adequate drainage.[101,102] The blind use of antibiotics to treat what appears to be cellulitis of the wound without adequately determining the need for drainage is to be discouraged. For most patients who have had their wounds opened and adequately drained, antibiotic therapy is unnecessary. One recommendation is to use antibiotics only when there are significant systemic signs of infection (temperature higher than 38.5°C or heart rate greater than 100 beats/min) or when erythema extends more than 5 cm from the incision.[101] When antibiotics are used, selection should be based on the likely pathogens for a given operative procedure; thus, gram-positive organisms would be suspected following a clean orthopedic procedure, but involvement of gram-negative and anaerobic organisms would be expected if the infection followed a colorectal procedure. As with all soft tissue infections, the possibility that MRSA is involved in the infection needs to be kept in mind when choosing the empiric regimen. Although it has not necessarily been routine to culture most SSIs, this should be strongly considered in patients who will be treated with antibiotics, so that resistant microorganisms can be adequately treated.[101,102]

For patients with complicated skin and soft tissue infections, antibiotic therapy is generally used. Thus, most patients with deep SSI who have elements of tissue necrosis should be treated with antibiotics. Antibiotic selection should follow the general guidelines established for the treatment of complicated skin and soft tissue infections.[101] Patients who develop the rare early infections due to streptococci or clostridial organisms are usually treated with penicillin with or without clindamycin, and aggressive surgical debridement.

SUMMARY

SSI remains an important issue for surgeons, hospitals, and health care delivery systems. Despite encouraging trends in reduction of other nosocomial infections, there is little indication that much progress has been made in preventing SSI. In part, this may relate to the perceived trivial nature of this infection for many surgeons, despite the catastrophic consequences that occasionally follow the development of a SSI. A number of initiatives, some voluntary and others required by regulatory agencies, have been undertaken to improve surgical outcomes in recent years. The SCIP initiative[44] and the National Surgical Quality Improvement Program [103] include prevention of SSI as an important facet of their overall efforts to decrease surgical morbidity and mortality. These efforts to prevent SSI are handicapped, however, because many of the current recommendations regarding prevention are based on investigations performed several decades ago, when patient comorbidities were lower and pathogens were less resistant. To realize the full potential of these programs with respect to prevention of SSI, new research needs to be performed, and investigators need to be reinvigorated to find better approaches to prevent this common complication of surgical therapy.

REFERENCES

1. Klevens RM, Edwards JR, Richards CL Jr, et al. Estimating health care-associated infections and deaths in U.S. hospitals, 2002. Public Health Rep 2007;122:160–6.
2. Barie PS. Surgical site infections: epidemiology and prevention. Surg Infect (Larchmt) 2002;3(Suppl 1):S9–21.
3. Fry DE. The economic costs of surgical site infection. Surg Infect (Larchmt) 2002;3(Suppl 1):S37–43.
4. Horan TC, Andrus M, Dudeck MA. CDC/NHSN surveillance definition of health care-associated infection and criteria for specific types of infections in the acute care setting. Am J Infect Control 2008;36:309–32.
5. Simmons BP. CDC guidelines on infection control. Infect Control 1982; 3(Suppl 2):187–96.
6. Garner JS. CDC guideline for prevention of surgical wound infections, 1985. Supersedes guideline for prevention of surgical wound infections published in 1982. (Originally published in November 1985). Infect Control 1986;7:193–200.
7. Mangram AJ, Horan TC, Pearson ML, et al. Guideline for prevention of surgical site infection, 1999. Infect Control Hosp Epidemiol 1999;20:250–78.
8. Haley RW, Culver DH, Morgan WM, et al. Identifying patients at high risk of surgical wound infection. A simple multivariate index of patient susceptibility and wound contamination. Am J Epidemiol 1985;121:206–15.
9. Culver DH, Horan TC, Gaynes RP, et al. Surgical wound infection rates by wound class, operative procedure, and patient risk index. Am J Med 1991;91(Suppl 3B):152S–7S.
10. Anonymous. National Nosocomial Infections Surveillance (NNIS) System Report, data summary from January 1992–June 2001, issued August 2001. Am J Infect Control 2001;29:404–21.
11. Edwards JR, Peterson KD, Andrus ML, et al. National Healthcare Safety Network (NHSN) Report, data summary for 2006 through 2007, issued November 2008. Am J Infect Control 2008;36:609–26.
12. Nichols RL. Preventing surgical site infections: a surgeon's perspective. Emerg Infect Dis 2001;7:220–4.
13. Anonymous. National Nosocomial Infections Surveillance (NNIS) report, data summary from October 1986-April 1996, issued May 1996. A report from the National Nosocomial Infections Surveillance (NNIS) System. Am J Infect Control 1996;24:380–8.
14. Anderson DJ, Sexton DJ, Kanafani ZA, et al. Severe surgical site infection in community hospitals: epidemiology, key procedures, and the changing prevalence of methicillin-resistant Staphylococcus aureus. Infect Control Hosp Epidemiol 2007;28:1047–53.
15. Weiss CA 3rd, Statz CL, Dahms RA, et al. Six years of surgical wound infection surveillance at a tertiary care center: review of the microbiologic and epidemiological aspects of 20,007 wounds. Arch Surg 1999;134:1041–8.
16. Cantlon CA, Stemper ME, Schwan W, et al. Significant pathogens isolated from surgical site infections at a community hospital in the Midwest. Am J Infect Control 2006;34:526–9.

17. L'Ecuyer PB, Murphy D, Little JR, et al. The epidemiology of chest and leg wound infections following cardiothoracic surgery. Clin Infect Dis 1996;22:424–9.

18. Itani KM, Wilson SE, Awad SS, et al. Ertapenem versus cefotetan prophylaxis in elective colorectal surgery. N Engl J Med 2006;355:2640–51.

19. García Prado ME, Matia EC, Ciuro FP, et al. Surgical site infection in liver transplant recipients: impact of the type of perioperative prophylaxis. Transplantation 2008;85:1849–54.

20. Jernigan JA. Is the burden of Staphylococcus aureus among patients with surgical-site infections growing? Infect Control Hosp Epidemiol 2004;25:457–60.

21. Naylor AR, Hayes PD, Darke S. A prospective audit of complex wound and graft infections in Great Britain and Ireland: the emergence of MRSA. Eur J Vasc Endovasc Surg 2001;21:289–94.

22. Sharma M, Berriel-Cass D, Baran J Jr. Sternal surgical-site infection following coronary artery bypass graft: prevalence, microbiology, and complications during a 42-month period. Infect Control Hosp Epidemiol 2004;25:468–71.

23. Kourbatova EV, Halvosa JS, King MD, et al. Emergence of community-associated methicillin-resistant Staphylococcus aureus USA 300 clone as a cause of health care-associated infections among patients with prosthetic joint infections. Am J Infect Control 2005;33:385–91.

24. Merrer J, Girou E, Lortat-Jacob A, et al. Surgical site infection after surgery to repair femoral neck fracture: a French multicenter retrospective study. Infect Control Hosp Epidemiol 2007;28:1169–74.

25. Zoumalan RA, Rosenberg DB. Methicillin-resistant Staphylococcus aureus-positive surgical site infections in face-lift surgery. Arch Facial Plast Surg 2008;10:116–23.

26. Davis SA, Rybak MJ, Muhammad A, et al. Characteristics of patients with healthcare-associated infection due to SCCmec Type IV methicillin-resistant Staphylococcus aureus. Infect Control Hosp Epidemiol 2006;27:1025–31.

27. Popovich KJ, Weinstein RA, Hota B. Are community-associated methicillin-resistant Staphylococcus aureus (MRSA) strains replacing traditional nosocomial MRSA strains? Clin Infect Dis 2008;46:787–94.

28. Manian FA, Griesnauer S. Community-associated methicillin-resistant Staphylococcus aureus (MRSA) is replacing traditional health care-associated MRSA strains in surgical-site infections among inpatients. Clin Infect Dis 2008;47:434–5.

29. Gaynes R, Edwards JR, National Nosocomial Infections Surveillance System. Overview of nosocomial infections caused by gram-negative bacilli. Clin Infect Dis 2005;41:848–54.

30. Kusachi S, Sumiyama Y, Arima Y, et al. Isolated bacteria and drug susceptibility associated with the course of surgical site infections. J Infect Chemother 2007;13:166–71.

31. Anonymous. National Nosocomial Infections Surveillance (NNIS) report, data summary from January 1992 through June 2004, issued October 2004. A report from the NNIS System. Am J Infect Control 2004;32:470–85.

32. Nichols FL, Florman S. Clinical presentations of soft-tissue infections and surgical site infections. Clin Infect Dis 2001;33(Suppl 2):S84–93.

33. Anderson DJ, Kaye KS, Classen D, et al. Strategies to prevent surgical site infections in acute care hospitals. Infect Control Hosp Epidemiol 2008;29(Suppl 1):S51–61.

34. Pessaux P, Msika S, Atalla D, et al. Risk factors for postoperative infectious complications in noncolorectal abdominal surgery: a multivariate analysis based

on a prospective multicenter study of 4718 patients. Arch Surg 2003;138: 314–24.

35. Raymond DP, Pelletier SJ, Crabtree TD, et al. Surgical infection and the aging population. Am Surg 2001;67:827–33.

36. Kaye KS, Schmit K, Pieper C, et al. The effect of increasing age on the risk of surgical site infection. J Infect Dis 2005;191:1056–62.

37. Dronge AS, Perkal MF, Kancir S, et al. Long-term glycemic control and postoperative infectious complications. Arch Surg 2006;141:375–80.

38. Forse RA, Karam B, MacLean LD, et al. Antibiotic prophylaxis for surgery in morbidly obese patients. Surgery 1989;106:750–7.

39. Bratzler DW, Houck PM. Surgical Infection Prevention Guidelines Writers Workgroup. Antimicrobial prophylaxis for surgery: an advisory statement from the National Surgical Infection Prevention Project. Clin Infect Dis 2004;38: 1706–15.

40. Weimann A, Braga M, Harsanyi L, et al. ESPEN guidelines on enteral nutrition: surgery including organ transplantation. Clin Nutr 2006;25:224–44.

41. Klein S, Kinney J, Jeejeebhoy K, et al. Nutrition support in clinical practice: review of published data and recommendations for future research directions. National Institutes of Health, American Society for Parenteral and Enteral Nutrition, and American Society for Clinical Nutrition. JPEN J Parenter Enteral Nutr 1997;21:133–56.

42. Anonymous. Perioperative total parenteral nutrition in surgical patients. The Veterans Affairs Total Parenteral Nutrition Cooperative Study Group. N Engl J Med 1991;325:525–32.

43. Kjønniksen I, Andersen BM, Søndenaa VG, et al. Preoperative hair removal–a systematic literature review. AORN J 2002;75:928–38, 940.

44. Bratzler DW, Hunt DR. The surgical infection prevention and surgical care improvement projects: national initiatives to improve outcomes for patients having surgery. Clin Infect Dis 2006;43:322–30.

45. Webster J, Osborne S. Preoperative bathing or showering with skin antiseptics to prevent surgical site infection. Cochrane Database Syst Rev 2007;2: CD004985.

46. Digison MB. A review of anti-septic agents for pre-operative skin preparation. Plast Surg Nurs 2007;27:185–9.

47. O'Grady NP, Alexander M, Dellinger EP, et al. Guidelines for the prevention of intravascular catheter–related infections. Clin Infect Dis 2002;35:1281–307.

48. Brandt C, Hott U, Sohr D, et al. Operating room ventilation with laminar airflow shows no protective effect on the surgical site infection rate in orthopedic and abdominal surgery. Ann Surg 2008;248:695–700.

49. Barie PS. Are we draining the life from our patients? Surg Infect (Larchmt) 2002; 3:159–60.

50. Brasel KJ, Borgstrom DC, Weigelt JA. Cost-utility analysis of contaminated appendectomy wounds. J Am Coll Surg 1997;184:23–30.

51. Cohn SM, Giannotti G, Ong AW, et al. Prospective randomized trial of two wound management strategies for dirty abdominal wounds. Ann Surg 2001;233: 409–13.

52. Bennett J, Boddy A, Rhodes M. Choice of approach for appendicectomy: a meta-analysis of open versus laparoscopic appendicectomy. Surg Laparosc Endosc Percutan Tech 2007;17:245–55.

53. Sessler DI, Akca O. Nonpharmacological prevention of surgical wound infections. Clin Infect Dis 2002;35:1397–404.

54. Kurz A, Sessler DI, Lenhardt R. Perioperative normothermia to reduce the incidence of surgical-wound infection and shorten hospitalization. N Engl J Med 1996;334:1209–15.

55. Barone JE, Tucker JB, Cecere J, et al. Hypothermia does not result in more complications after colon surgery. Am Surg 1999;65:356–9.

56. Walz JM, Paterson CA, Seligowski JM, et al. Surgical site infection following bowel surgery: a retrospective analysis of 1446 patients. Arch Surg 2006;141: 1014–8.

57. Greif R, Akça O, Horn EP, et al. Supplemental perioperative oxygen to reduce the incidence of surgical-wound infection. N Engl J Med 2000;342:161–7.

58. Pryor KO, Fahey TJ III, Lien CA, Goldstein PA. Surgical site infection and the routine use of perioperative hyperoxia in a general surgical population: a randomized controlled trial. JAMA 2004;291:79–87.

59. Belda FJ, Aguilera L, García de la Asunción J, et al. Supplemental perioperative oxygen and the risk of surgical wound infection: a randomized controlled trial. JAMA 2005;294:2035–42.

60. Mayzler O, Weksler N, Domchik S, et al. Does supplemental perioperative oxygen administration reduce the incidence of wound infection in elective colorectal surgery? Minerva Anestesiol 2005;71:21–5.

61. Chura JC, Byond A, Argenta PA. Surgical site infections and supplemental perioperative oxygen in colorectal surgery patients: a systematic review. Surg Infect (Larchmt) 2007;8:455–61.

62. Meyhoff CS, Wetterslev J, Jorgensen LN, et al. Perioperative oxygen fraction – effect on surgical site infection and pulmonary complications after abdominal surgery: a randomized clinical trial. Rationale and design of the PROXI-Trial. Trial 2008;9:58.

63. Zerr KJ, Furnary AP, Grunkemeier GL, et al. Glucose control lowers the risk of wound infection in diabetics after open heart operations. Ann Thorac Surg 1997;63:356–61.

64. Furnary AP, Zerr KJ, Grunkemeier GL, et al. Continuous intravenous insulin infusion reduces the incidence of deep sternal wound infection in diabetic patients after cardiac surgical procedures. Ann Thorac Surg 1999;67: 352–62.

65. Lazar HL, Chipkin SR, Fitzgerald CA, et al. Tight glycemic control in diabetic coronary artery bypass graft patients improves perioperative outcomes and decreases recurrent ischemic events. Circulation 2004;109:1497–502.

66. Carr JM, Sellke FW, Fey M, et al. Implementing tight glucose control after coronary artery bypass surgery. Ann Thorac Surg 2005;80:902–9.

67. Anonymous. ASHP Therapeutic guidelines on antimicrobial prophylaxis in surgery. Am J Health Syst Pharm 1999;56:1839–88.

68. Platt R, Zaleznik DF, Hopkins CC, et al. Perioperative antibiotic prophylaxis for herniorrhaphy and breast surgery. N Engl J Med 1990;322:153–60.

69. Nichols RL, Condon RE, Barie PS. Antibiotic prophylaxis in surgery–2005 and beyond. Surg Infect (Larchmt) 2005;6:349–61.

70. Springer R. The Surgical care improvement project-focusing on infection control. Plast Surg Nurs 2007;27:163–7.

71. Milsom JW, Smith DL, Corman ML, et al. Double-blind comparison of single-dose alatrofloxacin and cefotetan as prophylaxis of infection following elective colorectal surgery. Am J Surg 1998;176(Suppl 6A):46S–52S.

72. Burke JF. The effective period of preventive antibiotic action in experimental incisions and dermal lesions. Surgery 1961;50:161–8.

73. Classen DC, Evans RS, Pestotnik SL, et al. The timing of prophylactic administration of antibiotics and the risk of surgical-wound infection. N Engl J Med 1992; 326:281–6.
74. Scher K. Studies on the duration of antibiotic administration for surgical prophylaxis. Am Surg 1997;63:59–62.
75. Swoboda SM, Merz C, Kostuik J, et al. Does intraoperative blood loss affect antibiotic serum and tissue concentrations? Arch Surg 1996;131:1165–72.
76. Barie PS. Modern surgical antibiotic prophylaxis and therapy–less is more. Surg Infect (Larchmt) 2000;1:23–9.
77. DiPiro JT, Cheung RP, Bowden TA Jr, et al. Single dose systemic antibiotic prophylaxis of surgical wound infections. Am J Surg 1986;152:552–9.
78. McDonald M, Grabsch E, Marshall C, et al. Single- versus multiple-dose antimicrobial prophylaxis for major surgery: a systematic review. Aust N Z J Surg 1998; 68:388–96.
79. Rim JY, Bacon AE 3rd. Prevalence of community-acquired methicillin-resistant Staphylococcus aureus colonization in a random sample of healthy individuals. Infect Control Hosp Epidemiol 2007;28:1044–6.
80. Fritz SA, Garbutt J, Elward A, et al. Prevalence of and risk factors for community-acquired methicillin-resistant and methicillin-sensitive Staphylococcus aureus colonization in children seen in a practice-based research network. Pediatrics 2008;121:1090–8.
81. Gorwitz RJ, Kruszon-Moran D, McAllister SK, et al. Changes in the prevalence of nasal colonization with Staphylococcus aureus in the United States, 2001–2004. J Infect Dis 2008;197:1226–34.
82. Doebbeling BN, Breneman DL, Neu HC, et al. Elimination of Staphylococcus aureus nasal carriage in health care workers: analysis of six clinical trials with calcium mupirocin ointment. Clin Infect Dis 1993;17:466–74.
83. Kalmeijer MD, Coertjens H, van Nieuwland-Bollen PM, et al. Surgical site infections in orthopedic surgery: the effect of mupirocin nasal ointment in a double-blind, randomized, placebo-controlled study. Clin Infect Dis 2002;35: 353–8.
84. Perl TM, Cullen JJ, Wenzel RP, et al. Intranasal mupirocin to prevent postoperative Staphylococcus aureus infections. N Engl J Med 2002;346:1871–7.
85. Konvalinka A, Errett L, Fong IW. Impact of treating Staphylococcus aureus nasal carriers on wound infections in cardiac surgery. J Hosp Infect 2006;64:162–8.
86. Kluytmans JA, Mouton JW, VandenBergh MF, et al. Reduction of surgical-site infections in cardiothoracic surgery by elimination of nasal carriage of Staphylococcus aureus. Infect Control Hosp Epidemiol 1996;17:780–5.
87. Gernaat-van der Sluis AJ, Hoogenboom-Verdegaal AM, Edixhoven PJ, et al. Prophylactic mupirocin could reduce orthopedic wound infections: 1,044 patients treated with mupirocin compared with 1,260 historical controls. Acta Orthop Scand 1998;69:412–4.
88. Yano M, Doki Y, Inoue M, et al. Preoperative intranasal mupirocin ointment significantly reduces postoperative infection with Staphylococcus aureus in patients undergoing upper gastrointestinal surgery. Surg Today 2000;30:16–21.
89. Cimochowski GE, Harostock MD, Brown R, et al. Intranasal mupirocin reduces sternal wound infection after open heart surgery in diabetics and nondiabetics. Ann Thorac Surg 2001;71:1572–8.
90. Rao N, Cannella B, Crossett LS, et al. A preoperative decolonization protocol for Staphylococcus aureus prevents orthopaedic infections. Clin Orthop Relat Res 2008;466:1343–8.

91. Hacek DM, Robb WJ, Paule SM, et al. Staphylococcus aureus nasal decolonization in joint replacement surgery reduces infection. Clin Orthop Relat Res 2008; 466:1349–55.

92. Suzuki Y, Kamigaki T, Fujino Y, et al. Randomized clinical trial of preoperative intranasal mupirocin to reduce surgical-site infection after digestive surgery. Br J Surg 2003;90:1072–5.

93. Kallen AJ, Wilson CT, Larson RJ. Perioperative intranasal mupirocin for the prevention of surgical site infections: a systematic review of the literature and meta-analysis. Infect Control Hosp Epidemiol 2005;26:916–22.

94. Van Rijen MM, Bonten M, Wenzel RP, et al. Intranasal mupirocin for reduction of Staphylococcus aureus infections in surgical patients with nasal carriage: a systematic review. J Antimicrob Chemother 2008;61:254–61.

95. Laupland KB, Conly JM. Treatment of Staphylococcus aureus colonization and prophylaxis for infection with topical intranasal mupirocin: an evidence-based review. Clin Infect Dis 2003;37:933–8.

96. Bolon MK, Morlote M, Weber SG, et al. Glycopeptides are no more effective than β-lactam agents for prevention of surgical site infection after cardiac surgery: a meta-analysis. Clin Infect Dis 2004;38:1357–63.

97. Finkelstein R, Rabino G, Mashiah T, et al. Vancomycin versus cefazolin prophylaxis for cardiac surgery in the setting of a high prevalence of methicillin-resistant staphylococcal infections. J Thorac Cardiovasc Surg 2002;123:326–32.

98. Sivagnanam S, Deleu D. Red man syndrome. Crit Care 2003;7:119–21.

99. Martin C, Alaya M, Mallet MN, et al. Penetration of vancomycin into mediastinal and cardiac tissues in humans. Antimicrobial Agents Chemother 1994;38:396–9.

100. Dereskinski S. Counterpoint: vancomycin and Staphylococcus aureus—an antibiotic enters obsolescence. Clin Infect Dis 2007;44:1543–8.

101. Stevens DL, Bisno AL, Chambers HF, et al. Practice guidelines for the diagnosis and management of skin and soft-tissue infections. Clin Infect Dis 2005;41:1373–406.

102. Barie PS, Eachempati SR. Surgical site infections. Surg Clin North Am 2005;85:1115–35.

103. Khuri SF. Safety, quality, and the National Surgical Quality Improvement Program. Am Surg 2006;72:994–8.

Prosthetic Infection: Lessons from Treatment of the Infected Vascular Graft

Gabriel Herscu, MD[a],*, Samuel Eric Wilson, MD[b]

KEYWORDS

• Vascular • Prosthesis • Graft • Infection

Surgical prosthetic infections are a significant source of morbidity and mortality. In vascular surgery, infection of prosthetic grafts occurs in 1% to 6% of implanted conduits, with catastrophic consequences, including high amputation and mortality rates.[1] These outcomes, though infrequent, represent a significant health care cost to society (**Table 1**).[2] Research into the pathogenesis of graft infections, particularly in relation to biofilm formation, has broadened our understanding of prosthetic infection and alerted us to the contribution of antimicrobial-resistant bacteria. A thorough understanding of the etiology and presentation of a surgical prosthetic infection allows the surgeon to diagnose and treat infections more effectively. This article focuses on pathogenesis, diagnosis, and treatment of vascular graft infections as a model for infections of all surgical prosthetics, drawing on the extensive research on vascular prostheses. Over the past several decades there has been a paradigm shift in techniques for management of vascular infections, allowing graft preservation in selected patients with decreased morbidity. Attention has focused on prevention of infection during initial placement of the prostheses. Successful reduction in infection of vascular devices is most evident in central venous catheterization. Prosthetic infections, however, continue to present a challenge to the practicing surgeon, requiring early diagnosis and stratification of treatment methods based on the characteristics of the infection.

PATHOGENESIS

Our understanding of the pathogenesis of surgical prosthetic infection owes much to research on surface biofilms and their clinical sequelae. This section focuses on

[a] Department of Surgery, University of California, Irvine Medical Center, 333 City Boulevard West, Suite #705, Orange, CA 92868, USA
[b] Department of Surgery, University of California, Irvine Medical Center, 333 City Boulevard West, Suite #810, Orange, CA 92868, USA
* Corresponding author.
E-mail address: gherscu@uci.edu (G. Herscu).

Surg Clin N Am 89 (2009) 391–401
doi:10.1016/j.suc.2008.09.007
0039-6109/08/$ – see front matter © 2009 Elsevier Inc. All rights reserved.

Table 1
Clinical and economic consequences of infections associated with surgical implants

Implant	Implants Inserted in the United States Annually	Projected Infections of Implants Annually	Average Rate of Infection	Preferred Practice of Surgical Replacement	Estimated Average Cost of Combined Medical and Surgical Treatment
	Number		%	No. of stages	United States $
Cardiovascular					
Mechanical heart valve	85,000	3,400	4	1	50,000
Vascular graft	450,000	16,000	4	1 or 2	40,000
Pacemaker–defibrillator	300,000	12,000	4	2	35,000
Ventricular assist device	700	280	40	1	50,000
Orthopedic					
Joint prosthesis	600,000	12,000	2	2	30,000
Fracture-fixation device	2,000,000	100,000	5	1 or 2	15,000
Neurosurgical—ventricular shunt	40,000	2,400	6	2	50,000
Plastic—mammary implant (pair)	130,000	2,600	2	2	20,000
Urologic—inflatable penile implant	15,000	450	3	2	35,000

From Darouiche RO. Treatment of infections associated with surgical implants. N Engl J Med 2004;350(14):1423; with permission.

fundamental concepts learned from central venous catheter infections, demonstrating the relevance of these infections to those developing in vascular devices and other prostheses.

A biofilm, commonly referred to as a "slime layer," which forms on the outside of a catheter or prosthesis, is a complex structure composed of selected species of bacteria and their secreted polysaccharide matrix, along with components deposited from serum that provide a nurturing and protective environment for growth of bacteria.[3,4]

Prosthetic infections begin with colonization of the external surface. This occurs most commonly on intravascular catheters, with invasion by bacteria colonizing the insertion site leading to ingress along the catheter tract. In addition, hematogenous spread from a distant infection site or infusion of contaminated fluid through the device may less frequently lead to infection.[3]

Microbial seeding of the catheter or device is followed by biofilm formation. When a prosthesis is placed, it has a clean, sterile surface. Immediately following implantation, it is surrounded by tissue fluid and blood, which deposit a proteinaceous film. Depending on the location, intravascular, musculoskeletal, or urinary bladder, the conditioning film will vary as will the initial microbial flora that attach to the device. The conditioning film alters the surface characteristics of implants, allowing adherence of bacteria that may otherwise not attach to the bare surface.[5] Adherence of *Staphylococcus aureus* is a result of the presence of host-tissue ligands in the conditioning film, including fibronectin, fibrinogen, and collagen. The adherence is mediated by microbial proteins known as "microbial surface components recognizing adhesive matrix molecules." The most important of these are FnbpA and FnbpB (which bind fibronectin), "clumping factor" (which binds fibrinogen), and collagen adhesion (which binds collagen). *Staphylococcus epidermidis* adherence to a catheter is characterized by an initial rapid attachment to the surface, mediated by nonspecific factors, such as surface tension, hydrophobicity, electrostatic forces, or by specific adhesions. This is followed by an accumulative phase during which bacteria adhere to each other, forming a biofilm. This phase is mediated by specific bacterial adhesive factors.[6]

Once adherence has taken place, the now sessile (or fixed) organisms divide and form microcolonies. Secretion of a polysaccharide matrix along with incorporation of new micro-organisms form the architecture of the biofilm. The ultimate three-dimensional structure is that of thick pillars separated by fluid-filled spaces. The fluid-filled spaces are used for diffusing waste products, receiving nutrients, and sending chemical signals between bacteria. Multiple species may exist in a single biofilm. Sessile organisms may detach and become planktonic (or free-floating), which may lead to bacteremia and symptomatic host infection.[4]

The clinical significance of biofilms is the physical barrier formed that limits natural defense mechanisms and effectiveness of antimicrobials. Laboratory results of bloodstream infections typically identify only planktonic organisms. Treatment may be aimed at these organisms while ignoring the sessile organisms dwelling on the implanted device or graft. In addition, plasmid exchange may occur in the biofilm, incurring further antimicrobial resistance.[4] Infection of implanted prostheses begins with biofilm formation as described above, followed by activation of host defenses (neutrophil chemotaxis, complement activation), and finally an inflammatory response in the perigraft tissues and at the graft-arterial anastamosis.[1]

Catheters and grafts have been designed to combat biofilm formation and subsequent septic complications. Strategies have included mechanical design alternatives, such as Dacron skin cuffs in the subcutaneous tissue, tethered anti-infective agents (antiseptic impregnated catheters), and release of soluble toxic agents (chlorhexidine, antibiotics) into the surrounding tissues. Infection of vascular grafts is also dependent upon the graft structure. Woven Dacron is 10 to 100 times more susceptible then polytetrafluoreothylene (PTFE) to becoming colonized.[7]

Development of new biofilm detection and treatment strategies are underway.[8] The most common pathogens involved in vascular graft infections were historically coagulase-positive staphylococci for early-onset infections and coagulase-negative staphylococci for late-onset infections. More recently, mixed pathogens have predominated as the causative organisms in these infections. *S aureus, S epidermidis,* and *E coli* currently constitute 75% of graft infections. *Proteus* and *Pseudomonas* have also been isolated (**Table 2**).[9] *S epidermidis* has low virulence, with limited tissue destruction, causing a prolonged smoldering infection, often presenting 1 to 5 years postoperatively as perigraft fluid, sinus tract, anastomotic false aneurysm, or aortoenteric fistula. The increased virulence of *S aureus, Pseudomonas* species, and gram-negative organisms predispose to prosthetic anastomoses disruption.[10] In particular, methicillin resistant *S aureus* (MRSA) infection of vascular grafts confers an increased risk of amputation and prolonged hospital stay.[11] Accordingly, the identity of the specific infecting organism exerts a strong influence on treatment.

AORTO-ILIAC GRAFT INFECTION

Infection of aortic grafts still represents one of the most trying postoperative complications encountered by both patient and vascular surgeon. It occurs in 1% to 3% of aortic prostheses. Aortic graft infection may present with gastrointestinal hemorrhage from aorto-enteric fistula or septicemia. Overall, the mortality is up to 20%, with amputation reported in 5% to 25% of patients.[1]

Table 2
Bacteriology of prosthetic vascular graft infections: incidence from 1,400 collected cases

Micro-Organism	Incidence(%)					
	AEF	AI	AF	FD	TA	ICS
Staphylococcus aureus	4	3	27	28	32	50
Staphylococcus epidermidis	2	3	34	11	20	15
Streptococcus species	9	3	8	11	2	3
Escherichia coli	28	30	12	7	2	5
Pseudomonas species	3	7	6	16	10	6
Klebsiella species	5	10	5	2	2	4
Enterobacter species	5	13	2	2	2	–
Enterococcus species	8	10	2	7	6	–
Bacteroides species	8	3	3	2	–	–
Proteus species	4	–	4	7	2	–
Candida species	3	–	2	1	4	5
Serratia species	1	–	1	2	–	–
Other species	3	2	3	6	2	–
No growth culture	8	13	2	2	9	12

Abbreviations: AEF, aortoenteric fistula or erosion (*n* = 450); AI, aortoiliac or aortic tube graft (*n* = 54); AF, aortobifemoral or iliofemoral graft (*n* = 460); FD, femoropopliteal, femorotibial, axillofemoral, or femorofemoral graft (*n* = 285); ICS, innominate, carotid, or subclavian bypass graft or carotid patch following endarterectomy (*n* = 90); TA, thoracic aorta graft (*n* = 65).

From Bandyk DF, Back MR. Infection in prosthetic vascular grafts. *In* Rutherford RB, editor. Vascular surgery, Vol. 1. Philadelphia: Saunders; 2005. p. 880; with permission.

Diagnosis of aortic graft infection is often difficult, requiring a high index of suspicion and aggressive investigation. Temporally, it may present up to 10 years after operation. Median time to manifestation of a graft infection is 3 years.[12] Presenting symptoms include recurrent fever or chills, new back or groin pain, erythema, swelling or a pulsatile mass in the groin, or hematemesis. Conclusive evidence of an infection may be obtained by image-guided aspiration of pus from perigraft tissues with positive cultures, radiologic demonstration of a graft-cutaneous sinus draining pus, or endoscopic identification of a graft-enteric fistula.[13]

CT is an accurate imaging modality for diagnosis of a graft infection. For advanced graft infection, the sensitivity and specificity approach 100%. Overall, diagnosis of low-grade infection yields a specificity of 100% and a sensitivity of 55.5%.[12] Persistence of perigraft fluid or perigraft soft-tissue attenuation beyond 3 months or perigraft air beyond 4 to 7 weeks should be presumed to be infection and perigraft fluid should be aspirated using an image-guided technique and characterized for pathogens. MRI has been less extensively studied but most likely has the same accuracy in identifying infection as computed tomography. CT has the advantage of allowing simultaneous image-guided aspiration of fluid collections. MRI is limited by great-vessel motion artifact. Nuclear medicine studies (radiolabeled white blood cells) are occasionally helpful if other imaging studies are negative, but caution is urged in the first 6 weeks postoperatively because of false-positive studies.[12,14]

Ultrasound is useful for evaluation of the inguinal areas. It may detect perigraft fluid or gas outside the expected postoperative timeframe (3 months for fluid and 2 months for gas), which would alert the clinician to possible infection. For aortic evaluation, it is limited by body habitus and bowel gas. Ultrasound may also be used for following known fluid collections with serial examinations. It is not adequate as a sole imaging study in planning an operative intervention in the presence of graft infection.[12]

An expectation that graft infection would disappear with endovascular techniques of aortic aneurysm repair has not been realized. A recent retrospective cohort study of over 13,000 patients undergoing aortic aneurysm repair found a similar rate of infection for endovascular and open initial aneurysm repair, with the primary risk for subsequent infection being postoperative (nosocomial) infection. Specifically, pneumonia, bloodstream septicemia, and surgical site infection were major predictors of aortic graft infection. Primary endovascular repair appeared to have the same, albeit low-infection rate, as open surgery (0.44%).[15]

Traditional management of aortic graft infection has consisted of extra-anatomic bypass, specifically axillo-femoral bypass, with complete removal of the infected aortic graft. More recently, methods have included debridement of infected tissue, with in situ replacement using cryopreserved allograft, autogenous vein, or rifampicin-bonded prostheses. A recent meta-analysis of in-situ replacement methods by O'Connor and colleagues[16] found these alternative techniques overall to be superior to the traditional method in terms of rates of reinfection, conduit failure, and early and late mortality and amputation rates. Rifampicin-bonded prosthetics were found to have the lowest rates of amputation, conduit failure, and early mortality. Paradoxically, the reinfection rate with rifampin-impregnated grafts was higher than that of other methods. Autogenous vein use had the lowest rate of reinfection, followed by cryopreserved allograft. Later mortality was lowest for autogenous vein and cryopreserved allograft reconstruction. When all outcomes were considered, in situ options for aortic graft infection have shown considerable promise.[16]

An early study of silver-coated prosthetic grafts had encouraging results for in situ management of aortic graft infection. This study showed it to be a safe and effective treatment modality, with a 3.7% reinfection rate at 16 months. A later study showed results similar to other in situ methods. The use of silver in prevention of infection is commonplace; however, in treatment of aortic graft infection, this modality requires further study.[17,18]

Treatment of primary endograft infections has been described in multiple anecdotal reports in the literature, with methods ranging from complete graft excision and extra-anatomic bypass to graft preservation with surgical drainage and antibiotics. This complication of a new modality has not yet provided adequate sample size to form a strong recommendation for treatment. Surgical treatment, although associated with a high mortality in this setting, seems to have better outcomes than conservative management.[19] Surgical methods described have been similar to those for treating infections associated with open aneurysm repairs.

Endovascular treatment of complicated aortic graft infection has been analyzed through anecdotal reports in the literature. A review of cases of aortoesophageal and aortoenteric fistulas by Gonzalez-Fajardo and colleagues[20] in 2005 concluded that endoluminal techniques are useful only in select patients, specifically those with infection because of low virulence organisms, absence of gross purulence, and those at prohibitive operative risk for open surgery. Endoluminal methods also seem appropriate in unstable patients, as a bridge therapy to more definitive treatment after hemodynamic stabilization has been achieved.[20] Endovascular techniques have found use in primary treatment of mycotic organisms with fair results. Aneurysmal rupture and fever at presentation are the strongest predictors of recurrent infection.[21]

PERIPHERAL VASCULAR GRAFT INFECTION

The incidence of infection of vascular prosthetics implanted for peripheral arterial occlusive disease falls in the range of 1% to 5%.[10] Again, the virulence of the inoculated bacteria determines the clinical presentation of the infection. Early wound infection (within the first few weeks) is predominantly because of coagulase-positive staphylococci such as *S aureus*, along with *E coli, Proteus* spp, and *P aeruginosa*.[9] These early infecting organisms, especially *S aureus* and *Pseudomonas*, are associated with an increased risk of anastomotic disruption. This is in contrast to *S epidermidis*, the most common late-presenting (greater than 1 month) organism, which may produce an indolent infection presenting months to years after implantation (see **Table 2**). Early infections typically present with erythema, tenderness, drainage of purulent fluid and, in more advanced infection, with anastomotic disruption or septicemia. Late infections often present with a small draining sinus from the incision resembling a "stitch" abscess. Further investigation reveals a sinus tract leading to a fluid collection surrounding the graft.[10,22]

The extent of wound infection has been classified (Szilagyi grade 1–3) to distinguish overlying soft tissue infections from graft infection and to guide treatment.[23] A superficial (Szilagyi-1) infection may be observed and treated medically with a 5- to 7-day course of antibiotics effective against gram-positive organisms. In the setting of implanted PTFE grafts, occasionally this may represent an aseptic inflammatory response to a subcutaneous graft (foreign body). This is commonly seen after PTFE graft placement for hemodialysis.[10] Deeper infections involving the subcutaneous tissues and muscular layers (Szilagyi-2) may present as skin changes associated with an underlying fluid collection or drainage of purulent or serous fluid. These infections are assumed to be because of primary wound-healing problems and not an infected graft. In contrast, Szilagyi-3 infections have direct evidence of graft involvement. Traditional treatment of Szilagyi-3 infections includes complete graft excision with revascularization through an uninfected plane. Graft preservation techniques have been developed for infections that do not involve the entire graft. These techniques include local drainage, debridement of necrotic tissue with tissue culture, topical and intravenous antibiotics, and early autogenous tissue coverage.[22] Using this approach in patients with Szilagyi-2 and -3 infections, Calligaro and colleagues[24] reported a 71% healing rate for infected extracavitary graft site infections among survivors with a 4% amputation rate in 120 cases. Early drainage and debridement with skin closure over closed suction drainage was also shown to be effective for early graft exposure in one small series by Gordon and colleagues.[25] Muscle-flap coverage of the graft provides better obliteration of dead space, improved antibiotic and white blood cell delivery to the wound, and control of serous drainage.[26] Negative pressure dressings have been applied to periprosthetic wounds with encouraging results, including those with exposed graft and anastamosis.[27–30]

Early postoperative infection often precludes adequate graft incorporation into surrounding tissues. Septicemia, anastomotic hemorrhage, and pseudoaneurysm from infection in this timeframe are generally regarded as contraindications to graft preservation.[22] These are optimally managed with complete graft excision and revascularization through an uninfected plane. Selective in situ revascularization using autograft or homograft may be performed, but discretion should be used in determining appropriate candidates based upon evaluation of the wound bed and pathogens involved. Results of in situ methods have been positive.[31–33] Gram-negative pathogens, especially *Pseudomonas* and MRSA, are more virulent, involving more of the prosthesis and requiring aggressive conventional management.[10] Various revascularization routes through noninfected tissue planes are available in the groin area.[34] A staged approach beginning with removal of infected graft and staged revascularization may be used if limb viability is not in question after graft removal.[22]

Late (>1 month) infections are a diagnostic challenge that require prompt investigation. Injection of water-soluble contrast into a draining sinus outlining the graft may establish the diagnosis. Ultrasound-diagnosed fluid collections may be aspirated, providing a diagnosis and a culture specimen.[10] Computed tomography offers the added utility of CT-guided aspiration of fluid collections. Treatment of the infection proceeds by a similar paradigm as early graft infections, with the benefit of a trend toward low-virulence pathogens responsible for late graft infections.[10]

Antibiotic-loaded polymethylmethacrylate (PMMA) cement has been used by orthopedic surgeons in treatment of osteomyelitis and prosthetic joint infections. Recently it has been used as an adjunctive treatment for early and late vascular-site infections, allowing decontamination of the wound before in situ and graft preservation techniques. This has shown promising results, even against *S. aureus* and *Pseudomonas* species.[35]

HEMODIALYSIS GRAFT INFECTION

Infection of hemodialysis access PTFE grafts represents a significant source of morbidity and mortality. Early (<1 month) infection after graft placement is usually secondary to a postoperative incisional infection, whereas later infection is caused by local inoculation with bacteria at the site of graft puncture for routine hemodialysis. The infection rate of hemodialysis access grafts ranges from 3% to 35%, second only to thrombosis as a complication of this procedure.[36,37] The most common presentation of infection is an exposed graft or draining sinus tract. Less commonly, patients present with hemorrhage, pain, erythema, or sepsis. Traditional management of these infections has consisted of complete graft excision and new permanent access placement at another site. Temporary venous access placement was also necessary as the new fistula matured. These methods are still applicable to the patient with bacteremia. More recently, investigations have been performed to identify patients that may benefit from partial or subtotal graft excision in the face of late infection. Subtotal graft excision involves leaving the cuff of graft at a well-incorporated arterial anastomosis, thereby avoiding the often difficult arterial dissection and patch repair. This management is appropriate only if the arterial anastomosis is well incorporated, thereby excluding infection of this segment. It avoids the risk of nerve or vein injury during excision of well-incorporated graft segments. Partial graft excision involves placing an occlusive dressing over the infected area and performing a segmental bypass of the infected portion through uninfected tissue, followed by removal of the infected segment of graft as a single or two-stage operation. This method allows select patients to maintain the same access site without need for temporary venous access. Previous studies found a high rate of reinfection with partial graft excision.[38] Ryan and colleagues[39] outlined a management scheme used for graft infection management with 51 graft infections over a 7-year period. By performing partial graft excision for localized infection without sepsis and without fluid surrounding the uninfected portions of graft, they attained a 74% success rate for partial graft excision. In 2007, Schutte and colleagues[40] examined 111 infected hemodialysis grafts over a 10-year period and found a similar postoperative infection rate of 19.8% with partial graft excision. Walz and Ladowski[41] found a significantly increased infection rate (46%), with no increase in mortality for patients undergoing partial graft excision. Patency of the graft was 50% at 1 year and 44% at 2 years, without need for venous catheters or new distant vascular access. Continued use of the same access site completes the argument for partial graft excision over complete excision.

Hemodialysis access prosthetics represent an added challenge to vascular surgeons because of the continual risk of inoculation of the graft during scheduled hemodialysis and the immune hyporesponsiveness of the uremic state.[42] Increased colonization with phagocytic bacteria, particularly *S aureus*, breakdown of innate immunity, aberrant acquired immunity, and the regular need to access the graft put uremic, hemodialysis patients at a greater increased risk of graft infection.[37]

PREVENTION OF GRAFT INFECTION

Graft infection is thought to occur most commonly by inoculation of bacteria from the patient's skin at the time of surgery or by direct spread in the perioperative period, often secondary to wound breakdown. Laboratory and clinical research has focused on methods to decrease graft infection rates, including perioperative antibiotic regimens, preoperative skin antisepsis, antibiotic-bonded grafts, and antibiotic "lock" solutions for central venous catheters. Because of the difficulty in design of clinical trials, particularly the large number of patients required, robust evidence in support of a certain technique is scant. However, meta-analyses of these methods found that immediate preoperative antibiotics had the most substantial impact on wound infection rates with a relative risk (RR) for early infection of 31% (RR = 0.31).[43] There was no evidence of additional benefit based upon choice of comparable first- or second-generation cephalosporins, penicillin/β-lactamase inhibitor, aminoglycoside, vancomycin, or teicoplanin. Use of antibiotics beyond 24 hours postoperatively did not confer any additional benefit.[43] Postoperative administration of antibiotics may increase antibiotic-associated morbidity, resistant nosocomial bacteria, and cost.[9]

Established methods for prevention of infection include skin preparation with 10% povidone-iodine solution and application of an iodine-impregnated drape to the skin, avoidance of prolonged preoperative hospital stay (to prevent acquisition of antibiotic resistant skin flora), removal of operative site hair at the time of operation using clippers rather than a razor, protecting the graft from contact with contaminating surface, especially the surrounding skin, and avoidance of simultaneous gastrointestinal procedures.[1,10] Chlorhexidine gluconate skin preparation and application of liquid cyanoacrylate skin sealant to prevent carriage of skin flora into the wound are recently introduced techniques. Recently, skin preparation with chlorhexidine gluconate was shown to significantly reduce early infection after central venous catheter insertion,[44] although it is unknown if this applies to grafts placed during surgical procedures.

Some methods do not appear to impact rates of graft infection. Use of closed-suction wound drainage at time of initial surgery did not confer any benefit in reduction of wound infection rates. Review of studies involving preoperative antisepsis bathing regimens with chlorhexidine or povidone-iodine solutions also showed no benefit in reducing wound infection rates.[43]

Topical applications of antibiotics to prosthetic materials have also been studied in attempts to reduce rates of infection. The use of rifampicin-bonding to gelatin-coated Dacron grafts did not result in reduction in graft infection at 1 month or 2 years.[43] However, a well-studied successful application of this technique is the use of catheter lock (antibiotic left in the catheter for a period of time) and catheter flush (antibiotic flushed through the catheter) for central venous catheters. The rationale for this use is that this may prevent internal microbial colonization of the catheter and ultimately bloodstream dissemination of bacteria. Several meta-analyses of flush and lock solutions in neonates, oncology, and hemodialysis patients have suggested that risk of wound and bloodstream infections is decreased by more than 50%, with an even greater effect seen when focusing only on the lock treatment regimen. Additionally, there was a very low emergence of resistant bacteria in the studies.[45–47]

SUMMARY

Future development of detection and treatment methods will require a focus on the changing characteristics of bacterial virulence and antibiotic resistance while maintaining strict adherence to a prevention regimen. A high index of suspicion for these infections with a thorough understanding of the pathogenesis of the disease may guide the clinician. In situ methods in selected patients have been shown to be a viable treatment option, yet require further study and design. The optimal treatment regimen has not been clearly defined. Given the significant cost of these infections to society, however, further study is clearly warranted.

REFERENCES

1. Bandyk DF, Back MR. Infection in prosthetic vascular grafts. In: Rutherford RB, editor, Vascular surgery, vol. 1. Philadelphia: Saunders; 2005. p. 875–94.
2. Darouiche RO. Treatment of infections associated with surgical implants. N Engl J Med 2004;350(14):1422–9.
3. Trautner BW, Darouiche RO. Catheter-associated infections: pathogenesis affects prevention. Arch Intern Med 2004;164(8):842–50.
4. Watnick P, Kolter R. Biofilm, city of microbes. J Bacteriol 2000;182(10):2675–9.
5. Habash M, Reid G. Microbial biofilms: their development and significance for medical device-related infections. J Clin Pharmacol 1999;39(9):887–98.
6. Darouiche RO. Device-associated infections: a macroproblem that starts with microadherence. Clin Infect Dis 2001;33(9):1567–72.
7. Sugarman B. In vitro adherence of bacteria to prosthetic vascular grafts. Infection 1982;10(1):9–14.

8. Bryers JD. Medical biofilms. Biotechnol Bioeng 2008;100(1):1–18.
9. Homer-Vanniasinkam S. Surgical site and vascular infections: treatment and prophylaxis. Int J Infect Dis 2007;11(Suppl 1)):S17–22.
10. Wilson SE. New alternatives in management of the infected vascular prosthesis. Surg Infect (Larchmt) 2001;2(2):171–5 [discussion: 175–7].
11. Earnshaw JJ. Methicillin-resistant *Staphylococcus aureus*: vascular surgeons should fight back. Eur J Vasc Endovasc Surg 2002;24(4):283–6.
12. Orton DF, LeVeen RF, Saigh JA, et al. Aortic prosthetic graft infections: radiologic manifestations and implications for management. Radiographics 2000;20(4): 977–93.
13. Swain TW 3rd, Calligaro KD, Dougherty MD. Management of infected aortic prosthetic grafts. Vasc Endovascular Surg 2004;38(1):75–82.
14. Serota AI, Williams RA, Rose JG, et al. Uptake of radiolabeled leukocytes in prosthetic graft infection. Surgery 1981;90(1):35–40.
15. Vogel TR, Symons R, Flum DR. The incidence and factors associated with graft infection after aortic aneurysm repair. J Vasc Surg 2008;47(2):264–9.
16. O'Connor S, Andrew P, Batt M, et al. A systematic review and meta-analysis of treatments for aortic graft infection. J Vasc Surg 2006;44(1):38–45.
17. Batt M, Magne JL, Alric P, et al. In situ revascularization with silver-coated polyester grafts to treat aortic infection: early and midterm results. J Vasc Surg 2003; 38(5):983–9.
18. Batt M, Jean-Baptiste E, O'Connor S, et al. In-situ revascularisation for patients with aortic graft infection: a single centre experience with silver coated polyester grafts. Eur J Vasc Endovasc Surg 2008;36:182–8.
19. Fiorani P, Speziale F, Calisti A, et al. Endovascular graft infection: preliminary results of an international enquiry. J Endovasc Ther 2003;10(5):919–27.
20. Gonzalez-Fajardo JA, Gutierrez V, Martin-Pedrosa M, et al. Endovascular repair in the presence of aortic infection. Ann Vasc Surg 2005;19(1):94–8.
21. Kan CD, Lee HL, Yang YJ. Outcome after endovascular stent graft treatment for mycotic aortic aneurysm: a systematic review. J Vasc Surg 2007;46(5):906–12.
22. Piano G. Infections in lower extremity vascular grafts. Surg Clin North Am 1995; 75(4):799–809.
23. Szilagyi DE, Smith RF, Elliott JP, et al. Infection in arterial reconstruction with synthetic grafts. Ann Surg 1972;176(3):321–33.
24. Calligaro KD, Veith FJ, Schwartz ML, et al. Selective preservation of infected prosthetic arterial grafts. Analysis of a 20-year experience with 120 extracavitary-infected grafts. Ann Surg 1994;220(4):461–9 [discussion: 469–71].
25. Gordon IL, Pousti TJ, Stemmer EA, et al. Inguinal wound fluid collections after vascular surgery: management by early reoperation. South Med J 1995;88(4): 433–6.
26. Illig KA, Alkon JE, Smith A, et al. Rotational muscle flap closure for acute groin wound infections following vascular surgery. Ann Vasc Surg 2004;18(6):661–8.
27. Dosluoglu HH, Schimpf DK, Schultz R, et al. Preservation of infected and exposed vascular grafts using vacuum assisted closure without muscle flap coverage. J Vasc Surg 2005;42(5):989–92.
28. Kotsis T, Lioupis C. Use of vacuum assisted closure in vascular graft infection confined to the groin. Acta Chir Belg 2007;107(1):37–44.
29. Pinocy J, Albes JM, Wicke C, et al. Treatment of periprosthetic soft tissue infection of the groin following vascular surgical procedures by means of a polyvinyl alcohol-vacuum sponge system. Wound Repair Regen 2003;11(2):104–9.

30. Svensson S, Monsen C, Kolbel T, et al. Predictors for outcome after vacuum assisted closure therapy of peri-vascular surgical site infections in the groin. Eur J Vasc Endovasc Surg 2008;36(1):84–9.
31. Fujitani RM, Bassiouny HS, Gewertz BL, et al. Cryopreserved saphenous vein allogenic homografts: an alternative conduit in lower extremity arterial reconstruction in infected fields. J Vasc Surg 1992;15(3):519–26.
32. Dosluoglu HH, Kittredge J, Cherr GS. Use of cryopreserved femoral vein for in situ replacement of infected femorofemoral prosthetic artery bypass. Vasc Endovascular Surg 2008;42(1):74–8.
33. Castier Y, Francis F, Cerceau P, et al. Cryopreserved arterial allograft reconstruction for peripheral graft infection. J Vasc Surg 2005;41(1):30–7.
34. Hopkins SP, Kazmers A. Management of vascular infections in the groin. Ann Vasc Surg 2000;14(5):532–9.
35. Stone PA, Armstrong PA, Bandyk DF, et al. Use of antibiotic-loaded polymethyl-methacrylate beads for the treatment of extracavitary prosthetic vascular graft infections. J Vasc Surg 2006;44(4):757–61.
36. Anderson JE, Chang AS, Anstadt MP. Polytetrafluoroethylene hemoaccess site infections. ASAIO J 2000;46(6):S18–21.
37. Ready AR, Buckels JAC, Wilson SE. Infection in vascular access procedures. In: Wilson SE, editor. Vascular access: principles and practice. St. Louis: Mosby; 2002. p. xiv, p. 289.
38. Tabbara MR, O'Hara PJ, Hertzer NR, et al. Surgical management of infected PTFE hemodialysis grafts: analysis of a 15-year experience. Ann Vasc Surg 1995;9(4):378–84.
39. Ryan SV, Calligaro KD, Scharff J, et al. Management of infected prosthetic dialysis arteriovenous grafts. J Vasc Surg 2004;39(1):73–8.
40. Schutte WP, Helmer SD, Salazar L, et al. Surgical treatment of infected prosthetic dialysis arteriovenous grafts: total versus partial graft excision. Am J Surg 2007; 193(3):385–8 [discussion: 388].
41. Walz P, Ladowski JS. Partial excision of infected fistula results in increased patency at the cost of increased risk of recurrent infection. Ann Vasc Surg 2005;19(1):84–9.
42. Foley RN. Infections in patients with chronic kidney disease. Infect Dis Clin North Am 2007;21(3):659–72, viii.
43. Stewart A, Eyers PS, Earnshaw JJ. Prevention of infection in arterial reconstruction. Cochrane Database Syst Rev 2006;3:CD003073.
44. Chaiyakunapruk N, Veenstra DL, Lipsky BA, et al. Chlorhexidine compared with povidone-iodine solution for vascular catheter-site care: a meta-analysis. Ann Intern Med 2002;136(11):792–801.
45. van de Wetering MD, van Woensel JB, Kremer LC, et al. Prophylactic antibiotics for preventing early Gram-positive central venous catheter infections in oncology patients, a Cochrane systematic review. Cancer Treat Rev 2005;31(3):186–96.
46. Safdar N, Maki DG. Use of vancomycin-containing lock or flush solutions for prevention of bloodstream infection associated with central venous access devices: a meta-analysis of prospective, randomized trials. Clin Infect Dis 2006;43(4): 474–84.
47. Yahav D, Rozen-Zvi B, Gafter-Gvili A, et al. Antimicrobial lock solutions for the prevention of infections associated with intravascular catheters in patients undergoing hemodialysis: systematic review and meta-analysis of randomized, controlled trials. Clin Infect Dis 2008;47(1):83–93.

Skin and Soft Tissue Infections

Addison K. May, MD

KEYWORDS

- Skin and soft tissue infection • Skin and skin structure infection
- Necrotizing soft tissue infection • Necrotizing fasciitis

Skin and soft tissue infections (SSTIs) are a common cause of hospitalization, disability, and antibiotic therapy. Less severe infections are typically managed without the need for surgical intervention or the involvement of surgeons. SSTI may be more severe and invasive, however, placing patients at risk of soft tissue loss, limb amputation, and death. Recognition of the extent, depth, and severity of the skin and soft tissue infection is paramount if appropriate and timely therapeutic intervention is to be achieved. For more severe necrotizing infections, rapid and aggressive surgical debridement, appropriate antibiotic therapy, and supportive critical care management may be required.

TERMINOLOGY AND DEFINITIONS

A variety of terms are applied to infections of the skin and underlying soft tissue structures. For the purpose of therapeutic clinical trials, the Food and Drug Administration (FDA) uses the term "skin and skin structure infections."[1] The FDA specifically excludes necrotizing deep space infections from clinical trials, however, excluding infections involving the fascial planes and muscle and those infections with the greatest likelihood of adverse outcome.

Additionally, skin and skin structure infections are classified by the FDA as either "uncomplicated" or "complicated." Uncomplicated skin and skin structure infections are defined as those that respond to either a simple course of antibiotics alone or simple drainage alone and include superficial cellulitis, folliculitis, furunculosis, simple abscesses, and minor wound infections.[1–3] Complicated skin and skin structure infections are defined as those that involve the invasion of deeper tissues or require significant surgical intervention or occur in the presence of a significant underlying disease state that complicates the response to therapy. These infections include complicated abscesses, infected burn wounds, infected ulcers, infections in diabetics, and deep space wound infections.[1]

Division of Trauma and Surgical Critical Care, Department of Surgery, Vanderbilt University Medical Center, 1211 21st Avenue South, 404 Medical Arts Building, Nashville, TN 37212, USA
E-mail address: addison.may@vanderbilt.edu

Surg Clin N Am 89 (2009) 403–420
doi:10.1016/j.suc.2008.09.006   **surgical.theclinics.com**
0039-6109/08/$ – see front matter © 2009 Elsevier Inc. All rights reserved.

With the exception of cases of minor cellulitis that may occur at incision sites, SSTI that require intervention by surgeons include both complicated skin and skin structure infections and necrotizing soft tissue infections (NSTI). NSTIs by definition include the presence of devitalized or necrotic tissue as part of their pathophysiology. The presence of devitalized or necrotic tissue not only provides growth medium for bacteria but also precludes the delivery of host cellular and humoral defense mechanisms and antimicrobial agents. NSTIs may involve the dermal and subcutaneous layers (necrotizing cellulitis); fascia (necrotizing fasciitis); the muscle (pyomyositis and myonecrosis); or any combination of these.[3]

The author prefers the inclusive term "skin and soft tissue infection" to include uncomplicated, nonnecrotizing complicated, and necrotizing infections that may involve skin, subcutaneous tissues, fascia, or muscle. At presentation, the depth, severity, and specific tissues involved are frequently uncertain and at times difficult to establish. Additionally, the definitions of the various categories of these infections are indistinct and overlapping. This article discusses the diagnosis and management of complicated SSTI and NSTI.

NONNECROTIZING SKIN AND SOFT TISSUE INFECTIONS

SSTI may occur with a wide variety of clinical presentations and in numerous clinical settings, with diverse etiologic processes, and with varying severities. Numerous bacteria may be involved in SSTI, with the likelihood of individual pathogens being altered by factors including the inciting disease process and the clinical presentation and setting. Most SSTI infections are generally mild to moderate in severity and include simple cellulitis, folliculitis, furunculosis, and minor trauma-related wound infections.[2,3] Antibiotic therapy for most complicated SSTI is typically initiated empirically, hours to days before appropriate culture and sensitivity data are available. Selection of appropriate antibiotic therapy is based on knowledge of the likely pathogens involved in the particular infection episode.

Overall, *Staphylococcus aureus* is the most common pathogen isolated from SSTI, isolated in roughly one quarter to one half of all infections.[2,4,5] The most frequent pathogens identified in the SENTRY Antimicrobial Surveillance Program for the United States and Canada for SSTI collected from participating medical centers in five provinces in Canada and 32 states within the United States between 1998 and 2004 are provided in **Table 1**.[5] A total of 5837 pathogens tested represent 50 consecutive cultures collected from hospitalized patients in participating centers determined to be significant causes of pyogenic soft tissue infections. These cultures include both SSTI and surgical site infections and community-acquired and nosocomial infections. These results represent mainly complicated infections. These data may underrepresent the total frequency of β-hemolytic streptococci in SSTI because superficial cellulitis may not require hospital admission and adequate cultures are difficult to obtain even in severe cases of β-hemolytic streptococcal infections. A slightly different frequency distribution of pathogens in SSTI is provided through analysis of culture data from hospitalized patients in 584 hospitals in North America and Europe during 2001 obtained through the Surveillance Network.[2] The most frequent pathogens within this study in order of frequency are *S aureus*, *Enterococcus* spp, coagulase-negative staphylococcal species, *Escherichia coli*, and *Pseudomonas aeruginosa*. Again, streptococcal species were rarely isolated, representing only 1% to 2% of all isolates.

Antibiotic resistance among isolates from SSTI has increased significantly over time. **Fig. 1** demonstrates the percentage of individual pathogens that were classified

Table 1			
Rank order of bacterial pathogens producing skin and soft tissue infections in North America for the years 1998 to 2004			
Rank	**Pathogen**	**Total Isolates**	**% of Isolates**
1	*Staphylococcus aureus*	2602	44.6
2	*Pseudomonas aeruginosa*	648	11.1
3	*Enterococcus* spp	542	9.3
4	*Escherichia coli*	422	7.2
5	*Enterobacter* spp	282	4.8
6	*Klebsiella* spp	248	4.2
7	β-*Streptococcus*	237	4.1
8	*Proteus mirabilis*	166	2.8
9	Coagulase-negative *Staphylococcus*	161	2.8
10	*Serratia* spp	125	2.1

Data from Moet GJ, Jones RN, Biedenbach DJ, et al. Contemporary causes of skin and soft tissue infections in North America, Latin America, and Europe: report from the SENTRY antimicrobial surveillance program (1998–2004). Diagn Microbiol Infect Dis 2007;57:7–13.

as resistant in the SENTRY program between 1998 and 2004.[5] During that time period there has been a rise in methicillin resistance among *S aureus* (from 26.2%–47.4%); vancomycin resistance among enterococcus (from 8.6%–14.8%); extended-spectrum β-lactamase production among *Klebsiella* spp (from 4.9%–16.3%) and *E coli* (from 3.5%–12.8%); and multidrug resistant (nonsusceptible to members of four drug classes) *P aeruginosa* (from 1.3%–3.9%). The increase in methicillin-resistant *S aureus* (MRSA) in part represents the changing epidemiology of community-acquired soft tissue infections because of recent dramatic increases in the incidence of community-acquired MRSA (CA-MRSA) SSTI. In many locations within the United States, CA-MRSA is now the single most frequent pathogen isolated from SSTI.[6–9]

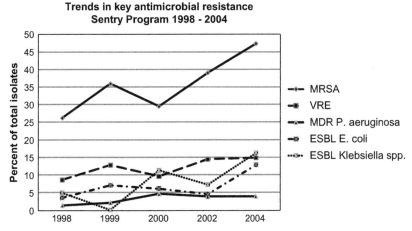

Fig. 1. Trends in key antimicrobial resistance Sentry Program 1998–2004. ESBL, extended spectrum β-lactamase; MDR, multidrug resistance; MRSA, methicillin-resistant *S aureus*; VRE, vancomycin-resistant enterococci.

Community-Acquired Methicillin-Resistant Staphylococcus Aureus Skin and Soft Tissue Infections

Staphylococcus aureus has consistently been the most common pathogen isolated from SSTI over the past decade or more.[5,10] Rapidly changing epidemiology now places CA-MRSA as one of the most common SSTI pathogens.[6–9] Historically, SSTIs caused by MRSA have generally been associated with nosocomial or chronic wound settings (hospital-acquired MRSA [HA-MRSA]), particularly when previous antibiotic selection pressure is present. Until recently, staphylococcal infections acquired outside of the health care setting have been frequently methicillin-sensitive and responsive to a wide range of antibiotics. As early as 1981, however, MRSA has been reported in community outbreaks in patients with and without risk factors for MRSA. These organisms have been called community-acquired or community-associated MRSA. Outbreaks have been reported in otherwise healthy Alaskan natives, children, inmates in correctional facilities, institutionalized adults with developmental disabilities, nursing homes, and athletes.[6] Most CA-MRSA infections are SSTI, although they may be associated with respiratory, bloodstream, and urinary tract infections.

CA-MRSA is more commonly associated with SSTI than HA-MRSA.[9,11] This association is likely related to the virulence factor Panton-Valentine leukocidin. This dermonecrotic cytotoxin may be carried by either methicillin-sensitive or methicillin-resistant strains of *S aureus,* but it is more commonly produced by certain clonal strains of CA-MRSA, particularly the USA 300 clone.[11,12] Enterotoxins and superantigens, such as toxic shock toxin–1, may also be produced by CA-MRSA and contribute to its virulence. Although most SSTI caused by CA-MRSA are associated with skin findings, such as furuncles and abscesses, they may also be associated with more serious findings, such as necrotizing fasciitis, invasive infections, toxic shock, and necrotizing pneumonia.[11,12]

CA-MRSA SSTI may involve previously healthy skin in an otherwise healthy adult. Patients may frequently believe that they have been bitten by a spider because of the character of the local wound involvement (a small central dark area surrounded by a firm indurated abscess and a variable degree of cellulitis). Although most cases of CA-MRSA SSTI may be considered uncomplicated infections, the toxin-related pathogenicity of CA-MRSA complicates the evaluation of depth and extent of tissue involvement in these infections and the possibility of an unsuspected necrotizing infection should be ruled out if unclear.

CA-MRSA isolates frequently have a different antibiotic susceptibility profile than HA-MRSA, although local patterns may be quite variable.[6–9,12] HA-MRSA is usually resistant to at least three β-lactam antibiotics and is usually susceptible to vancomycin, sulfamethoxazole, and nitrofurantoin. CA-MRSA is more likely to be susceptible to clindamycin and has varying susceptibility to tetracycline, fluoroquinolone, and erythromycin and vancomycin.[11]

Treatment of Nonnecrotizing Skin and Soft Tissue Infections

Most SSTIs treated by surgeons are classified as complicated infections and are more frequently severe in nature relative to those treated by nonsurgeons or treated on an outpatient basis. Uncomplicated skin and subcutaneous abscesses respond well to incision and drainage with appropriate wound care and do not require antibiotics.[13] Classification of an SSTI as uncomplicated is not always clear-cut, particularly with the involvement of CA-MRSA. The extent of the abscess must be appropriately evaluated during drainage to rule out underlying soft tissue involvement. Additionally, significant erythema, tenderness, or the presence of any systemic signs of infection should alert the clinician to the likelihood of a more complicated infection. More extensive cases of folliculitis and furunculosis may require treatment with antibiotics if the process is diffuse, has significant surrounding erythema, or the presence of fever.[2,3]

Nonnecrotizing cellulitis

Nonnecrotizing cellulitis by definition involves only the dermal layers and responds to antibiotic therapy without debridement. The term "nonnecrotizing cellulitis" incorporates two clinical entities, erysipelas and cellulitis, which are diffusely spreading skin infections not associated with underlying suppurative foci. The term "cellulitis" is frequently interchangeable with the term "erysipelas," and the latter term is frequently preferred in Europe. A fine distinction exists, however, between erysipelas and cellulitis. Erysipelas has two classic features of this skin infection: a clear line of demarcation between involved and uninvolved tissue, and lesions raised above the surrounding normal skin.[3] Cellulitis involves deeper layers of the dermis and subcutaneous tissue and has less distinctive features than erysipelas but both involve rapidly spreading areas of edema, erythema, and heat and may be accompanied by lymphangitis.[14] Establishing that the clinical signs and symptoms are indeed related to nonnecrotizing cellulitis or erysipelas rather than an underlying necrotizing infection is paramount but frequently inaccurate. Most cases of necrotizing fasciitis originally have an admitting diagnosis of cellulitis.[15–17] Several clinical and laboratory findings strongly suggest the presence of a necrotizing infection (see later) but careful clinical judgment is mandatory.

Nonnecrotizing cellulitis and erysipelas are most commonly caused by β-hemolytic streptococci (usually group A) but may also be caused by other streptococcal species.[14] In specific clinical situations, other bacterial species may cause a spreading, nonnecrotizing cellulitis, such as *Haemophilus influenzae* in children and pneumococcal cellulitis in the limbs of patients with altered immunity. Rarely, *S aureus* may be involved but these infections usually are more suppurative and less diffuse. Superficial, nonnecrotizing infections caused by certain strains of group A streptococci may also be associated with streptococcal toxic shock syndrome characterized by the rapid progression of septic shock and organ failure.[18]

Nonnecrotizing cellulitis and erysipelas generally arise when organisms enter through breaches in the skin. A number of predisposing factors for these infections broadly includes conditions involving alterations in integrity of the skin (ie, dermatoses, fungal infections, ulcerations); alterations in lymphatic and venous drainage (ie, saphenous vein harvest, lymph node dissections); alterations in vascularity of the skin; and alteration of host defenses (eg, diabetes mellitus).[19] Antibiotic therapy is most commonly based on empiric diagnosis established by clinical findings because cultures are most frequently negative. Blood cultures are positive in less than 5% of cases and positive results from either needle aspiration or punch biopsy range from less than or equal to 5% to 40%.

The treatment options for erysipelas and cellulitis have not been established through randomized, prospective studies but significant clinical practice has established standards of therapy. For cases of erysipelas and cellulitis caused by streptococci, penicillin given parentally (for severe infection) is the agent of choice.[3] Other regimens include antistaphylococcal penicillins, cefazolin, and ceftriaxone.[14] Teatment failures with β-lactam antibiotics do occur, however, despite in vitro microbial sensitivity to the agents used.[20,21] The mechanism of failure is believed to involve the failure of bacterial killing by cell wall–inhibiting agents when high numbers of bacteria in the static phase lead to decreased expression of penicillin-binding proteins.[21,22] Protein synthesis–inhibitory agents, such as macrolide and lincoamine antibiotics, may be as effective and potentially superior in certain settings.[20,21] Clindamycin either alone or in combination with a cell wall–inhibiting agent was found to be more effective than cell wall–inhibiting agents alone in a retrospective analysis of pediatric group A streptococcal infection.[21] Roxithromycin proved to be equivalent to penicillin for the treatment of erysipelas in a randomized, multicenter trial.[23] Increasing macrolide resistance among streptococci introduces concern for these agents, however, and local sensitivity patterns should be considered when using these agents alone for the treatment of complicated group A streptococcal infections.[21] Additionally, because clindamycin has been demonstrated to reduce exotoxin and superantigen production by pathogenic strains of group A streptococci, the drug is frequently used as an adjunct in the treatment of streptococcal toxic shock syndrome.[20] The most effective antibiotic regimen in this setting has not been established, however, in prospective studies. If methicillin-sensitive *S aureus* is suspected, the treatment of choice is a penicillinase-resistant semisynthetic penicillin or a first-generation cephalosporin for non–methicillin-resistant staphylococcal infections.[3,14] The recent dramatic increase in CA-MRSA makes the empiric treatment of staphylococcal infections with β-lactam antibiotics problematic, however, and other agents should be considered unless the risk of resistant staphylococcus is low (see later).[8,12]

Complicated skin and soft tissue infections

Complicated SSTIs may involve a variety of pathogens. They may involve only a single pathogen but are frequently polymicrobial in origin and may involve a number of organisms.[4,5,24–26] Initiating pathogens often vary on the originating site of the infection. Gram-positive aerobic pathogens are isolated in over 50% of all complicated abscesses and necrotizing infections and depending on the source of origin, anaerobes, *Pseudomonas* spp, gram-negative Enterobacteriaceae, and clostridial species may commonly be present. An accurate clinical history and examination should suggest the underlying etiology and direct empiric therapy. Complicated skin and subcutaneous abscesses are typically well circumscribed or walled off and respond to incision and drainage with adjuvant antibiotic therapy. Inadequate resolution should prompt consideration of further drainage, resistant pathogens, or host immune failure. During incision and drainage, appropriate examination must be undertaken to ensure that all loculations have been identified and that occult involvement of fascia or deeper tissue spaces is not involved. Certain areas, such as the perineum and perirectal space, may have deep space involvement that is very difficult to identify and CT imaging should be considered preoperatively to rule out occult, deep soft tissue involvement.

Empiric antibiotic therapy should be directed toward the likely pathogens involved. For polymicrobial infections, several classes of agents or combinations of agents provide adequate antibiotic coverage. Broad-spectrum agents with coverage of gram-positive, gram-negative, and anaerobic pathogens may be required depending on clinical setting. In nosocomial settings, coverage of resistant pathogens encountered locally should also be considered. De-escalation therapy should be considered and based on culture results. Given the high frequency of MRSA, this pathogen should be empirically covered unless specific data indicate otherwise. No randomized studies are available for the treatment of SSTI specifically caused by CA-MRSA. Sensitivity patterns are usually used to direct available options. A number of oral agents have been used for less severe infections treated as an outpatient.[11] In the patient with a simple abscess suspected to be caused by MRSA, incision and drainage of the abscess should be performed. The use of antibiotics as an adjunct to incision and drainage may be considered, particularly for those with significant cellulitis, and should be directed against MRSA. Although historically cultures of abscesses were not often obtained for simple SSTI, the increase in CA-MRSA prevalence suggests that this may be more clinically useful, particularly if there is no response to presumed adequate therapy. If CA-MRSA is suspected and the patient can be treated as an outpatient, oral antibiotics, such as clindamycin, tetracycline, trimethoprim-sulfame-thoxazole, erythromycin, and some quinolones, may be used. Other oral agents, such as linezolid, an oxazolidinone antibiotic that inhibits bacterial protein translation at the initial phase of protein synthesis, have been shown in randomized trials to be efficacious for MRSA.[27,28]

Complicated SSTI requiring hospital admission usually requires initiation of intrave-nous broad-spectrum antibiotics. Again, no randomized studies exist specifically for the treatment of CA-MRSA and therapeutic options are extrapolated from other stud-ies of soft tissue infections caused by MRSA. Although vancomycin has been the gold standard, one randomized study demonstrated superiority of linezolid in the treatment of complicated SSTI (88.6% versus 66.9% cured for linezolid versus vancomycin; P<.001).[28] Additionally, linezolid has been shown to inhibit toxin production in vitro providing theoretic advantage.[29] Other newer agents with activity against MRSA tested in randomized trials of complicated skin and skin structure infections include quinupristin-dalfopristin, daptomycin, and tigecycline.[6,30] Although each is approved for the treatment of complicated skin and skin structure infections, the randomized studies to evaluate the efficacy of these agents contained too few MRSA to draw con-clusions for recommendations. Quinupristin-dalfopristin is a combination of two strep-togramins that inhibit protein synthesis but requires central intravenous administration and has significant side effects, daptomycin is a lipopeptide with bactericidal activity against gram-positive pathogens including MRSA, and tigecycline is a broad-spec-trum glycylcycline antibiotic with activity against gram-positives including MRSA.[31] New agents currently being studied but not yet approved include dalbavancin, tela-vancin, and ceftobiprole. Another anti-MRSA cephalosporin, ceftaroline, has been shown to be effective in phase II trials and is currently undergoing further study.

NECROTIZING SKIN AND SOFT TISSUE INFECTIONS

NSTI are discussed separately because of (1) the increased severity; (2) the variation of pathogens relative to nonnecrotizing infections; (3) the difficulty and importance of establishing an early diagnosis; and (4) the impact of early, aggressive surgical debridement on outcome. NSTIs are serious infections, producing progressive tissue destruction with significant potential for soft tissue and limb loss and mortality. Despite advances in therapy over the past three decades, the mortality from NSTI remains sig-nificant. The overall published mortality in 67 studies of NSTI including 3302 patients between 1980 and 2008 (Table 2) is 23.5%.[4,15,16,24,32–94] Although the mortality has trended down slightly in published studies (27.8% mortality for studies from 1980–1999 versus 21.7% mortality since 1999), it still remains greater than 20%. NSTI may involve any combination of dermis, subcutaneous tissue, fascia, or muscle. Notably, each of these layers has varying degrees of intrinsic resistance to infectious processes. Blood supply to the fascia is typically more tenuous than that of muscle or healthy skin making the fascia more vulnerable to infectious processes. Additionally, the propensity for fluid to collect between involved fascia and adjacent tissues further weakens fascial immune function by altering host clearance of pathogens by decreas-ing phagocytic function. Necrotizing fasciitis is more common than necrotizing

Table 2
Outcome of necrotizing fasciitis

Authors	Year	Number of Cases	Percent Mortality	Authors	Year	Number of Cases	Percent Mortality
Casali[41]	1980	12	33	Gallup[54]	2002	23	13
Kaiser[61]	1981	20	40	Fustes-Morales[53]	2002	39	18
Freeman[51]	1981	14	29	Childers[44]	2002	163	28
Oh[73]	1982	28	36	Wong[16]	2003	89	21
Rouse[78]	1982	27	73	Tilou[85]	2004	46	17
Majeski[68]	1983	30	33	Qazi[77]	2004	25	24
Walker[88]	1983	8	38	Catena[42]	2004	11	64
Miller[71]	1983	15	27	Wilkinson[92]	2004	44	14
Adinolfi[33]	1983	11	27	Escobar[48]	2005	42	12
Spirnak[80]	1984	20	45	Kao[62]	2005	59	12
Stamenkovic[81]	1984	19	42	Legbo[65]	2005	24	17
Barzilai[37]	1985	11	36	Cheng[43]	2005	17	65
Pessa[76]	1985	33	33	Taviloglu[83]	2005	98	35
Freishlag[52]	1985	21	35	Endorf[47]	2005	65	17
Gozal[56]	1986	16	12	Tiu[86]	2005	48	29
Sudarsky[82]	1987	33	6	Anaya[34]	2005	166	17
Clayton[46]	1990	57	18	Bakleh[36]	2005	81	20
Asfar[35]	1991	10	30	Liu[67]	2005	87	33
Anaya[99]	1991	14	43	Kwan[63]	2006	36	36
Ward[91], Wang[90]	1992	18	33	Ozalay[74]	2006	22	14
Francis[49]	1993	25	24	Ogilvie[72]	2006	150	9
Chow[45]	1993	12	25	Yilmaziar[94]	2007	67	49
Brown[40]	1994	54	35	Lee[64]	2007	74	15
McHenry[69]	1995	65	29	Yaghoubian[93]	2007	124	17
Bosshardt[24]	1996	45	27	Peer[75]	2007	38	21
Elliot[4]	1996	198	25	Golger[55]	2007	99	20
Bilton[38]	1998	68	21	Tsai[87]	2007	32	31
Adant[32]	1998	7	14	Hefny[59]	2007	11	18
Hsiao[60]	1998	34	27	Miller[70]	2008	11	36
Haywood[58]	1999	20	20	Lui[66]	2008	118	22
Brandt[39]	2000	37	24	Frazee[50]	2008	122	16
Wall[89]	2000	21	29	Hsiao[15]	2008	128	19
Theis[84]	2002	13	31	Gunter[57]	2008	52	10
Singh[79]	2002	75	27	Total (N = 67 studies)		3302	23.5

processes involving other soft tissue layers because infection can spread widely across the fascial planes with minimal involvement of surrounding skin or muscle.

The pathogens involved in NSTIs differ somewhat from those isolated from nonnecrotizing infections, particularly those NSTIs that are rapidly progressive. In an analysis of 198 consecutive patients with necrotizing SSTI, Elliot and coworkers[4] documented a significant increase in the frequency of rapidly growing, virulent pathogens, particularly streptococcal and clostridial species (**Table 3**). In contrast to findings of the SENTRY program, which predominately includes nonnecrotizing, complicated SSTI, streptococcal species were the most commonly isolated organisms, occurring in greater than 50% of those patients in whom only one pathogen was isolated in this study. Streptococcal species were also the most frequent pathogens isolated from 707 patients included in six separate studies on NSTI, being isolated in 39.2% of patients, followed by S aureus, which was isolated from 30.1% of patients.[4,15,16,34,44,67] Most patients with necrotizing infections have polymicrobial infections with an average of 4.4 organisms isolated per infection in the study by Elliot and coworkers.[4] Such polymicrobial necrotizing infections arise from a number of inciting events including perirectal infection and Fournier's gangrene, trauma, intravenous drug abuse, chronic diabetic ulcerations, and surgical site infections.[4] An accurate clinical history and examination should be undertaken to identify the likely source and to identify the polymicrobial nature of these infections. Although these polymicrobial infections can spread widely and become both limb- and life-threatening, they tend to be much more indolent than infections caused by a fairly limited number of highly virulent pathogens. Such highly virulent pathogens may cause very rapidly spreading necrotizing infections in an immunologically intact host through production of exotoxins that contribute significantly to their pathogenicity. Such pathogens most commonly include *Streptococcus pyogenes* (group A β-hemolytic streptococcus), group B *Streptococcus*, CA-MRSA, and *Clostridium* spp. Other highly virulent species that can cause rapidly progressive NSTI with specific environmental exposures include *Pasteurella* spp (animal bites); *Vibrio* spp (shell fish or salt water exposure); and *Aeromonas hydrophila* (contaminated fresh water exposures).[95]

Table 3			
Microbiologic organisms recovered from original wounds			
Organism	**N**	**n**	**%**
Aerobic			
Streptococci	182	83	45.6
Enterococci	182	61	33.5
Staphylococci	182	64	35.2
Escherichia coli	182	57	31.3
Proteus sp	182	38	20.9
Other gram-negative rods[a]	182	76	41.8
Anaerobic			
Peptostreptococci	131	45	34.4
Bacteroides species	128	70	54.7
Clostridium perfringens	129	12	9.3
Other clostridial species	128	17	13.3
Other anaerobic species	128	27	21.1
Fungal species	171	9	5.3

N, number of cultures obtained; n, number of isolates.

[a]Including (in order of prevalence) *Klebsiella* spp, *Enterobacter* spp, *Pseudomonas*, *Acinetobacter* spp, *Eikenella corrodens*, *Citrobacterfreundii*.

Data from Elliott DC, Kufera JA, Myers RA. Necrotizing soft tissue infections: risk factors for mortality and strategies for management. Ann Surg 1996;224:672–83.

Diagnosis of Necrotizing Skin and Soft Tissue Infections

Early diagnosis of the presence of a necrotizing soft tissue infection is critical if optimal outcomes are to be achieved. Distinguishing a NSTI that necessitates surgical debridement from a nonnecrotizing cellulitis that responds solely to antibiotic therapy, however, can be difficult. Patients with NSTI have the diagnosis established on admission well less than 50% of the time.[15–17] Most patients are admitted with the diagnosis of cellulitis and a smaller number with the diagnosis of abscess. Unfortunately, any delay in diagnosis is potentially catastrophic, because the concomitant delay in appropriate surgical therapy has been shown to increase mortality.[4,24,26,38,69] Certain features of the disease presentation facilitate the detection of a necrotizing process. Pain, erythema, warmth, and swelling are present in most cases but are not specific to necrotizing infections and may not be universally present.[15,16] Several "hard" clinical signs are very specific to NSTI but occur late in the course. These include (1) the presence of bullae, (2) skin ecchymosis that precedes skin necrosis, (3) presence of gas in the tissues by examination or radiographic evaluation, and (4) cutaneous anesthesia. Although these findings are strongly suggestive of a necrotizing infection and should prompt immediate surgical exploration, these signs are present in the minority of cases (7%–44%).[16,69,93] Other clinical signs that are suggestive but less specific include (5) pain that is disproportionate to examination, (6) edema that extends beyond skin erythema, (7) systemic toxicity, and (8) progression of infection despite antibiotic therapy. The presence of gas in tissue by plain radiograph is more sensitive than detecting crepitance by physical examination.[69] CT scanning and MRI also assist in detecting the severe infections. These imaging techniques may detect fluid along fascial planes, edema within tissues, and gas not seen on plain radiographic evaluation. Notably, neither fluid nor edema is specific for the presence of necrotizing infection, and the sensitivity and specificity of these modalities have not been established.

Laboratory values may be useful to aid in the early diagnosis of NSTI. Two studies have examined the predictive value of standard laboratory tests to improve the diagnostic accuracy. In a study by Wall and colleagues,[89] 21 patients with necrotizing fasciitis were matched with 21 patients with nonnecrotizing infections. By multivariate analysis admission white blood cell count of greater than 14×10^9/L, serum sodium of less than 135 mmol/L, and blood-urea-nitrogen of greater than 15 mg/dL all discriminated necrotizing from nonnecrotizing infection with acceptable predictive ability. The small numbers of patients, however, limits the power required to evaluate a number of parameters of interest in this setting. More recently, Wong and colleagues[17] evaluated the predictive capability of various laboratory parameters in a larger population of patients (89 patients with NSTI, 225 with cellulitis or abscess). By multivariate analysis, they created the Laboratory Risk Indicator for Necrotizing Fasciitis score, which can classify patients as low, intermediate, and high risk for NSTI (**Tables 4** and **5**). This score should be applied to those patients without "hard" signs of necrotizing infection or in whom the diagnosis is uncertain. It use, however, has not been prospectively validated in other cohorts. The use of full-thickness biopsy and frozen section has been advocated but neither has been adequately evaluated or widely adopted.[81] If the presence of a necrotizing infection cannot be excluded, surgical exploration is indicated.

Therapeutic Approach for Necrotizing Infections

Aggressive and timely resuscitation, timely administration of appropriate antibiotic therapy, certain adjunctive therapies, and timely surgical debridement all may be required for optimal outcome. Of these interventions, surgical intervention is the mainstay of treatment. A number of studies demonstrate that time to first debridement

Table 4 Laboratory Risk Indicator for Necrotizing Fasciitis score	
Value	Score, Points
C-reactive protein, mg/L	
<150	0
>150	4
WBC count, cells/mm3	
<15	0
15–25	1
>25	2
Hemoglobin level, g/dL	
>13.5	0
11–13.5	1
<11	2
Sodium level, mmol/L	
≥135	0
<135	2
Creatinine level, mg/dL	
≤1.6	0
>1.6	2
Glucose level, mg/dL	
≤180	0
>180	1

Data from Wong CH, Khin LW, Heng KS, et al. The LRINEC (Laboratory Risk Indicator for Necrotizing Fasciitis) score: a tool for distinguishing necrotizing fasciitis from other soft tissue infections. Crit Care Med 2004;32:1535–41.

and adequacy of first debridement are important and alterable predictors of survival.[4,24,38,44,52,67–69,78,82,89] Unfortunately, definitions for delayed or inadequate initial therapy were not clearly described by the authors. In most studies, a delay in surgical debridement of greater than 24 hours after admission is associated with a significant increase in mortality. Surgical drainage and debridement at the earliest possible time, however, almost certainly improves outcome. In a recent report of 52 patients with NSTI managed by a dedicated acute care surgery service with in-house faculty, the median time from diagnosis to operative debridement was 8.6 hours with an overall mortality of 9.6%.[57] This mortality rate compares favorably with the combined published mortality rate in 67 studies since 1980 that is 23.5% (see **Table 2**). These data suggest that early recognition and adequate surgical management could reduce mortality to less than 10%.

Surgical Therapy for Necrotizing Infections

Surgical drainage and debridement of involved tissues is the mainstay of therapy in NSTI. No randomized studies or significant case series are available, however, to direct the actual surgical approach. Although retrospective reviews identify adequate and early surgical debridement as predictors of survival, they do not report quantifiable methods of defining adequate debridement.[4,24,38,44,52,67–69,78,82,89] Several issues should be considered: (1) determining the extent of resection, (2) full-thickness versus fascial excision for necrotizing fasciitis, (3) serial wound examination and

Table 5
Probability of necrotizing soft-tissue infection based on Laboratory Risk Indicator for Necrotizing Fasciitis score categories

Risk Category	Points by Score	Probability
Low	≤5	<50%
Intermediate	6–7	50%–75%
High	≥8	>75%

Data from Wong CH, Khin LW, Heng KS, et al. The LRINEC (Laboratory Risk Indicator for Necrotizing Fasciitis) score: a tool for distinguishing necrotizing fasciitis from other soft tissue infections. Crit Care Med 2004;32:1535–41; and Anaya DA, Dellinger EP. Necrotizing soft-tissue infection: diagnosis and management. Clin Infect Dis 2007;44:705–10.

debridement, and (4) diverting colostomy versus other methods of control of the fecal stream for perineal and scrotal infectious processes. The determination of extent of resection is most commonly based on clinical judgment and the gross appearance of tissues involved. Fascial layers, skin, subcutaneous fat, and muscle may each be involved in the infectious process with their involvement varying depending on the clinical setting, bacteriology, and inciting insult. The most common clinical entity is necrotizing fasciitis with involvement and spread along the fascial planes, frequently with little involvement of surrounding tissues. The ability to separate fascia easily from the normally adherent surrounding tissue strongly suggests involvement with infection.[26,69,82] In elderly and critically ill patients with extensive edema, however, the ease of separation can be difficult to distinguish from noninfected fascia and the previous necrotizing infection still requires considerable clinical judgment. For skin, fat, and muscle involvement, the lack of inflammation and purulence and the presence of normal bleeding at the line of incision are commonly used to determine adequacy of debridement. Additionally, muscle should demonstrate contractility. For fasciitis without involvement of surrounding tissues, debridement and drainage of involved fascia through a series of parallel incisions without resection of overlying tissue may be successful and preserve overlying tissues.[96] If surrounding tissues are involved, however, full-thickness excision is required.

Necrotizing infections have the potential for rapid and continued progression despite surgical debridement. Frequent re-evaluation of the wound should be undertaken. Many authors recommend return to the operating room within 24 hours to ensure adequacy of debridement and lack of progression,[26,38,69] and the average number of operative procedures is typically three to four per patient.[4,24,38,69,82] Prevention of heavy and recurrent contamination of dressings may be problematic in patients with perineal, perianal, or scrotal involvement. When fecal soilage of dressings is problematic, diverting colostomy is recommended.[97] Recently, the development of a specifically designed rectal system to control the fecal stream has been used successfully to avoid diverting colostomy.[98] In summary, the surgical management of necrotizing soft tissues continues to be driven by clinical experience and expertise. Early and adequate surgical debridement is linked to improved outcomes but remain poorly defined.

Antibiotic Therapy for Necrotizing Infections

As with surgical therapy, very limited prospective data exist to guide antibiotic therapy for necrotizing infections. As indicated earlier, FDA guidelines for the study of soft tissue infections exclude patients with these more severe infections from prospective trials.[1] Most randomized studies evaluating complicated skin and skin structure infections report clinical success rates ranging from 75% to 90% or greater, depending on the study population and analysis group. Typically, mortality for the populations included in these studies is well less than 1%. Because studies examining the outcome of NSTI identify mortality rates of 6% to greater than 70% (see **Table 2**), there may be little applicability of the data from randomized studies of complicated skin and skin structure infections to treatment of severe necrotizing infections. The current recommendations are garnered from limited data on seriously ill patients available from prospective studies of patients with complicated skin and skin structure infections; prospective studies of clinical problems involving similar pathogens (eg, intra-abdominal infection trials); and interpretation of current sensitivity patterns of the pathogens most typically involved in these infections. Because most of these infections are mixed infections and may involve aerobic and anaerobic gram-negative and gram-positive pathogens, broad antibiotic coverage of these pathogens is indicated in most cases. The clinical presentation and physical findings, along with the rapidity with which the pathologic process evolves, should alert the practitioner to the potential presence of specific, highly virulent pathogens, such as group A streptococci, *Clostridium* spp, and *Vibrio* spp, as discussed next. If such pathogens are suspected, then antibiotic therapy should be altered accordingly.

For most complicated and NSTI, a number of single-agent or combination regimens that provide anaerobic, gram-positive, and enteric gram-negative coverage may be effective. Several single-agent regimens have been evaluated in prospective, randomized trials of complicated skin and skin structure infections including imipenem-cilastatin, meropenem, ertapenem, piperacillin-tazobactam, ticarcillin-clavulanate, levofloxacin, and tigecycline. Ampicillin-sulbactam has been shown to be effective in complicated skin and skin structure infections; however, recent increases in resistance among gram-negative rods introduce concern about selecting this as a single agent. Numerous combination regimens are recommended by different sources, but have not been studied rigorously. These combinations typically include penicillins or cephalosporins with either an aminoglycoside or fluoroquinolone and an anaerobic agent, such as clindamycin or metronidazole. There are inadequate data comparing regimens to support the use of any one antimicrobial regimen over another for the treatment of these severe infections. For nonrapidly progressive soft tissue infections, use of one of the single agents or combination regimens noted previously, along with an anti-MRSA drug if suspicion of this pathogen is present, is the general recommendation.

Antibiotic Therapy for Necrotizing Skin and Soft Tissue Infections Caused by Highly Virulent Pathogens

As noted previously, some pathogens, such as *S pyogenes* (group A β-hemolytic streptococcus), group B *Streptococcus*, CA-MRSA, *Clostridium* spp, *Pasteurella* spp, *Vibrio* spp, and *A hydrophila*, can cause rapidly progressive soft tissue infections, even in intact hosts.[4,12,15,34,95] These pathogens generally produce a variety of exotoxins that contribute to their rapid growth and tissue invasion. The rapidity of clinical deterioration and high mortality for this group of necrotizing infections warrants special consideration. Although no prospective studies examine antibiotic efficacy in these settings, animal and retrospective human data support the use of protein synthesis–inhibiting antibiotics in combination with cell wall–active agents, particularly if toxin production is important pathogenically or if a high inoculum is present. The choice of protein synthesis–inhibiting agent should be based on the known or predicted sensitivity of the organisms to the agents considered. Recommended agents include clindamycin (if resistance is not of concern) or linezolid for gram-positive infections (*Streptococcus*,

CA-MRSA, and *Clostridium* spp), and members of the tetracycline class for the gram-negative pathogens *Vibrio* spp and *Aeromonas* spp.

REFERENCES

1. Guidance for Industry: Uncomplicated and complicated skin and skin structure infections: developing antimicrobial drugs treatment. US Dept of Health and Human Services, Food and Drug Administration, Center for Drug Evaluation and Research, 1998. Available at: http://www.fda.gov/CDER/guidance/2566dft. pdf. Accessed October 17, 2008.
2. Jones ME, Karlowsky JA, Draghi DC, et al. Epidemiology and antibiotic susceptibility of bacteria causing skin and soft tissue infections in the USA and Europe: a guide to appropriate antimicrobial therapy. Int J Antimicrob Agents 2003;22:406–19.
3. Stevens DL, Bisno AL, Chambers HF, et al. Practice guidelines for the diagnosis and management of skin and soft-tissue infections. Clin Infect Dis 2005;41:1373–406.
4. Elliott DC, Kufera JA, Myers RA. Necrotizing soft tissue infections: risk factors for mortality and strategies for management. Ann Surg 1996;224:672–83.
5. Moet GJ, Jones RN, Biedenbach DJ, et al. Contemporary causes of skin and soft tissue infections in North America, Latin America, and Europe: report from the SENTRY antimicrobial surveillance program (1998–2004). Diagn Microbiol Infect Dis 2007;57:7–13.
6. Deresinski S. Methicillin-resistant *Staphylococcus aureus*: an evolutionary, epidemiologic, and therapeutic odyssey. Clin Infect Dis 2005;40:562–73.
7. Fridkin SK, Hageman JC, Morrison M, et al. Methicillin-resistant *Staphylococcus aureus* disease in three communities. N Engl J Med 2005;352:1436–44.
8. King MD, Humphrey BJ, Wang YF, et al. Emergence of community-acquired methicillin-resistant *Staphylococcus aureus* USA 300 clone as the predominant cause of skin and soft-tissue infections. Ann Intern Med. 2006;144:309–17.
9. Moran GJ, Amii RN, Abrahamian FM, et al. Methicillin-resistant *Staphylococcus aureus* in community-acquired skin infections. Emerg Infect Dis 2005;11:928–30.
10. Doern GV, Jones RN, Pfaller MA, et al. Bacterial pathogens isolated from patients with skin and soft tissue infections: frequency of occurrence and antimicrobial susceptibility patterns from the sentry antimicrobial surveillance program (United States and Canada, 1997). Sentry Study Group (North America). Diagn Microbiol Infect Dis 1999;34:65–72.
11. Naimi TS, LeDell KH, Como-Sabetti K, et al. Comparison of community- and health care-associated methicillin-resistant *Staphylococcus aureus* infection. JAMA 2003;290:2976–84.
12. Miller LG, Perdreau-Remington F, Rieg G, et al. Necrotizing fasciitis caused by community-associated methicillin-resistant *Staphylococcus aureus* in Los Angeles. N Engl J Med 2005;352:1445–53.
13. Llera JL, Levy RC. Treatment of cutaneous abscess: a double-blind clinical study. Ann Emerg Med 1985;14:15–9.
14. Swartz MN. Clinical practice. Cellulitis. N Engl J Med 2004;350:904–12.
15. Hsiao CT, Weng HH, Yuan YD, et al. Predictors of mortality in patients with necrotizing fasciitis. Am J Ethics Med 2008;26:170–5.
16. Wong CH, Chang HC, Pasupathy S, et al. Necrotizing fasciitis: clinical presentation, microbiology, and determinants of mortality. J Bone Joint Surg Am 2003; 85-A:1454–60.

17. Wong CH, Khin LW, Heng KS, et al. The LRINEC (Laboratory Risk Indicator for Necrotizing Fasciitis) score: a tool for distinguishing necrotizing fasciitis from other soft tissue infections. Crit Care Med 2004;32:1535–41.
18. Defining the group A streptococcal toxic shock syndrome. Rationale and consensus definition. The Working Group on Severe Streptococcal Infections. JAMA 1993;269:390–1.
19. Dupuy A, Benchikhi H, Roujeau JC, et al. Risk factors for erysipelas of the leg (cellulitis): case-control study. BMJ 1999;318:1591–4.
20. Mascini EM, Jansze M, Schouls LM, et al. Penicillin and clindamycin differentially inhibit the production of pyrogenic exotoxins A and B by group A streptococci. Int J Antimicrob Agents 2001;18:395–8.
21. Zimbelman J, Palmer A, Todd J. Improved outcome of clindamycin compared with beta-lactam antibiotic treatment for invasive *Streptococcus pyogenes* infection. Pediatr Infect Dis J 1999;18:1096–100.
22. Stevens DL, Gibbons AE, Bergstrom R, et al. The Eagle effect revisited: efficacy of clindamycin, erythromycin, and penicillin in the treatment of streptococcal myositis. J Infect Dis 1988;158:23–8.
23. Bernard P, Plantin P, Roger H, et al. Roxithromycin versus penicillin in the treatment of erysipelas in adults: a comparative study. Br J Dermatol 1992;127:155–9.
24. Bosshardt TL, Henderson VJ, Organ CH Jr. Necrotizing soft-tissue infections. Arch Surg 1996;131:846–52.
25. Brook I, Frazier EH. Aerobic and anaerobic bacteriology of wounds and cutaneous abscesses. Arch Surg 1990;125:1445–51.
26. Green RJ, Dafoe DC, Raffin TA. Necrotizing fasciitis. Chest 1996;110:219–29.
27. Stevens DL, Herr D, Lampiris H, et al. Linezolid versus vancomycin for the treatment of methicillin-resistant *Staphylococcus aureus* infections. Clin Infect Dis 2002;34:1481–90.
28. Weigelt J, Itani K, Stevens D, et al. Linezolid versus vancomycin in treatment of complicated skin and soft tissue infections. Antimicrobial Agents Chemother 2005;49:2260–6.
29. Stevens DL, Wallace RJ, Hamilton SM, et al. Successful treatment of staphylococcal toxic shock syndrome with linezolid: a case report and in vitro evaluation of the production of toxic shock syndrome toxin type 1 in the presence of antibiotics. Clin Infect Dis 2006;42:729–30.
30. Ellis-Grosse EJ, Babinchak T, Dartois N, et al. The efficacy and safety of tigecycline in the treatment of skin and skin-structure infections: results of 2 double-blind phase 3 comparison studies with vancomycin-aztreonam. Clin Infect Dis 2005;5(41 Suppl):S341–53.
31. Raghavan M, Linden PK. Newer treatment options for skin and soft tissue infections. Drugs 2004;64:1621–42.
32. Adant JP, Bluth F, Fissette J. Necrotizing fasciitis: a life-threatening infection. Acta Chir Belg 1998;98:102–6.
33. Adinolfi MF, Voros DC, Moustoukas NM, et al. Severe systemic sepsis resulting from neglected perineal infections. South Med J 1983;76:746–9.
34. Anaya DA, McMahon K, Nathens AB, et al. Predictors of mortality and limb loss in necrotizing soft tissue infections. Arch Surg 2005;140:151–7.
35. Asfar SK, Baraka A, Juma T, et al. Necrotizing fasciitis. Br J Surg 1991;78:838–40.
36. Bakleh M, Wold LE, Mandrekar JN, et al. Correlation of histopathologic findings with clinical outcome in necrotizing fasciitis. Clin Infect Dis 2005;40:410–4.
37. Barzilai A, Zaaroor M, Toledano C. Necrotizing fasciitis: early awareness and principles of treatment. Isr J Med Sci 1985;21:127–32.

38. Bilton BD, Zibari GB, McMillan RW, et al. Aggressive surgical management of necrotizing fasciitis serves to decrease mortality: a retrospective study. Am Surg 1998;64:397–400.
39. Brandt MM, Corpron CA, Wahl WL. Necrotizing soft tissue infections: a surgical disease. Am Surg 2000;66:967–70.
40. Brown DR, Davis NL, Lepawsky M, et al. A multicenter review of the treatment of major truncal necrotizing infections with and without hyperbaric oxygen therapy. Am J Surg 1994;167:485–9.
41. Casali RE, Tucker WE, Petrino RA, et al. Postoperative necrotizing fasciitis of the abdominal wall. Am J Surg 1980;140:787–90.
42. Catena F, La Donna M, Ansaloni L, et al. Necrotizing fasciitis: a dramatic surgical emergency. Eur J Emerg Med 2004;11:44–8.
43. Cheng NC, Tai HC, Tang YB, et al. Necrotising fasciitis: clinical features in patients with liver cirrhosis. Br J Plast Surg 2005;58:702–7.
44. Childers BJ, Potyondy LD, Nachreiner R, et al. Necrotizing fasciitis: a fourteen-year retrospective study of 163 consecutive patients. Am Surg 2002;68:109–16.
45. Chow LWC, Ong C, Damien JCP, et al. Necrotizing fasciitis revisited. Contemp Surg 1993;42:181–4.
46. Clayton MD, Fowler JE Jr, Sharifi R, et al. Causes, presentation and survival of fifty-seven patients with necrotizing fasciitis of the male genitalia. Surg Gynecol Obstet 1990;170:49–55.
47. Endorf FW, Supple KG, Gamelli RL. The evolving characteristics and care of necrotizing soft-tissue infections. Burns 2005;31:269–73.
48. Escobar SJ, Slade JB Jr, Hunt TK, et al. Adjuvant hyperbaric oxygen therapy (HBO$_2$) for treatment of necrotizing fasciitis reduces mortality and amputation rate. Undersea Hyperb Med 2005;32:437–43.
49. Francis KR, Lamaute HR, Davis JM, et al. Implications of risk factors in necrotizing fasciitis. Am Surg 1993;59:304–8.
50. Frazee BW, Fee C, Lynn J, et al. Community-acquired necrotizing soft tissue infections: a review of 122 cases presenting to a single emergency department over 12 years. J Emerg Med 2008;34:139–46.
51. Freeman HP, Oluwole SF, Ganepola GA, et al. Necrotizing fasciitis. Am J Surg 1981;142:377–83.
52. Freischlag JA, Ajalat G, Busuttil RW. Treatment of necrotizing soft tissue infections. the need for a new approach. Am J Surg 1985;149:751–5.
53. Fustes-Morales A, Gutierrez-Castrellon P, Duran-Mckinster C, et al. Necrotizing fasciitis: report of 39 pediatric cases. Arch Dermatol 2002;138:893–9.
54. Gallup DG, Freedman MA, Meguiar RV, et al. Necrotizing fasciitis in gynecologic and obstetric patients: a surgical emergency. Am J Obstet Gynecol 2002;187:305–10.
55. Golger A, Ching S, Goldsmith CH, et al. Mortality in patients with necrotizing fasciitis. Plast Reconstr Surg 2007;119:1803–7.
56. Gozal D, Ziser A, Shupak A, et al. Necrotizing fasciitis. Arch Surg 1986;121:233–5.
57. Gunter OL, Guillamondegui OD, May AK, et al. Improved outcome in necrotizing fasciitis; an Emergency General Surgery Service Experience. Presented at the 27th Annual Meeting of the Surgical Infection Society, Toronto. 2007.
58. Haywood CT, McGeer A, Low DE. Clinical experience with 20 cases of group A streptococcus necrotizing fasciitis and myonecrosis: 1995 to 1997. Plast Reconstr Surg 1999;103:1567–73.

59. Hefny AF, Eid HO, Al Hussona M, et al. Necrotizing fasciitis: a challenging diagnosis. Eur J Emerg Med 2007;14:50–2.
60. Hsiao GH, Chang CH, Hsiao CW, et al. Necrotizing soft tissue infections: surgical or conservative treatment? Dermatol Surg 1998;24:243–7.
61. Kaiser RE, Cerra FB. Progressive necrotizing surgical infections: a unified approach. J Trauma 1981;21:349–55.
62. Kao LS, Knight MT, Lally KP, et al. The impact of diabetes in patients with necrotizing soft tissue infections. Surg Infect (Larchmt) 2005;6:427–38.
63. Kwan MK, Saw A, Chee EK, et al. Necrotizing fasciitis of the lower limb: an outcome study of surgical treatment. Med J Malaysia 2006;61(Suppl A):17–20.
64. Lee TC, Carrick MM, Scott BG, et al. Incidence and clinical characteristics of methicillin-resistant *Staphylococcus aureus* necrotizing fasciitis in a large urban hospital. Am J Surg 2007;194:809–12.
65. Legbo JN, Shehu BB. Necrotizing fasciitis: a comparative analysis of 56 cases. J Natl Med Assoc 2005;97:1692–7.
66. Liu BM, Chung KJ, Chen CH, et al. Risk factors for the outcome of cirrhotic patients with soft tissue infections. J Clin Gastroenterol 2008;42:312–6.
67. Liu YM, Chi CY, Ho MW, et al. Microbiology and factors affecting mortality in necrotizing fasciitis. J Microbiol Immunol Infect 2005;38:430–5.
68. Majeski JA, Alexander JW. Early diagnosis, nutritional support, and immediate extensive debridement improve survival in necrotizing fasciitis. Am J Surg 1983;145:784–7.
69. McHenry CR, Piotrowski JJ, Petrinic D, et al. Determinants of mortality for necrotizing soft-tissue infections. Ann Surg 1995;221:558–63.
70. Miller AT, Saadai P, Greenstein A, et al. Postprocedural necrotizing fasciitis: a 10-year retrospective review. Am Surg 2008;74:405–9.
71. Miller JD. The importance of early diagnosis and surgical treatment of necrotizing fasciitis. Surg Gynecol Obstet 1983;157:197–200.
72. Ogilvie CM, Miclau T. Necrotizing soft tissue infections of the extremities and back. Clin Orthop Relat Res 2006;447:179–86.
73. Oh C, Lee C, Jacobson JH. Necrotizing fasciitis of perineum. Surgery 1982;91: 49–51.
74. Ozalay M, Ozkoc G, Akpinar S, et al. Necrotizing soft-tissue infection of a limb: clinical presentation and factors related to mortality. Foot Ankle Int 2006;27: 598–605.
75. Peer SM, Rodrigues G, Kumar S, et al. A clinicopathological study of necrotizing fasciitis: an institutional experience. J Coll Physicians Surg Pak 2007;17: 257–60.
76. Pessa ME, Howard RJ. Necrotizing fasciitis. Surg Gynecol Obstet 1985;161: 357–61.
77. Qazi SA, Mohammed AA, Saber EI, et al. Necrotizing fasciitis: role of early surgical intervention. Saudi Med J 2004;25:890–4.
78. Rouse TM, Malangoni MA, Schulte WJ. Necrotizing fasciitis: a preventable disaster. Surgery 1982;92:765–70.
79. Singh G, Sinha SK, Adhikary S, et al. Necrotising infections of soft tissues: a clinical profile. Eur J Surg 2002;168:366–71.
80. Spirnak JP, Resnick MI, Hampel N, et al. Fournier's gangrene: report of 20 patients. J Urol 1984;131:289–91.
81. Stamenkovic I, Lew PD. Early recognition of potentially fatal necrotizing fasciitis: the use of frozen-section biopsy. N Engl J Med 1984;310:1689–93.

82. Sudarsky LA, Laschinger JC, Coppa GF, et al. Improved results from a standard-ized approach in treating patients with necrotizing fasciitis. Ann Surg 1987;206: 661–5.
83. Taviloglu K, Cabioglu N, Cagatay A, et al. Idiopathic necrotizing fasciitis: risk fac-tors and strategies for management. Am Surg 2005;71:315–20.
84. Theis JC, Rietveld J, Danesh-Clough T. Severe necrotising soft tissue infections in orthopaedic surgery. J Orthop Surg (Hong Kong) 2002;10:108–13.
85. Tillou A, St Hill CR, Brown C, et al. Necrotizing soft tissue infections: improved outcomes with modern care. Am Surg 2004;70:841–4.
86. Tiu A, Martin R, Vanniasingham P, et al. Necrotizing fasciitis: analysis of 48 cases in South Auckland, New Zealand. ANZ J Surg 2005;75:32–4.
87. Tsai YH, Hsu RW, Huang TJ, et al. Necrotizing soft-tissue infections and sepsis caused by *Vibrio vulnificus* compared with those caused by *Aeromonas* species. J Bone Joint Surg Am 2007;89:631–6.
88. Walker M, Hall M Jr. Necrotizing fasciitis: the Howard University Hospital experience. J Natl Med Assoc 1983;75:159–63.
89. Wall DB, de Virgilio C, Black S, et al. Objective criteria may assist in distinguish-ing necrotizing fasciitis from nonnecrotizing soft tissue infection. Am J Surg 2000; 179:17–21.
90. Wang KC, Shih CH. Necrotizing fasciitis of the extremities. J Trauma 1992;32: 179–82.
91. Ward RG, Walsh MS. Necrotizing fasciitis: 10 years' experience in a district general hospital. Br J Surg 1991;78:488–9.
92. Wilkinson D, Doolette D. Hyperbaric oxygen treatment and survival from necrotizing soft tissue infection. Arch Surg 2004;139:1339–45.
93. Yaghoubian A, de Virgilio C, Dauphine C, et al. Use of admission serum lactate and sodium levels to predict mortality in necrotizing soft-tissue infections. Arch Surg 2007;142:840–6.
94. Yilmazlar T, Ozturk E, Alsoy A, et al. Necrotizing soft tissue infections: APACHE II score, dissemination, and survival. World J Surg 2007;31:1858–62.
95. Vinh DC, Embil JM. Rapidly progressive soft tissue infections. Lancet Infect Dis 2005;5:501–13.
96. Nichols RL, Florman S. Clinical presentations of soft-tissue infections and surgical site infections. Clin Infect Dis 2001;33(Suppl 2):S84–93.
97. Eke N. Fournier's gangrene: a review of 1726 cases. Br J Surg 2000;87:718–28.
98. Echols J, Friedman B, Mullins R, et al. Initial experience with a new system for the control and containment of fecal output for the protection of patients in a large burn center. Chest 2004;126:862S.
99. Anaya DA, Dellinger EP. Necrotizing soft-tissue infection: diagnosis and management. Clin Infect Dis 2007;44:705–10.

Intra-Abdominal Infections

John E. Mazuski, MD, PhD[a],*, Joseph S. Solomkin, MD[b]

KEYWORDS

- Intra-abdominal infection • Appendicitis • Secondary peritonitis
- Tertiary peritonitis • Intra-abdominal abscess • Source control
- Antimicrobial therapy

Intra-abdominal infections are generally the result of invasion and multiplication of enteric bacteria in the wall of a hollow viscus or beyond. When the infection extends into the peritoneal cavity or another normally sterile region of the abdominal cavity, the infection is described as a "complicated" intra-abdominal infection.[1,2] Complicated intra-abdominal infections are usually treated with an invasive procedure for source control; this use of a source control procedure has been included as part of the operational definition of a complicated intra-abdominal infection.[3] The term "uncomplicated" intra-abdominal infection is less well defined; usually, it refers to an inflammatory process or infection in the wall of an abdominal organ, which may result in the development of a complicated intra-abdominal infection if not treated expeditiously. Thus, pathologic processes such as acute appendicitis or cholecystitis have been considered examples of uncomplicated intra-abdominal infections.

The use of this terminology is problematic. For instance, acute appendicitis and cholecystitis are initially inflammatory disorders related to obstruction, and are not infectious in nature until later in their course. Moreover, even at the time of surgical treatment, most cases of acute cholecystitis are still sterile inflammatory processes rather than overt infections. The distinction between uncomplicated and complicated intra-abdominal infections becomes further muddled when one attempts to classify acute diverticulitis. Acute diverticulitis may be due to obstruction and bacterial multiplication within the diverticulum itself, in which case it could be considered an uncomplicated infection. However, it may also be due to a microperforation resulting in extension of the infection into the mesentery, and thus could be considered a complicated intra-abdominal infection. However, because most cases of diverticulitis are managed nonoperatively, without a source control procedure, they are considered uncomplicated according to the operational version of the definition. Thus, in

[a] Department of Surgery, Washington University School of Medicine, Campus Box 8109, 660 S. Euclid Avenue, Saint Louis, MO 63110-1093, USA
[b] Department of Surgery, University of Cincinnati College of Medicine, 231 Albert B. Sabin Way, Cincinnati, OH 45267-0558, USA
* Corresponding author.
E-mail address: mazuskij@wustl.edu (J.E. Mazuski).

Surg Clin N Am 89 (2009) 421–437
doi:10.1016/j.suc.2008.12.001
0039-6109/08/$ – see front matter © 2009 Elsevier Inc. All rights reserved.

surgical.theclinics.com

describing intra-abdominal infections, it is probably preferable to describe the source and extent of spread of the infection rather than rely on the nonspecific and confusing terms, "uncomplicated" and "complicated" intra-abdominal infections.

Most of the complicated intra-abdominal infections treated by surgeons involve peritonitis or intra-abdominal abscesses. Peritonitis is subdivided into primary, secondary, and tertiary varieties (**Table 1**). Primary peritonitis is a monomicrobial infection in which the integrity of the gastrointestinal tract has not been violated.[2] The most common manifestation is "spontaneous bacterial peritonitis," and is typically identified in patients who have ascites due to end-stage liver disease.[4] Historically, primary streptococcal or pneumococcal infections of the peritoneal cavity were common, although these entities are rarely seen in the current era. Peritonitis may also develop in conjunction with the use of indwelling peritoneal catheters, such as peritoneal dialysis catheters; this type of peritonitis is sometimes considered a form of primary peritonitis, or may be described as a separate entity.[2,5] Primary and catheter-associated peritonitis are usually monomicrobial infections treated medically, and are not considered further here.

Secondary peritonitis results from the perforation of a hollow viscus, and is the most common type of complicated intra-abdominal infection managed by surgeons. Tertiary peritonitis is a poorly defined entity. At a minimum, it is a diffuse infection developing after the failure of initial management of secondary peritonitis. However, it is generally recognized in patients who have failed several previous attempts at control of an intra-abdominal infection.[2,6,7] Many of these patients have impaired host defenses because of ongoing infection or pre-existing comorbid conditions.

Intra-abdominal abscesses may develop following secondary peritonitis. In reality, intra-abdominal abscesses are the end result of the host's response to secondary peritonitis, and represent the temporal evolution of that infection rather than a distinct pathologic process. Thus, following contamination of the peritoneal cavity as a result of perforation of a hollow viscus, normal host defense mechanisms are invoked, which serve to limit the development and spread of an infection. Bacteria and other particulate matter are rapidly removed from the peritoneal cavity through the process

Table 1
Classification of peritonitis

Type	Definition	Microbiology
Primary	A peritoneal infection developing in the absence of a break in the integrity of the gastrointestinal tract, as a result of hematogenous or lymphatic seeding, or bacterial translocation	Monomicrobial infection due to gram-negative *Enterobacteriaceae* or streptococci
Secondary	A peritoneal infection developing in conjunction with an inflammatory process of the gastrointestinal tract or its extensions, usually associated with microscopic or macroscopic perforation	Polymicrobial infection due to aerobic gram-negative bacilli, gram-positive cocci, and enteric anaerobes
Tertiary	A persistent or recurrent peritoneal infection developing after initial treatment of secondary peritonitis	Nosocomial organisms, including resistant gram negative-bacilli, enterococci, staphylococci, and yeast

of mechanical clearance, in which peritoneal fluid circulates within the peritoneal cavity as a result of diaphragmatic contractions and is absorbed into the lymphatic system through specialized stomata on the undersurface of the diaphragm. This process results in the elimination of a significant portion of the bacterial inoculum. In addition to mechanical clearance, an inflammatory reaction is rapidly generated within the peritoneal cavity to aid in removal of infective material. This reaction involves recognition of pathologic microbial molecules by pattern recognition receptors on resident macrophages within the peritoneal cavity, and the triggering of signals that promote the rapid ingress of polymorphonuclear leukocytes and subsequently mononuclear cells into the peritoneal cavity. These phagocytic cells further eliminate pathogenic organisms from the peritoneal cavity. Finally, the process of sequestration results in limitation of the infection. Microscopic sequestration results from the generation of fibrin and other macromolecules that trap populations of microorganisms and may also seal small gastrointestinal tract perforations. These adhesive molecules also promote adherence of the omentum, loops of bowel, the mesentery, and the abdominal wall to each other, which results in macroscopic restriction of the infectious process. Overall, these mechanisms result in either complete clearance of the infection or in the formation of a localized infection, now recognized as an intra-abdominal abscess.[1,8] In this sense, then, an intra-abdominal abscess represents a success of the usual host defense mechanisms. In contrast, the poorly localized, diffuse infections characteristic of tertiary peritonitis represent a failure of these normal host defenses.

In addition to primary and catheter-associated peritonitis, certain types of infections found in the abdominal region are usually excluded from consideration in descriptions of intra-abdominal infections. Many of these infections arise from the genitourinary tract, including gynecologic infections such as tubo-ovarian abscesses, and perirenal infections, extending into the surrounding tissues from an infected kidney. Abscesses in solid organs such as the liver and spleen, which develop as a result of hematogenous seeding, are also generally considered apart from other types of intra-abdominal infections. These infections are not the focus of this discussion, which will be restricted to the pathologic processes arising from the gastrointestinal tract and its appendages.

MICROBIOLOGY

The resident gastrointestinal flora are the cause of most intra-abdominal infections. Because the microbiology of the gastrointestinal tract changes markedly with location, the types of microorganisms isolated in these infections may also vary, depending on the source of the infecting inoculum. As one progresses down the gastrointestinal tract in the normal individual, the number of microorganisms increases and their character changes. Few microorganisms are found in the normal stomach and proximal small intestine, typically less than 10^3 to 10^4 organisms per gram of contents. Most of these are gram-positive cocci, particularly streptococci, or lactobacilli. These microorganisms are considered by many to represent "transients" from the oral cavity, and not true colonizers of the upper gastrointestinal tract. In the more distal small intestine, gram-positive cocci continue to be present, but enteric gram-negative aerobic/facultative anaerobic bacilli begin to make an appearance. In the terminal ileum, bacterial counts may reach 10^8 organisms per gram of contents, and many anaerobic organisms are present in addition to the aerobic organisms. In the colon, 10^{10} to 10^{11} microorganisms are present per gram of contents, and obligate anaerobic microorganisms predominate by as much as 100 to 1000 fold over the aerobic and facultative anaerobic microorganisms.[9–12]

Most intra-abdominal infections resulting from perforations of the gastrointestinal tract or its appendages are polymicrobial. Enteric gram-negative bacilli, gram-positive cocci, and anaerobic microorganisms are the predominant pathogens. Only a few of these microorganisms are typically identified by most clinical laboratories. In research studies, five to ten bacterial isolates may be isolated from each clinical sample,[13,14] with anaerobic species predominating over aerobic ones. However, clinical laboratories may report only one or two organisms per sample, with 25% to 50% of the samples showing no growth;[2,15] full characterization of anaerobic isolates is typically not done by most clinical laboratories.

Escherichia coli is the most common organism isolated from patients who have intra-abdominal infections. Usually, 50% or more of patients are found to be infected with this organism.[1,13,14] Several other enteric gram-negative bacilli may also be isolated, including *Klebsiella* sp, which is probably the next most common isolate, and *Enterobacter* sp, although these are generally encountered much less frequently. Noncoliform gram-negative bacilli, particularly *Pseudomonas aeruginosa*, may also be isolated from some of these infections.

Gram-positive cocci are frequently components of intra-abdominal infections. The most common gram-positive organisms isolated are streptococci, predominately of the viridans type.[1,14] *Enterococcus* sp is isolated much less frequently than streptococci, being reported in 10% to 20% of patients.[1,14,16] Most of the enterococcal strains isolated from patients who have community-acquired intra-abdominal infections are penicillin-susceptible strains of *Enterococcus faecalis*.[17] The role of *Enterococcus* in intra-abdominal infections, particularly those acquired in the community, remains controversial.[16]

Obligate anaerobic organisms are important components of most intra-abdominal infections, even though clinical laboratories may not recover or report these organisms. The most prevalent anaerobic organism in intra-abdominal infections is *Bacteroides fragilis*, likely present in one third to one half of these infections. Other members of the *B fragilis* group, including *B thetaiotaomicron, B distasonis, B vulgatus, B ovatus,* and *B uniformis*, can probably be found in an equivalent percentage of patients. Anaerobic microorganisms that also contribute to these infections include *Peptostreptococcus, Peptococcus, Eubacteria, Fusobacterium*, and *Clostridia* sp, among others.[1,13,14,18]

The microbiology of intra-abdominal infections is significantly altered in patients who have been exposed to the health care setting. This alteration may be due to the acquisition of nosocomial pathogens or may reflect prior antimicrobial therapy that has selected for resistant organisms. Even the normal gastrointestinal flora is altered significantly in patients who have been hospitalized. Reddy and colleagues[19] found gastric colonization with *Enterobacteriaceae* and *Candida* in 16% and 31% of unselected patients undergoing surgical procedures. Marshall and colleagues[20] demonstrated near universal colonization of the upper gastrointestinal tract in critically ill surgical patients; the pathogenic organisms encountered included *Enterobacteriaceae*, gram-positive cocci, and yeast.

Thus, compared with patients who have community-acquired intra-abdominal infections, patients who have acquired their intra-abdominal infections postoperatively have a shift in the relative frequency of the gram-negative isolates, with *E coli* being isolated less often, and *Enterobacter* and *Pseudomonas* more often. Similarly, isolation of streptococci is decreased, whereas isolation of *Enterococcus* is increased in these patients.[15,21] Fungal organisms, predominantly *Candida albicans*, are also encountered with some frequency in hospitalized patients who have intra-abdominal infections.[22,23]

This shift toward a more resistant group of microorganisms reaches its zenith in patients who have tertiary peritonitis, who have likely been treated with multiple courses of antibiotics.[6,7] These patients may have intra-abdominal infections due to multiply-resistant gram-negative pathogens, such as *Pseudomonas* and *Acinetobacter*; enterococci, particularly the more resistant *E faecium*, with strains of vancomycin-resistant *E faecium* occasionally surfacing; staphylococci, including coagulase-negative staphylococci and *Staphylococcus aureus*, most of which are resistant to methicillin; and yeast, including some non–*C albicans* species.[24–26]

SOURCE CONTROL

Source control is the general term for the interventional procedures used to control or eliminate the focus of an intra-abdominal infection. Marshall[1] has described source control as "drainage of abscesses or infected fluid collections, debridement of necrotic infected tissue, and definitive measures to control a source of ongoing microbial contamination and to restore anatomy and function." Source control of uncomplicated intra-abdominal infections, such as nonperforated appendicitis or cholecystitis, should serve to eliminate the infective focus completely and thereby prevent dissemination of pathogenic microorganisms into the peritoneal cavity. With complicated intra-abdominal infections, however, source control procedures by themselves cannot completely eliminate all infected material, although the goal should be to reduce the infective inoculum sufficiently such that additional anti-infective therapy will lead to complete resolution of the infection. Given the importance of source control in the management of intra-abdominal infections, the failure or inability to achieve adequate source control is associated with a worse clinical outcome in terms of increased rates of treatment failure and increased mortality.[27,28]

Despite the perceived primacy of source control in the management of intra-abdominal infections, there has been a trend toward the use of less aggressive forms of source control or even deferral or avoidance of source control procedures altogether under selected circumstances. Thus, minimally invasive surgical procedures are widely used for managing acute appendicitis and cholecystitis, and percutaneous, image-guided drainage procedures are the standard for treatment of most intra-abdominal abscesses.[29,30] Initial nonoperative management has long been the standard for most patients who have localized acute diverticulitis. Many patients who have perforated appendicitis who present with an inflammatory phlegmon or small abscess can be managed nonoperatively in an analogous fashion. These less invasive approaches have the potential to reduce the complications associated with major surgical procedures. Nonetheless, avoiding operative complications will have little benefit if the patient ultimately succumbs to an inadequately treated intra-abdominal infection. Therefore, carefully performed research studies are needed to identify the appropriate patients for management using this approach, and to further delineate the relative risks and benefits of deferral or elimination of definitive source control as part of their overall therapy.

Source Control for Appendicitis

Treatment of appendicitis represents a good example of a potential paradigm shift in the approach to source control. Appendicitis is the most common intra-abdominal infection treated by surgeons. For at least the past century, early appendectomy has been considered essential for the treatment of this disease. In part, this practice was based on the view that there was inexorable progression from obstruction of the appendiceal lumen with an appendicolith, through subsequent distention and bacterial overgrowth within the lumen of the appendix, to gangrene or perforation of the appendix with the development of severe peritonitis. However, this concept of the pathophysiology of appendicitis has been challenged, and the results of recent clinical trials question whether the natural history of the disease is truly inevitable progression to perforation and potentially fatal peritonitis.[31,32]

Deferral of appendectomy for acute appendicitis has been intermittently described in the surgical literature as an option for treatment of acute appendicitis, although generally in the context of a treatment to be used under extraordinary circumstances. A commonly cited reference refers to a case series of nine military patients who had acute appendicitis who were successfully managed nonoperatively using antibiotic therapy alone.[33] Subsequently, a small prospective randomized pilot study demonstrated that most patients who had acute appendicitis could be managed nonoperatively with antibiotic therapy only, although late recurrence of the disease was frequent.[34] A follow-up prospective randomized controlled trial of nonoperative management of appendicitis was reported in 2005.[35] This trial enrolled 252 Swedish male patients who had acute appendicitis, who were not believed to have perforated appendicitis based on clinical findings. This study compared immediate surgical management in 124 patients with initial nonoperative therapy in 128; the latter patients received 2 days of intravenous antibiotic therapy followed by 10 days of outpatient oral antibiotic therapy, and only underwent operative management if their clinical picture had not improved 24 hours after admission. Overall, 15 patients (12%) of those randomized to initial nonoperative therapy underwent early appendectomy. Seven patients in this group (5% of the overall group) were found to have perforated appendicitis at the time of the operation. In the patients randomized to undergo immediate operation, six (5%) had perforated appendicitis. Therefore, perforation did not appear to increase dramatically as a result of a 24-hour delay in undertaking operative management in nonresponding patients. By the time of the 1-year follow-up, 16 additional patients (15%) randomized to initial nonoperative management had undergone appendectomy because of recurrent appendicitis; this procedure occurred an average of 4 months after initial enrollment in the study. Thus, at 1 year, nonoperative management had been successful in 76% (97/128) of the patients randomized to initial nonoperative management.

Although these data suggest that nonoperative management of acute appendicitis is safe, extensive data also document that appendectomy is a safe procedure for patients who have this disease. In the Swedish population, the overall mortality rate was 0.8 per 1000 for patients who underwent appendectomy for nonperforated appendicitis; this rate was greater than 10 per 1000 (1%) only in patients 70 years of age or older.[36] For patients aged 20 to 59, mortality was increased 1.8 fold compared with the general population, but this increase was not statistically significant. The incidence of operatively managed small bowel obstruction after appendectomy was examined using a case-control design in another study of the Swedish population.[37] At the 30-year time point, an operation for small bowel obstruction had only been noted in 0.75% of the patients who had undergone appendectomy for nonperforated appendicitis; in matched control patients who had not undergone appendectomy, the corresponding rate was 0.21%. The corresponding rate in patients being managed nonoperatively for acute appendicitis is unknown. These data suggest, then, that the traditional operative approach and the initial nonoperative approach are viable options for treating patients who have acute nonperforated appendicitis.

The therapy of perforated appendicitis is also undergoing evolution. Traditionally, appendectomy had been recommended for all patients who had perforated appendicitis, except for those who had a periappendiceal abscess; in those patients, treatment with antimicrobial therapy and drainage of the abscess, with subsequent interval appendectomy, was recommended. Many aspects of this treatment approach have now been questioned, particularly for patients who have perforated appendicitis who develop a periappendiceal phlegmon or inflammatory mass in the region of the appendix.

In a recent meta-analysis by Andersson and Petzold,[38] this pathology was estimated to occur in 3.8% of patients who had appendicitis. Usually, such patients have had symptoms for several days, and do not present acutely. Because of extensive inflammation around the cecum, operative therapy of such patients may necessitate a more complicated procedure than simple appendectomy (eg, an ileocecectomy or right hemicolectomy). Therefore, interest has grown in treating such patients with antibiotics alone, in a manner analogous to that used for acute diverticulitis, in the hope of avoiding a more morbid and difficult operative procedure.

In their meta-analysis reviewing nonsurgical management of perforated appendicitis with appendiceal abscess or phlegmon, Andersson and Petzold[38] found that 19.7% of these patients underwent drainage of an abscess associated with the process, but that more than 80% were treated without any source control procedure, in many cases because no abscess existed or it was too small or inaccessible for drainage. Nevertheless, the failure rate for this initial nonoperative approach was only 7.2% in the combined series. In studies that compared use of an initial nonoperative approach with immediate operation, the former was associated with a nearly threefold decrease in morbidity compared with the latter (13.5% versus 35.6%). Thus, these results suggest that the nonoperative approach is appropriate and may be preferable for patients who have perforated appendicitis presenting with an abscess or phlegmon.

In the meta-analysis by Andersson and Petzold,[38] centers that practiced routine interval appendectomy reported a morbidity of that procedure of 11%. However, in those centers that did not schedule routine interval appendectomy, recurrent appendicitis developed in 7.4% of the non–surgically managed patients; most of these recurrences occurred within 6 months. Thus, the low risk for recurrent appendicitis and the morbidity of interval appendectomy argue against the use of routine interval appendectomy in most patients following successful nonoperative management of a periappendiceal abscess or phlegmon.

Source Control for Severe, Diffuse Peritonitis

At the opposite end of the spectrum from good-risk patients who have a localized process such as appendicitis are patients who have severe, diffuse peritonitis. Such patients should undergo emergency abdominal exploration to control the source of their infection. Increasingly, though, a "damage control" approach has been advocated for such patients, with a plan for subsequent relaparotomy. Thus, if the patient has septic shock or other significant physiologic derangements, placement of anastomoses or ostomies may be deferred to a later operation. Additionally, with aggressive fluid resuscitation, some of these patients are at risk for developing abdominal compartment syndrome, and definitive closure of the abdomen might be delayed for this reason. Finally, for patients who have questionable bowel viability, a second-look laparotomy may be advisable. Thus, performing a limited initial operation with a plan for relaparotomy may be a useful approach for some severely ill patients who have intra-abdominal infections. Much more controversial, however, is the use of scheduled relaparotomy for patients who have diffuse peritonitis but who lack any of these indications for relaparotomy. Van Ruler and colleagues[39] recently reported the results of a prospective trial comparing scheduled relaparotomy every 36 to 48 hours with repeat laparotomy based on clinical indications in 232 patients who had secondary peritonitis and an Acute Physiology and Chronic Health Evaluation (APACHE)-II score greater than 10. Scheduled relaparotomy did not result in decreased mortality or major morbidity, and was associated with increased costs and use of health care resources. Thus, mandatory relaparotomy does not appear to be beneficial for most patients who have diffuse, secondary peritonitis in the absence of a clear indication for the procedure.

ANTIMICROBIAL THERAPY

Antimicrobial therapy is generally considered an adjunct to the use of appropriate source control in the treatment of intra-abdominal infections. However, in patients in whom source control is deferred, antimicrobial therapy plays a more definitive role.

The general principle underlying antimicrobial therapy for patients who have intra-abdominal infections is to use agents effective against the aerobic/facultative anaerobic gram-negative bacilli, aerobic gram-positive cocci, and obligate anaerobic organisms commonly encountered with these infections.[40–42] The importance of anaerobic coverage has been verified in two recent studies, which found higher failure rates when patients were treated with regimens lacking anaerobic coverage.[43,44] Several single antimicrobial agents or combinations of agents have reasonable activity against common aerobic and anaerobic enteric bacteria, and can potentially be used for this indication. Regimens that have this activity and have been used for the treatment of intra-abdominal infections are listed in **Box 1**.

Several factors should be taken into account when selecting specific antimicrobial regimens for the treatment of patients who have intra-abdominal infections, including considerations of efficacy, toxicity, prevention of "collateral damage," and cost. The most important of these is efficacy. However, despite numerous prospective trials comparing various antimicrobial regimens, little evidence indicates that any particular regimen is more effective than any other for the treatment of patients who have intra-abdominal infections.[40–42]

The inability to identify superior regimens could reflect the limited power of these prospective trials to detect true differences in efficacy. Generally, the subjects enrolled in clinical trials have a low acuity of illness and a good prognosis[45] and the trials themselves are designed as "noninferiority" trials, which makes it unlikely that significant differences in efficacy between regimens can be uncovered.[46] Nonetheless, the similarity in the efficacy of various antimicrobial regimens does not appear to be simply a question of inadequate data. A recent large multi-institutional database study of 6056 patients who had complicated intra-abdominal infections also revealed little difference in efficacy among different regimens, with the exception of those that lacked effective anaerobic coverage.[44]

Other data, however, suggest that some caution should be paid to the use of certain antimicrobial agents. For instance, the use of aminoglycoside-based regimens, the historic "gold standard" for the treatment of patients who have intra-abdominal infections, was called into question in a meta-analysis, which suggested that these regimens were actually inferior to most other comparator regimens.[47] The increased development of resistance in bacteria, including those acquired in the community, might also lead one to avoid the use of certain antimicrobials. In vitro resistance of *E coli* to this antibiotic was identified in 45% of the isolates obtained worldwide from patients who had intra-abdominal infections; this high level of resistance was also present in patients who likely had community-acquired intra-abdominal

Box 1
Antimicrobial agents for patients who have intra-abdominal infections

Single agents

β-lactam/β-lactamase inhibitor combinations

    Ampicillin/sulbactam[a,b]

    Piperacillin/tazobactam[c]

    Ticarcillin/clavulanic acid

Carbapenems

    Doripenem[c]

    Ertapenem

    Imipenem/cilastatin[c]

    Meropenem[c]

Anaerobic cephalosporins

    Cefotetan[b]

    Cefoxitin[b]

Fluoroquinolone

    Moxifloxacin

Glycylcycline

    Tigecycline

Combination regimens

Cephalosporin-based regimens

    First- or second-generation cephalosporin (cefazolin or cefuroxime) plus metronidazole

    Third- or fourth-generation cephalosporin (cefotaxime, ceftriaxone, ceftazidime,[c] cefepime[c]) plus metronidazole or clindamycin[b]

Monobactam-based regimens

    Aztreonam[d] plus clindamycin[b] or aztreonam plus metronidazole plus vancomycin

Fluoroquinolone-based regimens

    Ciprofloxacin[c] or levofloxcin plus metronidazole

Aminoglycoside-based regimens[e]

    Amikacin, gentamicin, netilmicin, or tobramycin plus metronidazole or clindamycin[b]

[a] This agent may not be optimal because of increasing resistance of *E coli.*
[b] Increased resistance of *B fragilis* and other anaerobes has been observed with this agent.
[c] This broad-spectrum agent is most appropriate for use in patients who have higher severity infections.
[d] Because aztreonam lacks appreciable activity against gram-positive organisms, it should be used in conjunction with an agent with such activity (clindamycin or vancomycin).
[e] Because of toxicity and possible lower efficacy, these are no longer considered first-line agents for treatment of intra-abdominal infections.

infections. Increasing resistance of E coli to ciprofloxacin was also documented in this study, although this issue may not be as important in North America and Europe as it is in other parts of the world.[48] Emergence of gram-negative isolates with high-level resistance to several antibiotics is frequently observed in patients who have nosocomial intra-abdominal infections, but these problematic organisms are also being encountered with community-acquired infections in certain locales.[48,49] In vitro resistance of B fragilis to several agents, such as clindamycin and anaerobic cephalosporins, also appears to be widespread, although the clinical importance of this is still debated.[46,50,51]

Retrospective studies have identified bacterial resistance as a risk factor for treatment failure and mortality in patients who have complicated intra-abdominal infections. Krobot and colleagues[52] found that 26% of all isolates, 26% of gram-negative isolates, and 22% of E coli isolates from patients who had community-acquired infections were resistant to some commonly used antimicrobial agents. Moreover, the use of an empiric regimen that did not cover these resistant bacteria was associated with a greater than twofold increase in the risk for treatment failure, although it did not result in any increase in mortality. In an older study of critically ill patients who had postoperative infections, however, Montravers and colleagues[53] found that mortality increased twofold when the initial empiric regimen was determined retrospectively to be "inadequate" (ie, it failed to have in vitro activity against some of the microbial pathogens eventually isolated). This twofold increase in mortality with inadequate therapy is similar to that observed in studies monitoring the efficacy of empiric antimicrobial regimens for other indications, particularly for ventilator-associated pneumonia.[54]

Thus, the data regarding the importance of antimicrobial selection seem at first glance to be contradictory. Many of the studies suggest little influence of the antimicrobial regimen on the ultimate outcome of patients who have intra-abdominal infections, whereas others indicate that an inadequate initial empiric antimicrobial regimen can have a deleterious effect on outcome. This contradiction may be explained to some extent by considering the dichotomous nature of these infections. At first approximation, two groups of patients who have intra-abdominal infections exist. One group includes many patients who have a localized disease process, such as perforated appendicitis. These patients typically have community-acquired intra-abdominal infections. The bacteria involved in these infections are generally susceptible to most antimicrobial agents, with the exception of certain resistant bacterial strains already established in the community, such as ampicillin/sulbactam–resistant E coli. These patients are at a low risk for treatment failure and mortality. For these patients, the selection of specific antimicrobial agents is likely to play a minor role in the ultimate success or failure of the overall therapeutic program.[55]

In contrast to these lower-risk patients, a few higher-risk patients typically have severe, diffuse peritonitis, postoperative peritonitis, or tertiary peritonitis. These patients are much more likely to have an adverse outcome as a result of their infection. Multivariate analyses have attempted to identify the risk factors that characterize this group of higher-risk patients. In these analyses, however, the most important risk factors are usually related to the patient's underlying medical conditions and to his or her physiologic response to the infection.[46,56] Thus, APACHE II-scores, which are based on both of these components, have generally been the most reproducible markers of treatment failure and death in patients who have intra-abdominal infections.[46] Unfortunately, this score provides little information as to how treatment might be altered in the higher-risk patient. However, the recognition that higher-risk patients who have intra-abdominal infections are much more likely to have infections due to resistant organisms, and that these resistant organisms place these patients at higher risk for treatment failure and death, suggest that altering empiric antimicrobial therapy to better cover these potentially resistant organisms may prove advantageous.[52,53,57–60]

Published guidelines have therefore recommended different approaches to antimicrobial therapy for the lower and higher-risk patients who have intra-abdominal infections. For patients who have community-acquired intra-abdominal infections who are considered to be at mild-to-moderate risk for treatment failure, the guidelines recommend using narrower-spectrum antimicrobial agents as first-line therapy. The selected regimen should satisfy the principle of providing coverage of the typical aerobic and anaerobic pathogens involved in these infections, such as *E coli* and *B fragilis*. In addition, if a bacterial pathogen resistant to a certain antibiotic is frequently isolated in the local community, that antibiotic should be avoided for initial empiric therapy. The goal of using narrower-spectrum agents for this group of patients is to preserve the usefulness of the broader-spectrum agents listed in **Box 1** for the higher-risk patients who are more likely to have resistant and difficult-to-treat pathogens.[40,41]

For these higher-risk patients, the recommended approach is to use an agent or agents with activity against a wide range of gram-negative bacilli and anaerobic organisms. These regimens include piperacillin/tazobactam; broad-spectrum carbapenems, including imipenem/cilastatin, meropenem, and doripenem; third- or fourth-generation cephalosporins plus metronidazole; and ciprofloxacin plus metronidazole. This regimen may be further broadened in selected patients to provide coverage of *Enterococcus*, yeast, and resistant gram-positive cocci.[40,41]

Empiric treatment of *Enterococcus* sp is not routinely recommended for the patients who have community-acquired intra-abdominal infections. However, isolation of *Enterococcus* is more common in patients who have hospital-acquired intra-abdominal infections, and is a risk factor for treatment failure and death in those patients.[15,21,53,61,62] Thus, coverage of *Enterococcus* sp should be considered for higher-risk patients, particularly those who have postoperative infections and those who have had recent exposure to broad-spectrum antimicrobial agents.[40,41,63]

Postoperative patients, especially those who have been treated with broad-spectrum antibiotics, are also at risk for the development of invasive infections due to *Candida*.[64] Patients at a particularly high risk for *Candida* peritonitis include those who have recurrent gastrointestinal perforations and those who have surgically treated pancreatitis.[22,23] Empiric use of fluconazole was shown to be of benefit in one prospective trial performed in such higher-risk patients.[65] In general, empiric antifungal therapy is unnecessary in patients who have community-acquired intra-abdominal infections[40,41] but can be considered in patients whose underlying medical conditions and history of prior infections and antimicrobial exposure place them at significant risk for a nosocomial intra-abdominal infection secondary to *Candida*.

Finally, patients who develop tertiary peritonitis may have infections due to highly resistant organisms, including methicillin-resistant coagulase-negative and coagulase-positive staphylococci, vancomycin-resistant enterococci, multiply-resistant gram-negative bacteria, and non–*C albicans* candidal species. Such patients typically need multiple drug regimens. Agents should be selected empirically, based on knowledge of the likely nosocomial organisms present in the local setting.[40,41,60] A reasonable approach in such patients is to provide broad-spectrum empiric antimicrobial therapy initially but then to de-escalate or narrow that therapy based on definitive culture results.[66]

Beyond efficacy considerations, other factors that play a role in antimicrobial selection include the toxicity of a given regimen and its propensity for creation of "collateral damage." Concerns regarding the ototoxicity and nephrotoxicity of aminoglycosides have led to limitations in their use for the treatment of patients who have intra-abdominal infections.[47] In the case of an individual patient, a history of a reaction to an antibiotic of a certain class, such as a penicillin, should lead to the use of an alternative agent. The question of "collateral damage," referring to the development of resistant or superinfecting bacteria in the patient and the institution, is more difficult to evaluate. Emergence of resistant bacteria and epidemics of *Clostridium difficile*–associated disease have been attributed to overuse of certain antibiotics[67] but these may be specific to an individual institution or locale. Nonetheless, if epidemiologic evidence indicates that a given antimicrobial agent is associated with the spread of resistant organisms or the development of significant superinfections, it would be prudent to limit its use at that site.

One of the most important ways to limit "collateral damage" is to curtail the unnecessary use of antibiotics.[68–70] For most patients who have intra-abdominal infections, evidence is increasing that prolonged antimicrobial therapy is unnecessary.[40,41,71] One approach to limiting antibiotics is to discontinue them once the patient has defervesced, has a normalizing white blood cell count, and has had return of gastrointestinal activity.[72,73] An alternative approach it to set the maximum duration of therapy to no more than 4 days, rather than the traditional 7 or more days. Prospective trials have indicated that this approach also allows for a reduction in the days of antibiotic therapy without impacting clinical outcome.[74–76] Thus, expeditious discontinuation of antimicrobial therapy may contribute to an improvement in the outcome of patients who have intra-abdominal infections by limiting the "collateral damage" associated with excessive antimicrobial therapy.

CLINICAL OUTCOMES

Treatment of patients who have complicated intra-abdominal infections using a combination of adequate source control and appropriate antimicrobial therapy has generally been thought to produce satisfactory results. Contemporary clinical trials have demonstrated cure in 78% to 86% of patients who were considered clinically evaluable, with an overall mortality of 2% to 3% among all enrolled patients.[77–79] However, results from published clinical trials are not representative of the true morbidity and mortality of these infections. Patients who have perforated appendicitis are usually overrepresented in clinical trials;[46] mortality from perforated appendicitis is low compared with that observed in patients who have intra-abdominal infections from other sources.[36,56,80] The patient enrolled in a clinical trial who has an infection from a source other than the appendix also likely has a better prognosis than the typical patient who has that intra-abdominal infection. After excluding patients who have perforated appendicitis, Merlino and colleagues[45] found that the cure rate among patients who had intra-abdominal infections and were enrolled in clinical trials was much higher than that of patients who were not enrolled (79% versus 41%) and that the mortality rate was much lower (10% versus 33%). Epidemiologic studies of patients who have intra-abdominal infections that include severely ill patients have demonstrated mortality rates of 17% to 32%.[46] A statewide survey of patients who had complicated intra-abdominal infections in New Mexico found an overall mortality rate of 6%, a postoperative abscess rate of 10%, and a reoperation rate of 13%; mortality was 1% among patients with perforated appendicitis, but 13% among patients who had a non-appendiceal source of their intra-abdominal infection.[81] Thus, despite the seemingly good results identified in clinical trials, complicated intra-abdominal infections are still responsible for considerable morbidity and mortality, particularly among patients who have a nonappendiceal source of infection and other risk factors contributing to a poorer prognosis.

SUMMARY

"Intra-abdominal infection" is a term that is applied to various infections usually described as peritonitis or intra-abdominal abscess. The prognosis of these infections varies widely, depending on the source of the infection, the patient's underlying physiologic reserves, and the extent of prior treatment. The principles of therapy remain restoration of systemic perfusion through fluid resuscitation and adjunctive measures for managing sepsis, source control to prevent ongoing microbial contamination, and the use of appropriate antimicrobial therapy directed against enteric bacteria. In recent years, few changes have been made to this treatment paradigm, although nonoperative management for highly selected patients who have a well-controlled focus of infection is gaining favor. Antimicrobial therapy should be stratified to the individual patient. Patients who have community-acquired intra-abdominal infections should receive narrower-spectrum agents that provide coverage against the common gram-negative and gram-positive aerobic and obligate anaerobic micro-organisms typically found with these infections. In contrast, higher-risk patients, especially those who have nosocomial intra-abdominal infections, may benefit from a broader-spectrum empiric regimen, which includes selective use of agents effective against resistant gram-negative organisms, *Enterococcus* sp, and *Candida* sp. Such a regimen can be de-escalated once definitive culture results are available. Antimicrobial therapy should generally be limited to no more than 4 to 5 days in most patients who have a satisfactory clinical response, to lower the risk for superinfection and the emergence of highly resistant bacteria.

REFERENCES

1. Marshall JC. Intra-abdominal infections. Microbes Infect 2004;6:1015–25.
2. Blot S, De Waele JJ. Critical issues in the clinical management of complicated intra-abdominal infections. Drugs 2005;65:1611–20.
3. Solomkin JS, Hemsell DL, Sweet R, et al. Evaluation of new anti-infective drugs for the treatment of intra-abdominal infections. Clin Infect Dis 1992;15:S33–42.
4. Strauss E, Caly WR. Spontaneous bacterial peritonitis: a therapeutic update. Expert Rev Anti Infect Ther 2006;4:248–60.
5. Faber MD, Yee J. Diagnosis and management of enteric disease and abdominal catastrophe in peritoneal dialysis patients with peritonitis. Adv Chronic Kidney Dis 2006;13:271–9.
6. Buijk SE, Bruining HA. Future directions in the management of tertiary peritonitis. Intensive Care Med 2002;28:1024–9.
7. Nathens AB, Rotstein OD, Marshall JC. Tertiary peritonitis: clinical features of a complex nosocomial infection. World J Surg 1998;22:158–63.
8. Cheadle WG, Spain DA. The continuing challenge of intra-abdominal infections. Am J Surg 2003;186:15S–22S.
9. Savage DC. Microbial ecology of the gastrointestinal tract. Annu Rev Microbiol 1977;31:107–33.
10. Mackowiak PA. The normal microbial flora. N Engl J Med 1982;307:83–93.
11. Berg RD. The indigenous gastrointestinal microflora. Trends Microbiol 1996;4:430–5.
12. Tappenden KA, Deutsch AS. The physiological relevance of the intestinal microbiota – contributions to human health. J Am Coll Nutr 2007;26:679S–83S.
13. Brook I. Microbiology of polymicrobial abscesses and implications for therapy. J Antimicrob Chemother 2002;50:805–10.

14. Goldstein EJC, Snydman DR. Intra-abdominal infections: review of the bacteriology, antimicrobial susceptibility and the role of ertapenem in their therapy. J Antimicrob Chemother 2004;53:ii29–36.
15. Roehrborn A, Thomas L, Potreck O, et al. The microbiology of postoperative peritonitis. Clin Infect Dis 2003;33:1513–9.
16. Waites KB, Duffy LB, Dowzicky MJ. Antimicrobial susceptibility among pathogens collected from hospitalized patients in the United States and in vitro activity of tigecycline, a new glycylcycline antimicrobial. Antimicrobial Agents Chemother 2006;50:3479–84.
17. Teppler H, McCarroll K, Gesser RM, et al. Surgical infections with *Enterococcus*: outcome in patients treated with ertapenem versus piperacillin-tazobactam. Surg Infect (Larchmt) 2002;3:337–49.
18. Goldstein EJC. Intra-abdominal anaerobic infections: bacteriology and therapeutic potential of newer antimicrobial carbapenem, fluoroquinolone, and desfluoroquinolone therapeutic agents. Clin Infect Dis 2002;35(Suppl 1):S106–11.
19. Reddy BS, Gatt M, Sowdi R, et al. Gastric colonization predisposes to septic morbidity in surgical patients: a prospective study. Nutrition 2008;24:632–7.
20. Marshall JC, Christou NV, Meakins JL. The gastrointestinal tract. The "undrained abscess"of multiple organ failure. Ann Surg 1993;218:111–9.
21. Sitges-Serra A, Lopez MJ, Girvent M, et al. Postoperative enterococcal infection after treatment of complicated intra-abdominal sepsis. Br J Surg 2002;89:361–7.
22. Calandra T, Bille J, Schneider R, et al. Clinical significance of Candida isolated from peritoneum in surgical patients. Lancet 1989;2(8677):1437–40.
23. Sandven P, Giercksky KE. NORGAS Group, Norwegian Yeast Study Group. Yeast colonization in surgical patients with intra-abdominal perforations. Eur J Clin Microbiol Infect Dis 2001;20:475–81.
24. DeLisle S, Perl TM. Vancomycin-resistant enterococci: a road map on how to prevent the emergency and transmission of antimicrobial resistance. Chest 2003;123:504S–18S.
25. Trick WE, Fridkin SK, Edwards JR, et al. Secular trend of hospital-acquired candidemia among intensive care unit patients in the United States during 1989–1999. Clin Infect Dis 2002;35:627–30.
26. Pfaller MA, Kiekema DJ, Rinaldi MG, et al. Results from the ARTEMIS DISK Global Antifungal Surveillance Study: a 6.5-year analysis of susceptibilities of Candida and other yeast species to fluconazole and voriconazole by standardized disk diffusion testing. J Clin Microbiol 2005;43:5848–59.
27. Wacha H, Hau T, Dittmer R, et al. Risk factors associated with intra-abdominal infections: a prospective multicenter study. Langenbecks Arch Surg 1999;384:24–32.
28. Mulier S, Penninckx F, Verwaest C, et al. Factors affecting mortality in generalized postoperative peritonitis: multivariate analysis in 96 patients. World J Surg 2003;27:379–84.
29. Betsch A, Wiskirchen J, Trübenbach J, et al. CT-guided percutaneous drainage of intra-abdominal abscesses: APACHE III score stratification of 1-year results. Eur Radiol 2002;12:2883–9.
30. Theisen J, Bartels H, Weiss W, et al. Current concepts of percutaneous abscess drainage in postoperative retention. J Gastrointest Surg 2005;9:280–3.
31. Watters JM. Acute appendicitis. In: Schein M, Marshall JC, editors. Source control. Berlin: Springer-Verlag; 2003. p. 124–30.
32. Mason RJ. Surgery for appendicitis: is it necessary? Surg Infect (Larchmt) 2008; 9:481–8.
33. Adams ML. The medical management of acute appendicitis in a nonsurgical environment: a retrospective case review. Mil Med 1990;155:345–7.

34. Eriksson S, Granström L. Randomized controlled trial of appendicectomy versus antibiotic therapy for acute appendicitis. Br J Surg 1995;82:166–9.
35. Styrud J, Eriksson S, Nilsson I, et al. Appendectomy versus antibiotic treatment in acute appendicitis. A prospective multicenter randomized controlled trial. World J Surg 2006;30:1033–7.
36. Blomqvist PG, Andersson RE, Granath F, et al. Mortality after appendectomy in Sweden, 1987–1996. Ann Surg 2001;233:455–60.
37. Andersson RE. Small bowel obstruction after appendicectomy. Br J Surg 2001; 88:1387–91.
38. Andersson RE, Petzold MG. Nonsurgical treatment of appendiceal abscess or phlegmon: a systematic review and meta-analysis. Ann Surg 2007;246:741–8.
39. Van Ruler O, Mahler CW, Boer KR, et al. Comparison of on-demand vs planned relaparotomy strategy in patients with severe peritonitis. A randomized trial. JAMA 2007;298:865–73.
40. Mazuski JE, Sawyer RG, Nathens AB, et al. The Surgical Infection Society guidelines on antimicrobial therapy for intra-abdominal infections: an executive summary. Surg Infect (Larchmt) 2002;3:161–73.
41. Solomkin JS, Mazuski JE, Baron EJ, et al. Guidelines for the selection of anti-infective agents for intra-abdominal infections. Clin Infect Dis 2003;37:997–1005.
42. Wong PF, Gilliam AD, Kumar S, et al. Antibiotic regimens for secondary peritonitis of gastrointestinal origin in adults. Cochrane Database Syst Rev 2005;2: CD004539.
43. Sturkenboom MCJM, Goettsch WG, Picelli G, et al. Inappropriate initial treatment of secondary intra-abdominal infections leads to increased risk of clinical failure and costs. Br J Clin Pharmacol 2005;60:438–43.
44. Edelsberg J, Berger A, Schell S. Economic consequences of failure of initial antibiotic therapy in hospitalized adults with complicated intra-abdominal infections. Surg Infect (Larchmt) 2008;9:335–47.
45. Merlino JI, Malangoni MA, Smith CM, et al. Prospective randomized trials affect the outcomes of intraabdominal infection. Ann Surg 2001;233:859–66.
46. Mazuski JE, Sawyer RG, Nathens AB, et al. The Surgical Infection Society guide-lines on antimicrobial therapy for intra-abdominal infections: evidence for the recommendations. Surg Infect (Larchmt) 2002;3:175–233.
47. Bailey JA, Virgo KS, DiPiro JT, et al. Aminoglycosides for intra-abdominal infection: equal to the challenge? Surg Infect (Larchmt) 2002;3:315–35.
48. Chow JW, Satishchandran V, Snyder TA, et al. In vitro susceptibilities of aerobic and facultative gram-negative bacilli isolated from patients with intra-abdominal infections worldwide: the 2002 Study for Monitoring Antimicrobial Resistance Trends (SMART). Surg Infect (Larchmt) 2005;6:439–48.
49. Dupont H. The empiric treatment of nosocomial intra-abdominal infections. Int J Infect Dis 2007;11:S1–6.
50. Snydman DR, Jacobus NV, McDermott LA, et al. Multicenter study of in vitro susceptibility of the *Bacteroides fragilis* group, 1995 to 1996, with comparison of resistance trends from 1990 to 1996. Antimicrobial Agents Chemother 1999;43:2417–22.
51. Aldridge KE, Ashcraft D, Cambre K, et al. Multicenter survey of the changing in vitro antimicrobial susceptibilities of clinical isolates of *Bacteroides fragilis* group, *Prevotella, Fusobacterium, Porphyromonas,* and *Peptostreptococcus* species. Antimicrobial Agents Chemother 2001;45:1238–43.
52. Krobot K, Yin D, Zhang Q, et al. Effect of inappropriate initial empiric antibiotic therapy on outcome of patients with community-acquired intra-abdominal infections requiring surgery. Eur J Clin Microbiol Infect Dis 2004;23:682–7.

53. Montravers P, Gauzit R, Muller C, et al. Emergence of antibiotic-resistant bacteria in cases of peritonitis after intra-abdominal surgery affects the efficacy of empirical antimicrobial therapy. Clin Infect Dis 1996;23:486–94.

54. Chastre J, Fagon JY. Ventilator-associated pneumonia. Am J Respir Crit Care Med 2002;165:867–903.

55. Mazuski JE. Clinical challenges and unmet needs in the management of complicated intra-abdominal infections. Surg Infect (Larchmt) 2005;6:S49–69.

56. Anaya DA, Nathens AB. Risk factors for severe sepsis in secondary peritonitis. Surg Infect (Larchmt) 2003;4:355–62.

57. Hopkins JA, Lee JCH, Wilson SE. Susceptibility of intra-abdominal isolates at operation: a predictor of postoperative infection. Am Surg 1993;59:791–6.

58. Christou NV, Turgeon P, Wassef R, et al. Management of intra-abdominal infections. The case for intraoperative cultures and comprehensive broad-spectrum antibiotic coverage. Arch Surg 1996;131:1193–201.

59. Barie PS, Vogel SB, Dellinger EP, et al. A randomized, double-blind clinical trial comparing cefepime plus metronidazole with imipenem-cilastatin in the treatment of complicated intra-abdominal infections. Arch Surg 1997;132:1294–302.

60. Solomkin JS. Antibiotic resistance in postoperative infections. Crit Care Med 2001;29:N97–9.

61. Burnett RJ, Haverstock DC, Dellinger EP, et al. Definition of the role of enterococcus in intra-abdominal infection: analysis of a prospective randomized trial. Surgery 1995;118:716–23.

62. Sotto A, Lefrant JY, Fabbro-Peray P, et al. Evaluation of antimicrobial therapy management of 120 consecutive patients with secondary peritonitis. J Antimicrob Chemother 2002;50:569–76.

63. Harbarth S, Uckay I. Are there patients with peritonitis who require empiric therapy for Enterococcus? Eur J Clin Microbiol Infect Dis 2004;23:73–7.

64. Solomkin JS, Flohr AB, Quie PG, et al. The role of *Candida* in intraperitoneal infections. Surgery 1980;88:524–30.

65. Eggiman P, Francioli P, Bille J, et al. Fluconazole prophylaxis prevents intra-abdominal candidiasis in high-risk surgical patients. Crit Care Med 1999;27:1066–72.

66. Mazuski JE. Antimicrobial treatment for intra-abdominal infections. Expert Opin Pharmacother 2007;8:2933–45.

67. Paterson DL. "Collateral damage" from cephalosporin or quinolone antibiotic therapy. Clin Infect Dis 2004;38(Suppl 4):S341–5.

68. Raymond DP, Kuehnert MJ, Sawyer RG. Preventing antimicrobial-resistant bacterial infections in surgical patients. Surg Infect (Larchmt) 2002;3:375–85.

69. Davey P, Brown E, Fenelon L. Interventions to improve antibiotic prescribing practices for hospital inpatients. Cochrane Database Syst Rev 2005;4:CD003543.

70. Dellit TH, Owens RC, McGowan JE Jr, et al. Guidelines for developing an institutional program to enhance antimicrobial stewardship. Clin Infect Dis 2007;44:159–77.

71. Gleisner AL, Argenta R, Pimentel M, et al. Infective complications according to duration of antibiotic treatment in acute abdomen. Int J Infect Dis 2004;8:155–62.

72. Smith JA, Bell GA, Murphy J, et al. Evaluation of the use of a protocol in the antimicrobial treatment of intra-abdominal sepsis. J Hosp Infect 1985;6:60–4.

73. Taylor E, Dev V, Shah D, et al. Complicated appendicitis: is there a minimum intravenous antibiotic requirement? A prospective randomized trial. Am Surg 2000;66:887–90.

74. Schein M, Assalia A, Bachus H. Minimal antibiotic therapy after emergency abdominal surgery: a prospective study. Br J Surg 1994;81:989–91.

75. Andåker L, Höjer H, Kihlström E, et al. Stratified duration of prophylactic antimicrobial treatment in emergency abdominal surgery. Metronidazole-fosfomycin vs. metronidazole-gentamicin in 381 patients. Acta Chir Scand 1987;153:185–92.

76. Basoli A, Chirletti P, Cirino E, et al. A prospective, double-blind, multicenter, randomized trial comparing ertapenem 3 vs. ≥5 days in community-acquired intraabdominal infection. J Gastrointest Surg 2008;12:592–600.

77. Malangoni MA, Song J, Herrington J, et al. Randomized controlled trial of moxifloxacin compared with piperacillin-tazobactam and amoxicillin-clavulanate for the treatment of complicated intra-abdominal infections. Ann Surg 2006; 244:204–11.

78. Babinchak T, Ellis-Grosse E, Dartois N, et al. The efficacy and safety of tigecycline for the treatment of complicated intra-abdominal infections: analysis of pooled clinical data. Clin Infect Dis 2005;41(Suppl 5):S354–67.

79. Lucasti C, Abel Jasovich A, Umeh O, et al. Efficacy and tolerability of IV doripenem versus meropenem in adults with complicated intra-abdominal infection: a phase III, prospective, multicenter, randomized, double-blind, noninferiority study. Clin Ther 2008;30:868–83.

80. Wilson SE, Faulkner K. Impact of anatomical site on bacteriological and clinical outcome in the management of intra-abdominal infections. Am Surg 1998;64: 402–7.

81. Mosdell DM, Morris DM, Voltura A, et al. Antibiotic treatment for surgical peritonitis. Ann Surg 1991;214:543–9.

Hospital-Acquired Pneumonia: Pathophysiology, Diagnosis, and Treatment

Alicia N. Kieninger, MD[a], Pamela A. Lipsett, MD[b],*

KEYWORDS

- Pneumonia • Ventilator • Nosocomial infection
- Diagnosis • Pathophysiology • Epidemiology

Pneumonia is one of the most common nosocomial infections occurring in hospitalized patients. Hospital-acquired pneumonia (HAP) is pneumonia that occurs more than 48 hours after admission[1] and without any antecedent signs of infection at the time of hospital admission. The distinction of HAP from community-acquired pneumonia is important, as patients with HAP are susceptible to pneumonia from a different and potentially more virulent spectrum of organisms. Health care–associated pneumonia is a similar entity, occurring in patients who have been hospitalized in the last 90 days; live in nursing facilities; have received recent intravenous antibiotics, chemotherapy, or wound care; or who attend a hemodialysis clinic.[2] Based on their prior exposures, these patients have been found to be at risk for the same pathogens prevalent in HAP, and clinicians consider them the same disease. Treatment recommendations then take these risks into account. Ventilator-associated pneumonia (VAP), a subset of HAP, is pneumonia that stems from extended mechanical ventilation. Normally, pneumonia is categorized as VAP if it occurs after 48 hours of mechanical ventilation, but within 72 hours of the start of ventilation. If pneumonia occurs before 48 hours or after 72 hours, the cause is presumed to be unrelated to mechanical ventilation.

The impact of pneumonia on health care is significant in terms of morbidity, cost, and likely patient mortality.[3–5] To best prevent and treat HAP, it is important to have an understanding of the risk factors and pathophysiology leading to HAP. In addition,

[a] Department of Surgery, Johns Hopkins University School of Medicine, 600 North Wolfe Street, Osler 603, Baltimore, MD 21287-4685, USA
[b] Department of Surgery, Anesthesiology and Critical Care Medicine, and Nursing, Johns Hopkins University Schools of Medicine and Nursing, 600 North Wolfe Street, Osler 603, Baltimore, MD 21287, USA
* Corresponding author.
E-mail address: plipsett@jhmi.edu (P.A. Lipsett).

Surg Clin N Am 89 (2009) 439–461
doi:10.1016/j.suc.2008.11.001
0039-6109/08/$ – see front matter © 2009 Elsevier Inc. All rights reserved.
surgical.theclinics.com

knowledge of the varying diagnostic and treatment regimens may lead to improvements in patient care and outcomes. This understanding takes on increased importance as the focus of medicine shifts toward decreasing preventable complications.

EPIDEMIOLOGY
Incidence

HAP represents one of the most common nosocomial infections, with significant impact on patient morbidity and mortality, as well as on the cost of health care. Accounting for 15% of all hospital-acquired infections, nosocomial pneumonia is a frequent lethal complication of hospitalization.[6] At a rate of 3 to 10 cases per 1000 hospital admissions, HAP may increase a patient's hospital stay by more than a week, resulting in up to $40,000 in additional costs and a threefold increase in mortality.[1,3,5,7] VAP represents a large and important subset of HAP. The overall risk of VAP is estimated at 3% per day for the first 5 days of mechanical ventilation, 2% per day for days 6 through 10, and 1% per day for every day beyond 10 days of mechanical ventilation, with each day of mechanical ventilation adding infectious risk.[1]

Risk Factors

The pathogenesis of HAP is multifactorial. The concomitant illnesses of hospitalized patients place them at risk for nosocomial infections. Alterations in patient immune function allow pathogens to cause invasive infections that would not occur in healthy individuals. Many hospitalized patients experience poor nutrition, increasing their risk of infection.[8] Severe illness and hemodynamic compromise have also been associated with increased rates of HAP.[9]

Aspiration of oropharyngeal secretions plays a significant role in the development of HAP.[10] As many as 45% of all healthy individuals may aspirate during sleep. However, the combination of depressed immune function, impaired mucocilliary clearance of the respiratory tract, and the presence of more pathogenic organisms makes aspiration a significant contributor to HAP.[6,11] Supine positioning contributes greatly to this aspiration risk and has been demonstrated to increase the rate of HAP among hospitalized patients.[12,13]

The oropharynx of hospitalized patients is colonized by enteric gram-negative pathogens. Risk factors for these pathogens include prolonged hospital length of stay, cigarette smoking, increasing age, uremia, prior antibiotic exposure, alcohol consumption, endotracheal intubation, coma, major surgery, malnutrition, multiple organ-system failure, and neutropenia.[6] Additionally, the use of stress ulcer prophylaxis, such as histamine blockers and proton pump inhibitors, is now a mainstay treatment for intensive care unit (ICU) patients. While histamine blockers and proton pump inhibitors are effective in preventing gastrointestinal bleeding, their use is also associated with increased gram-negative colonization of the aerodigestive tract,[1] increasing the risk of HAP due to these organisms. Finally, foreign bodies, such as endotracheal and nasogastric tubes, provide a source for further colonization and act as physical conduits for the migration of pathogens to the lower respiratory tract.[1]

PATHOPHYSIOLOGY
Microbiology

The causative organisms for HAP differ significantly from those typically responsible for community-acquired pneumonia.[1,14–16] The clinical setting in which HAP arises is likely to influence the likely causative organisms. Not only does this change in microbiology affect the appropriate treatment, but it also has implications on morbidity and mortality. HAP arising early (<5 days) in the hospital course is associated with a better prognosis than late-onset HAP.[1] Thus, HAP can be divided into two categories: early onset (arising less than 5 days into a hospital course) and late onset (arising 5 days or later into a hospital course). These two categories can then be further subdivided into categories of patients with prior antibiotic exposure and patients without prior antibiotic exposure.

Early-onset HAP in patients with no prior antibiotic exposure tends to mirror community-acquired pneumonia. The most common pathogens include *Enterobacteraciea, Haemophilus influenzae, Streptococcus pneumonia,* and methicillin-sensitive *Staphyloccous aureus.*[15] Patients with recent antibiotic exposures are susceptible to the above organisms, in addition to non–lactose fermenting gram-negative bacilli. Late-onset HAP in patients with no prior antibiotic exposure presents with similar bacteria. However, occasionally these patients present with gram-negative bacilli resistant to first-generation cephalosporins. The preceding three categories of microbes involve generally antibiotic-sensitive organisms. The final category, late-onset HAP with prior antibiotic exposure, presents a greater problem in both the prediction of and empiric treatment of likely pathogens. As many as 40% of these patients present with potentially multidrug-resistant pathogens, including *Pseudomonas aeruginosa, Acinetobacter baumannii,* and methicillin-resistant *Staphylococcus aureus* (MRSA).[15]

Gram-Positive Bacteria

The common gram-positive cocci causing pneumonia in hospitalized patients are *S pneumoniae* and *S aureus. S pneumoniae* colonizes the upper airways and is a common causative organism of community-acquired pneumonia.[16] For this reason, *S pneumoniae* is more likely to be associated with early-onset HAP than late-onset HAP.[15,17] *S pneumoniae* is rarely resistant to traditional beta-lactam antibiotics. *S aureus* also frequently colonizes the upper airways, particularly the nasal passages. Younger patients hospitalized with traumatic brain injuries are at increased risk of pneumonia due to *S aureus.*[18] This organism can cause pneumonia at any point in the hospital course. Early on, most isolates are sensitive to penicllinase-resistant beta-lactam antimicrobials (methicillin-sensitive *S aureus*). However, patients who have been hospitalized for longer periods or exposed to prior antimicrobial therapy are at increased risk for MRSA.[18]

MRSA is a gram-positive coccus that frequently colonizes the nares of hospitalized patients and is seen even now as a community-acquired pathogen. Risk factors for MRSA pneumonia include chronic obstructive pulmonary disease (COPD), longer duration of mechanical ventilation, prior antibiotic exposure, prior use of corticosteroids, and prior bronchoscopy.[16] Its resistance mechanisms develop via a penicillin-binding protein that causes decreased affinity for beta-lactam antimicrobials, leaving a narrow spectrum of treatment options for MRSA.[1]

Gram-Negative Bacteria

Early-onset HAP is associated with *Hemophilus influenzae* and lactose-fermenting gram-negative bacilli, such as *Enterobacteraciae.* As with *S pneumoniae, H influenzae* is a common cause of community-acquired pneumonia and is easily eradicated when treated.[17] *Enterobacteraciae* are lactose-fermenting enteric gram-negative bacilli. This group of organisms includes *Echerichia coli, Klebsiella* spp and *Enterobacter* spp. Overgrowth of these organisms can be associated with prior antibiotic therapy, and their virulence may increase in critical illness. *Enterobacteraciae* spp are increasingly demonstrating extended-spectrum beta-lactamase activity (ESBL). While these organisms were frequently treated with broad-spectrum beta-lactam antimicrobials, plasmid-mediated resistance to these agents is increasing.[19] ESBL-producing strains are considered resistant to all beta-lactam agents.[20] They additionally demonstrate a high rate of concomitant resistance to fluoroquinolones, making carbapenems the recommended first-line agents for ESBL-producing strains.[19,20]

P aeruginosa is the most common multidrug-resistant gram-negative bacillus causing HAP/VAP[1,16] and is the most frequent VAP isolate in patients on mechanical ventilation for more than 4 days.[7] Risk factors are similar to those of MRSA. Resistance is acquired via the formation of multiple efflux pumps that force antibiotics back out of the cell. Pseudomonas also develops increased resistance to many different types of beta-lactam antimicrobials. Patients with pneumonia caused by multidrug-resistant P aeruginosa are at increased risk of severe sepsis and death.[21] Specifically, infection with non–lactose-fermenting gram-negative bacilli, of which Pseudomonas is the most common, has been suggested to be an independent predictor of death and recurrence.[22]

A baumannii represents an emerging pathogen in the care of critically ill patients with pneumonia. The rates of infection among injured military personnel in the Middle East are high.[23] Moreover, epidemiologic studies examining the military health system indicate that outbreaks stem from contamination of hospital equipment rather than inoculation of wounds from the environment.[23,24] Acinetobacter spp are aerobic, non–lactose-fermenting gram-negative bacilli frequently found in soil and fresh water.[16] While normally of low virulence, those strains recovered in injured and hospitalized patients have intrinsic resistance to many antibiotics, and cause nosocomial infections that may spread rapidly among hospitalized patients.[16,24] Mechanisms of antimicrobial resistance of Acinetobacter spp are threefold, and several mechanisms may be at work in any given strain.[24,25] Due to its ability to rapidly acquire resistance to many drugs, prior antibiotic exposure is a significant risk factor for resistance.[26]

PREVENTION
Patient Risk Modification

Preoperative risk factors to help stratify and modify risk in patients have been widely applied in cardiac prediction models.[27] Several substantial studies have attempted to create a similar pulmonary risk index.[28–31] The National Surgical Quality Improvement Program (NSQIP) and the Patient Safety in Surgery (PSS) study are national collaborative efforts that have sought to decrease complications among surgical patients. Using data from the NSQIP and PSS, Johnson developed the Respiratory Risk Index, which may be more broadly applicable.[32] This index is a scoring system that categorizes patients as low, medium, or high risk for postoperative respiratory failure, based on such factors as emergency and complex surgeries, American Society of Anesthesiologists (ASA) status, and patient comorbidities (eg, COPD, ascites, renal failure). While these studies focus on respiratory failure in general, they likely correlate with risk factors for HAP specifically.

Targeting modifiable risk factors can decrease rates of postoperative pneumonia. Current smoking increases the risk for postoperative pulmonary complications threefold[33–37] even in patients without chronic lung disease. Paradoxically, patients who stop smoking immediately before surgery appear to be at a higher risk of pulmonary complications than those who are still smoking and those who have quit for a longer period of time.[34,36] While this finding is unexplained and somewhat paradoxical, patients who smoke and will undergo elective surgery should be encouraged to stop smoking at least 8 weeks before surgery whenever possible. In patients with COPD and asthma, as well as congestive heart failure, it is important to optimize their treatment preoperatively. For patients with asthma and COPD, preoperative steroids and measurement of peak inspiratory flow may dictate when a patient is in his or her personal best condition. This should be the goal for elective preoperative therapy.

Postoperative pain control is essential to decrease pulmonary complications. Neuraxial anesthesia may have a 20% absolute reduction in risk of pulmonary complications.[38] Procedure site and its relation to postoperative pain also have a significant impact on respiratory complications. There is an inverse relationship between pulmonary complications and distance of the incision from the diaphragm,[39] making postoperative pain control a significant modifiable risk factor.

Minimizing Aspiration Risk

As previously described, aspiration of oropharyngeal and gastric secretions contributes greatly to nosocomial pneumonia. Hospitalized patients frequently have nasogastric and nasoenteric tubes placed for various reasons, such as for decompression of the digestive tract or facilitation of enteral feedings. Patients with nasogastric tubes in place demonstrate increased rates of pharyngeal aspiration, regardless of the size of the tube.[40] The role of percutaneous endoscopic gastrostomy versus nasogastric tube feedings has been debated with no clear evidence-based conclusion about whether one is better than the other.[41,42] Realistically, the elimination the use of nasogastric tubes in hospitalized patients is impossible. The clinician must carefully evaluate the need for enteral access and perhaps consider solutions that eliminate nasal tubes for patients who require long-term enteral access.

Patient positioning can also have a significant impact on rates of pneumonia. Among 86 patients randomized to the semirecumbent position (45°) versus supine position (0°), patients in the supine position had significantly higher rates of pneumonia.[13] Similarly, Metheny[10] demonstrated that patients who had more frequent aspiration events were more likely to have been maintained with their head of bed at less than 30°. Current guidelines for prevention of VAP recommend semirecumbent positioning for all patients without contraindications to doing so.[1,28,43] Diligence is required in this endeavor, as the goal of 45% head-of-bed elevation is not reached as much 85% of the time.[44]

Decontamination of Digestive Tract

Organisms colonizing the upper aerodigestive tract in hospitalized patients are frequently associated with HAP. Elimination of these colonizing organisms may significantly impact the rates of HAP. The majority of the research into this area has focused on its effect on nosocomial infections and colonization with drug-resistant bacteria.[15,45] Poor oral hygiene contributes significantly to the incidence of VAP in intubated patients. Nurses must understand their important role in improving oral hygiene and its effect on rates of pneumonia. Education and diligence with current patient care standards can be a powerful starting point for decreasing rates of VAP. An education program focusing on the role of oral hygiene in prevention of VAP was accompanied by a reported 50% decrease in institutional VAP rates.[46] Good oral hygiene alone will not eliminate VAP, however. For this reason, there is interest in the effects of eliminating colonizing organisms from the oropharynx with the use of antimicrobial solutions. A large prospective, randomized, double-blind, placebo-controlled trial of more than 900 patients using a chlorhexidine oral rinse and nasal gel to decrease rates of nosocomial infections in cardiac surgery patients found a significantly lower rate of lower respiratory tract infections in the treatment group.[47] While this study focuses purely on cardiac surgery patients, the large sample size makes the results very compelling. In a recent meta-analysis, the use of chlorhexidine resulted in a 59% relative risk reduction for VAP in surgical patients.[48] However, the findings of this study were limited by significant heterogeneity among the trials examined.

Aspiration of gastric contents has also been felt to contribute to nosocomial pneumonia. Selective decontamination of the digestive tract (SDD) involves, in addition to topical antimicrobials, an oral antibiotic regimen and possibly a brief course of systemic antibiotics. A meta-analysis published in 1994 included 2270 patients in randomized trials and attempted to assess the impact of SDD on mortality and rates of respiratory tract infections.[49] While investigators found a significant decrease in the rate of nosocomial pneumonia in the treatment group, specifically due to gram-negative bacteria, this study found no difference in overall mortality between the two groups. Additionally, the study noted several trials demonstrating trends toward increased colonization with drug-resistant organisms in the treatment group.

More recently, de Jonge and colleagues[45] re-examined the effect of SDD on colonization with drug-resistant organisms. They found no difference in ICU or hospital mortality between control patients and those randomized to SDD. The rate of acquired colonization of gram-negative bacteria was 16% in the treatment group versus 26% in the control group. While this study did not demonstrate a negative impact of SDD with respect to antibiotic resistance, concern for this outcome remains. Current clinical practice guidelines recommend that topical antibiotics not be used alone. There is insufficient data regarding the cost-effectiveness of intravenous antibiotics or regarding their impact on antibiotic resistance to make any recommendations about their use for SDD.[43]

Finally, an important contributor to upper digestive tract colonization in critically ill patients is stress ulcer prophylaxis. Many ICU patients are at increased risk of upper gastrointestinal bleeding secondary to stress ulceration, with an associated increase in morbidity and mortality.[50,51] For this reason, these patients are frequently treated with such medications as histamine blockers and proton pump inhibitors to curb their risk of bleeding. The normal acidic environment of the stomach renders it essentially sterile. Today's antacid medications are able to decrease gastric acid secretion by approximately 80%. This alteration in the acid content of gastric secretions is likely to promote rather than inhibit bacterial colonization. The question of whether or not agents that increase gastric pH and control stress ulcer bleeding are associated with increased rates of nosocomial pneumonia when compared with agents that reduce bleeding but do not affect pH has been the subject of much debate and some study. Decreased rates of nosocomial pneumonia have been shown in patients treated with sucralfate as compared with antacid medications or ranitidine.[33,52] However, these decreased rates of pneumonia may come at the cost of increased gastrointestinal bleeding.[52] As it stands, patients felt to be at high risk for stress ulceration (eg, patients with head trauma, burns, prolonged mechanical ventilation, coagulopathy) should continue to be treated with medications that increase gastric pH. Consideration should be given to limiting the use of these medications in patients not truly at high risk for bleeding.[28,43]

Endotracheal Tube and Ventilator Management

The endotracheal tube and ventilator circuit present another area commonly targeted for risk reduction. Specifically, the endotracheal tube is a foreign body that forms a direct conduit from the heavily colonized oropharynx to the normally sterile trachea. The presence of an endotracheal tube allows biofilm formation and promotes entrapment and adherence of bacteria to the biofilm, where antibiotics do not penetrate well. Some investigators have suggested the use of specialized endotracheal tubes that resist the formation of biofilm, or the use of mucous shaving devices to remove biofilm from the interior of the tube.[53] Currently, the cost associated with implementing these measures has limited their use.

The route of endotracheal intubation has also been considered as a risk factor for VAP. Many investigators have suspected nasotracheal intubation to be associated with increased rates of nosocomial maxillary sinusitis. Results of studies examining this topic are not conclusive.[54–56] Of 399 nasotracheally intubated patients, those who underwent weekly screening and treatment where indicated for sinusitis, had a significantly decreased rate of VAP as compared with patients who were not screened for sinusitis (relative risk, 0.61; 95% CI, 0.4–0.93).[54] Whether or not such aggressive screening for sinusitis is cost-effective is not clear, but clinicians should maintain an appropriate index of suspicion for sinusitis, and investigate further when indicated.

The elimination of secretions pooling on the endotracheal tube cuff has been successful in clinical trials by reducing tracheal contamination.[57,58] A study randomizing cardiac surgery patients to traditional endotracheal tubes versus those with a subglottic suction port did not demonstrate a significant decrease in VAP. However, the time to VAP occurrence was 5.6 days in the treatment group, versus 2.9 days in the control group (P = .006).[57] This delay to onset of VAP has been echoed in a recent meta-analysis.[59] The additional cost for treatment is approximately $14 per tube. An endotracheal tube with a subglottic drainage port, as well as a polyurethane cuff, has also shown promising results. The high-volume, low-pressure cuff is designed to have fewer longitudinal channels that allow secretions to run down below the cuff, and may be associated with a more than 50% risk reduction for VAP.[58] Based on the above results, current evidence-based prevention guidelines advocate the use of subglottic secretion drainage.[2,28,43]

The method of endotracheal tube suctioning has not been shown to influence the rates of VAP.[60–64] Closed suctioning systems are thought to have several advantages:

Positive pressure in the ventilator circuit is maintained.
Exogenous contamination of the endotracheal tube is prevented.
The need for barrier precautions on performance of suctioning is eliminated.
The surrounding environment is left uncontaminated.

Studies looking at this topic are heterogeneous and inconclusive.[61–63] Current guidelines describe these techniques as equivalent for patient care, with a slight cost savings associated with the reusable closed suction techniques.[43]

Management of the ventilator circuit has been examined as a method to prevent VAP. Frequent changing of the ventilator circuit, while attractive theoretically, has not been shown to decrease rates of VAP.[65–67] Circuit changes should occur only when tubing is visibly soiled and, of course, between patients.[28,43,68]

Similarly, the method of humidification of the ventilator circuit has been targeted for risk reduction. Previous studies indicate that heat- and moisture-exchange filters may be associated with decreased rates of colonization of ventilator circuits when compared with heated humidifiers.[69] These results have led some to recommend the use of heated moisture exchangers to decrease the risk of VAP.[43] Recently, two large randomized studies compared rates of VAP for heated humidification systems versus those for heat- and moisture-exchange filters.[70,71] The studies found no difference between the groups in rates of pneumonia, rates of mortality, or length of mechanical ventilation. The current guidelines from the American Thoracic Society do not recommend the use of heated moisture exchange filters for VAP prevention.[1]

Sedation and Ventilator Weaning

Risk of VAP is associated with length of mechanical ventilation.[1] Mechanically ventilated patients are frequently given sedative infusions both for their comfort and to prevent self-injury. However, these medications depress levels of consciousness and respiration. Patients randomized to receive daily interruptions of their sedative medications spend fewer days on mechanical ventilation and fewer days in the ICU than those receiving traditional care.[72] Daily wake-ups are also associated with a decreased incidence of VAP as compared with control patients, whose sedation was interrupted only at the discretion of the clinician.[73] Efforts to improve the efficiency of ventilator weaning have also met with success. Patients randomized to a ventilator management protocol, including a daily spontaneous breathing trial, have been shown to spend fewer days on the ventilator.[74]

In a recent study by Girard and colleagues,[75] these efforts were implemented in a paired fashion. Patients were randomized to receive a daily spontaneous awakening trial followed by a spontaneous breathing trial, versus usual care with a daily spontaneous breathing trial. Study patients were found to have increased ventilator-free days, decreased ICU length of stay, and decreased mortality. The above studies have indicated that implementation of protocols designed to minimize mechanical ventilation can lead to decreased rates of VAP.

Pulmonary Hygiene

Pulmonary hygiene, or the ability to cough and clear secretions, plays an important role in the development of HAP. Surgical patients, in particular, suffer from an impaired ability to cough and deep breathe secondary to incisional pain leading to splinting. Thoracic and abdominal procedures are associated with the highest risk of pneumonia.[76] The use of incentive spirometry to improve patients' ability to cough and deep breathe is encouraged to decrease the risk of HAP. A recent Cochrane Review examined the use of incentive spirometry as a preventative measure in patients' status post–coronary artery bypass grafting with a single study demonstrating a nonsignificant reduction in pneumonia.[77] That being said, current guidelines still recommend the use of either incentive spirometry or cough and deep breathing exercises as a preventative measure.[2,39]

DIAGNOSIS
Clinical Evaluation

The method of establishing the diagnosis of HAP remains controversial and no method has emerged as the gold standard. A multitude of possible explanations exist for new-onset fevers and leukocytosis. Attempting to establish the diagnosis of pneumonia on radiological studies alone is similarly unreliable. For these reasons, clinical guidelines are available to aid in decision making about who does and does not have pneumonia. The Centers for Disease Control and Prevention and the National Healthcare Safety Network have developed criteria for the diagnosis of nosocomial pneumonia, taking into account clinical factors, such as fever and leukocytosis, as well as radiological criteria, including persistent new findings on chest radiograph (**Box 1**).[78] Physicians have used these types of clinical features to formulate the diagnosis of pneumonia for years. However, many investigators have questioned the reliability of the physician's clinical impression. Autopsy studies have shown that relying on a clinical diagnosis of pneumonia is unsatisfactory,[79,80] Many clinical circumstances make it difficult to determine the likelihood of pneumonia, and antibiotics are frequently used when pneumonia is not present. These results call into question the physician's ability to diagnose pneumonia based solely on clinical findings. The Clinical Pulmonary Infection Score (CPIS) was developed to help quantify clinical findings and minimize either the initiation of antibiotic therapy or to influence its duration. CPIS represents a "weighted

Box 1
Centers for Disease Control and Prevention criteria for nosocomial pneumonia (adult)

Radiology

Two or more serial chest radiographs[a] with at least one of the following:

New or progressive and persistent infiltrate

Consolidation

Cavitation

Signs/symptoms/laboratory

At least one of the following:

Fever (>38°C or >100.4°F) with no other recognized cause

Leukopenia (<4000 white blood cell count per microliter [WBC/μL] or leukocytosis (>12,000 WBC/μL)

For adults 70 years old or older, mental status changes with no other recognized cause

And at least two of the following:

New onset of purulent sputum, or change in character of sputum, or increased respiratory secretions, or increased suctioning requirements

New-onset or worsening cough, or dyspnea, or tachycardia

Rales or bronchial breath sounds

Worsening gas exchange (Pao_2/fraction of inspired oxygen [Fio_2] ≤240), increased oxygen requirements, or increased ventilation demand

[a] In patients with no underlying pulmonary or cardiac disease, one definitive radiograph is acceptable.

From Centers for Disease Control and Prevention. Available at: www.cdc.gov/ncidod/hop/nnis/members/pneumonia/final/pneumoniacriteriav1. Accessed May 1, 2008.

approach" to the clinical diagnosis.[81] This scoring system includes both clinical and radiological factors that increase the likelihood of the presence of pneumonia. Point values are assigned to each criteria and a sum is calculated. Traditionally, a threshold score of more than six has been used to diagnose pneumonia (**Table 1**).[82]

The clinical utility of this scoring system has been evaluated extensively. In a review of 40 specimens obtained from bronchoalveolar lavage (BAL), Pugin[82] compared the findings to clinical data. In this study, the CPIS correlated with BAL results in 80% of cases. In cases where the CPIS was more than six, 93% had bacteriologic evidence on pneumonia based on BAL. On the other hand, of cases where the CPIS was six or less, no patient satisfied the microbiologic criteria for pneumonia. These results indicate that the CPIS may be good predictor of the presence of pneumonia in mechanically ventilated patients.

On the other hand, some investigators suggest that the CPIS, while being very sensitive, lacks specificity and leads to unnecessary antimicrobial treatment. In a study of 201 patients who underwent an invasive diagnosis of pneumonia, patients with VAP had the same CPIS as patients without VAP. The CPIS strategy agreed with bronchoscopy findings in 65% of patients. In patients without VAP on BAL, 53% would have received antibiotics based on their CPIS. The CPIS strategy in these patients would have led to 840 days of empiric antibiotic treatment as compared with 424 days when the invasive strategy was used.[83]

Table 1
Modified Clinical Pulmonary Infection Score

Measurement	Points		
	0	1	2
Temperature (°C)	36.5–38.4	38.5–38.9	$\leq$36.4 or $\geq$39
Peripheral white blood cell count	4000–11,000	<4000 or >11,000 (>50% bands: add 1 extra point)	
Tracheal secretions	None	Nonpurulent	Purulent
Chest radiograph	No infiltrate	Diffuse or patchy infiltrate	Localized infiltrate
Progression of infiltrate from prior radiographs	None		Progression (acute respiratory distress syndrome or congestive heart failure thought unlikely)
Culture of endotracheal tube suction	No growth/light growth	Heavy growth (Some bacteria on gram stain: add 1 extra point)	
Oxygenation (Pao_2/ fraction of inspired oxygen [Fio_2])	>240 or acute respiratory distress syndrome		$\leq$240 and no acute respiratory distress syndrome

Adapted from Swoboda SM, Dixon T, Lipsett PA. Can the clinical pulmonary infection score impact ICU antibiotic days? Surg Infect (Larchmt) 2006;7:331–9; with permission.

While most studies indicate that clinical evaluation is extremely sensitive in identifying VAP, the specificity is quite low. Clinical diagnosis combined with short-course antibiotic therapy may be reasonable.[84] In a 2000 study, Singh[85] examined short-course empiric therapy for patients in the ICU with suspected VAP. Patients with a new pulmonary infiltrate and a CPIS of six or less were randomized to receive a standard 10 to 21 days of antimicrobial therapy versus 3 days of empiric ciprofloxacin. The CPIS was re-evaluated after 3 days and, if it remained six or less, patients in the experimental group had therapy discontinued. The rate of antimicrobial resistance or superinfection was significantly higher in patients receiving standard therapy. The duration of antimicrobial therapy was significantly lower in the experimental group, with no difference in mortality. This study suggested that patients with suspected VAP could be safely treated with an initial short course of antimicrobial therapy, followed by re-evaluation of their clinical status. However, while this strategy helps limit overall antibiotic exposure, patients will continue to be exposed patients to unnecessary antibiotics. Clinical guidelines can aid physicians in the diagnosis of suspected HAP, but clinical judgment remains somewhat unreliable.

BACTERIOLOGIC EVALUATION

The bacteriologic diagnosis of pneumonia involves sampling the lower airways to obtain quantitative cultures. Blind tracheobronchial aspiration (TBAS) is a noninvasive technique accomplished by inserting a flexible catheter into the distal trachea via the endotracheal tube. Suction samples are obtained and sent for quantitative culture. The typical threshold for diagnosis of pneumonia is growth of more than 10^5 colony forming units per milliliter (cfu/mL). This technique has the advantage of being relatively noninvasive and offers a distinct bacterial load to establish the diagnosis of pneumonia. However, the blind nature of the technique prevents directed sampling of specific lung segments known to have an infiltrate on radiograph, possibly increasing the false-negative rate. Additionally, contamination of the suction catheter is difficult to prevent as it traverses the endotracheal tube and more proximal airways, possibly increasing the false-positive rate.

More invasive techniques involve bronchoscopically guided sampling of the lower airways. BAL allows sampling of specific lung segments suspected to be involved with pneumonia. The bronchoscope is advanced and wedged in a distal airway. The airway is then irrigated with approximately 50 mL of sterile saline, which is retrieved after several seconds. This process is repeated and the samples are pooled. Bacterial growth of more than 10^4 cfu/mL is consistent with pneumonia.[1,86] The advantage of this technique is that it allows the clinician to perform directed sampling of the airway, ideally limiting the false-negative rate. It also provides a bacteriologic cut-off for the diagnosis of VAP. Unfortunately, the technique is highly operator dependent. Contamination of the bronchoscope and other technical problems can compromise the results. Some investigators have also questioned the accepted diagnostic cut-off of 10^4 cfu/mL, suggesting that the use of 10^5 cfu/mL provides fewer false positives and reduces the use of inappropriate antibiotic therapy.[87] Finally, BAL is an invasive procedure with possible complications. Use of the bronchoscope can cause alterations in oxygenation and ventilation that may be poorly tolerated by some patients. Additionally, bronchoscopy can be associated with such complications as bleeding, airway inflammation, and pneumothorax.

The final invasive microbiologic diagnostic technique is use of the protected specimen brush (PSB). The telescoping catheter brush is advanced blindly or through a bronchoscope directed in the suspected distal airway. Serial dilutions of the specimen are performed. A diagnostic cutoff of more than 10^3 cfu/mL is typically accepted as being consistent with HAP.[1,87] This technique has similar advantages and disadvantages to those of BAL. If bronchoscopy is used, PSB does offer the advantage that the specimen brush is protected from contamination with upper airway secretions, as it is not advanced until properly positioned in the distal airway. There is a concern that the risk of bleeding or pneumothorax as a complication may be higher with PSB, and thus patients with thrombocytopenia may be at slightly greater risk with this technique.

Many studies have looked at the utility of various quantitative culture techniques. Heyland[88] found that patients undergoing invasive testing with BAL or PSB were ultimately treated with fewer broad-spectrum antibiotics and fewer antimicrobials overall. Timsit[89] found that direct examination of BAL fluid had an overall sensitivity and specificity of 93.6% and 91.5% for the diagnosis of VAP, focusing on the intracellular organism count as a guide to diagnosis. He found that for patients who had empiric therapy started based on the results of BAL fluid examination, only 12% received incorrect empiric therapy. With early appropriate antibiotic therapy being an important predictor of mortality, a technique that facilitates early guidance of therapy may be very clinically useful.

Ruiz[90] compared invasive and noninvasive quantitative cultures in a randomized trial looking at PSB versus TBAS. This study showed no difference in ICU length of stay, length of mechanical ventilation, 30-day mortality, or attributable mortality between the two study groups. The cost was $29 per patient for PSB versus $368 per patient for TBAS. The only independent factor found to influence growth in culture was the presence of antimicrobial treatment at the time of sampling.

More recently, the Canadian Critical Care Trials group demonstrated similar findings in looking at BAL compared with TBAS.[91] They randomized 740 patients on mechanical ventilation for more than 4 days with a clinical suspicion of pneumonia to BAL with quantitative culture versus TBAS with qualitative culture. This study controlled for the time of initiation of empiric antibiotic therapy, which was after completion of the diagnostic study in both groups. The choice of empiric therapy was also considered. Investigators found no difference in 28-day mortality between patients undergoing BAL as compared with those undergoing TBAS. Additionally, there were no differences in the secondary outcomes of hospital and ICU length of stay, duration of mechanical ventilation, or ICU and hospital mortality.

These results are somewhat in contradistinction to the large randomized trial completed by Fagon and colleagues.[92] This study of 413 patients randomized to invasive versus noninvasive diagnosis of VAP found decreased 14-day mortality and improved organ function scores in patients undergoing invasive diagnosis. These patients also were subject to fewer days of antibiotic therapy and fewer numbers of antibiotics, and identification of pathogenic processes that required intervention, such as intra-abdominal infection. The hazard ratio for death at 28 days for patients who underwent noninvasive diagnosis and management was 1.54 (95% CI, 1.10–2.16).

Many authorities continue to recommend invasive techniques even though such techniques have yet to demonstrate that they reduce mortality rates. In patients with a high incidence of systemic inflammatory response syndrome, clinical criteria alone are associated with a high false-positive rate. These patients are frequently given antibiotic therapy based on clinical findings. With further evaluation of these patients by BAL, pneumonia can be frequently ruled out and antibiotics discontinued.[93] In another study, Croce[94] demonstrated that TBAS and gram stain provide inadequate data on which to base empiric treatment because of a poor correlation between findings on gram stain of BAL fluid versus results of quantitative culture. In this study, the best diagnostic yield was seen when clinical suspicion was used to prompt further testing by invasive techniques.

The utility of invasive culture techniques may not be found in the primary diagnosis of VAP. Shorr[95] evaluated four randomized trials of diagnostic techniques and found that invasive strategies do not ultimately affect mortality related to VAP. This is likely because empiric antibiotic choices must be made before knowing the results of quantitative cultures. However, invasive cultures may play an important role in decreasing antibiotic use, an effect that may have an indirect impact on mortality.

TREATMENT
Empiric Therapy

The most important factor influencing the mortality of HAP is prompt and adequate empiric treatment. Multiple studies have demonstrated that delays in appropriate antibiotic therapy are associated with increased mortality.[1,15,96,97] In a study looking at inadequate empiric therapy for VAP in trauma patients, Mueller[97] found that mortality, ICU length of stay, and duration of mechanical ventilation all increased with the number of episodes of inadequate empiric therapy. Treatment should be instituted immediately after specimen collection and should be directed against likely specific pathogens. The choice of empiric therapy should account for patient risk factors, such as length of hospital stay, duration of mechanical ventilation, previous culture results, previous antibiotic exposure, and immunosuppression. Specifically, the number of days spent on mechanical ventilation and prior antibiotic administration have both been demonstrated to be independent risk factors for HAP secondary to multidrug-resistant pathogens.[98] Local community- and hospital-resistance patterns should also be considered. In general, common hospital-acquired pathogens include MRSA, *P aeruginosa, Klebsiella*, and *Acinetobacter* sp.[16,87,99]

Vancomycin has become the most commonly used agent to treat MRSA in hospitalized patients. Pulmonary infections with MRSA present a particular problem because vancomycin has poor penetration of lung tissue. Higher plasma levels are required to achieve therapeutic concentrations in the lung, leading to potentially increased toxicity. Such difficulties in dosing also lead to increased recurrence rates after treatment with vancomycin.[22] An additional consideration is concern for emergence of vancomycin resistance. Recent studies have demonstrated a trend of increasing mean inhibitory concentration toward vancomycin (>2 μg/mL), indicating decreasing susceptibility.[100,101] Based on these trends, it is unclear if vancomycin remains the drug of choice for treating MRSA pneumonia. To ensure adequate antibiotic coverage at the start of treatment, alternative therapies have emerged for treatment of MRSA in the face of increasing concern for vancomycin resistance.[101–103] When compared with pneumonia caused by methicillin-sensitive *S aureus*, MRSA is associated with a prolonged ICU length of stay and increased hospital costs, despite appropriate initial therapy.[104]

Due to the incidence of resistance discussed previously, acinetobacter pneumonias may be particularly difficult to treat. Carbapenem agents are the initial drug of choice for *Acinetobacter* spp, if susceptibility is retained.[24] Beta-lactamase inhibitors, such as sulbactam, may also be considered, as these agents have intrinsic activity against *Acinetobacter*.[1] In as many as 50% of cases, acinetobacter isolates may be resistant to all antimicrobials except the polymyxins.[105,106] There is some evidence that treatment with intravenous or inhaled polymyxin E (Colistin) may be a safe and effective treatment for patients with pneumonia secondary to this highly resistant organism.[105,107]

The question of whether or not to cover potentially multidrug-resistant gram-negative pathogens, such as *P aeruginosa,* with two antimicrobials remains unanswered.[15,108] There has been considerable debate regarding combination therapy for nosocomial pneumonia, particularly when concern exists for potentially drug-resistant pathogens.[109,110] Those in support of combination therapy argue that synergy between agents with different mechanisms improves response to treatment and decreases the risk of developing antibiotic resistance.[109] In addition, with two drugs the probability that one of the drugs will cover the pathogen initially is increased. Others argue, however, that monotherapy is effective in most cases, and combination therapy results in unnecessary antibiotic exposure. In addition to placing patients at risk for antibiotic toxicity, this approach can also lead to antibiotic resistance.[110] In a study of trauma patients, Croce[111] found that patients treated with a combination of a third-generation cephalosporin and gentamicin actually had increased rates of treatment failure and superinfection compared with those treated with the cephalosporin alone.

In general, for patients who receive appropriate initial therapy, there is no proven benefit related specifically to combination therapy. However, recent investigations suggest that patients treated with initial combination therapy are more likely to receive appropriate empiric therapy, with an associated improved mortality.[112–114] In addition, pneumonia secondary to non–lactose-fermenting gram-negative bacilli is associated with increased rates of recurrence and mortality.[22,115] In a recent study by Heyland,[113] patients with suspected VAP were randomized to empiric monotherapy versus combination therapy. There was no improvement in mortality with combination therapy. However, the percentage of patients receiving effective empiric therapy was significantly higher in the combination-therapy group. In addition, for patients with one or more multidrug-resistant organism identified on enrollment cultures, empiric therapy was adequate only 19% of the time, versus 84% of the time for patients receiving combination therapy. For these reasons, current treatment guidelines recommend double coverage for multidrug-resistant gram-negative bacilli in patients critically ill with suspected pneumonia.[1,15]

De-Escalation of Treatment

Prolonged treatment with broad-spectrum antibiotics contributes to development of drug-resistant organisms.[15,116,117] While narrowing the spectrum of coverage based on culture results may not improve treatment of specific infections in individual patients, it can benefit the hospital as a whole by limiting development of bacterial resistance.[15] De-escalation of therapy is accomplished by changing to antibiotics with a narrower spectrum, by eliminating unnecessary antibiotics from the treatment regimen, or by changing to oral therapy as tolerated. Several recent studies have examined the use of de-escalation therapy for VAP. Up to 68% of ICU patients will have the spectrum of antibiotic therapy narrowed based on culture results.[9,118,119] However, patients with VAP secondary to multidrug-resistant pathogens have a significantly decreased rate of de-escalation therapy. In a recent observational study looking at empiric broad-spectrum therapy ICU patients with VAP, de-escalation was accomplished for only 23% of patients with multidrug-resistant pathogens, versus 68% of cases due to other pathogens. De-escalation was not associated with decreased response rates.[118] Gianstou and colleagues[120] examined outcomes in patients who undergo de-escalation of therapy after diagnosis with BAL or tracheal aspiration with quantitative culture. Patients who received adequate empiric therapy and underwent de-escalation had decreased 15- and 28-day mortality, and decreased ICU and hospital length of stay. De-escalation rates were significantly higher for patients undergoing diagnosis with BAL (66.1%) as compared with tracheal aspiration (21%). Again, while BAL has not been proven to be the gold standard for diagnosis of VAP, it may be helpful in guiding treatment.

Duration of Therapy

Recommendations for duration of antimicrobial therapy for nosocomial pneumonia have evolved significantly in recent years. As described previously, the study by Singh and colleagues[85] suggested that a shortened course of therapy may be acceptable for many patients if they demonstrate clinical improvement. As clinicians saw the results of short course of therapy in this unblinded study, the duration of antibiotic therapy given in the control group decreased significantly over the study period, resulting in an early termination of the study. These results gave an early indication that antibiotic duration could be safely limited in many patients.

The most significant impact on this topic likely came with Chastre's 2003 study[115] randomizing patients with VAP to 8 versus 15 days of antimicrobial therapy. Death from any cause was similar between the two groups (18.8% for 8 days versus 17.2% for 15 days, risk difference 1.6 [95% CI, -3.7–6.9]). Additionally, there was no difference in overall recurrence rate (28.9% versus 26.0%; risk difference, 2.9 [95% CI, -3.2–0.1]) for VAP. However, for patients with pneumonia caused specifically by non–lactose-fermenting gram-negative bacilli, the recurrence rate after 8 days of therapy was significantly higher. In a retrospective evaluation of the same study population, pneumonia secondary to non–lactose-fermenting gram-negative bacilli and

MRSA were both independently associated with recurrence.[22] While concern for recurrence is significant when treating drug-resistant infections, the results of these studies indicated that many patients could be safely and effectively treated with shortened courses of antibiotics.

The question remains: What is the shortest course of antimicrobial therapy appropriate for nosocomial pneumonia? Repeat BAL has been used as a method of assessing response to therapy and allowing for shorter duration of antibiotic therapy. Discontinuation of appropriate therapy after 4 days in patients with decreased bacterial growth on repeat BAL has shown a decrease in antibiotic duration and total antibiotic days, with no effect on mortality, length of stay, ventilator-free days, relapse rate, or rate of superinfection.[86] These data indicate that further shortening of antibiotic courses may be safely accomplished in appropriate patients.

In 2005, the American Thoracic Society published comprehensive guidelines for the management of HAP and VAP in adults.[1] Timing of onset of pneumonia and patient risk factors are important considerations. For patients with early-onset pneumonia and no additional risk factors, initial therapy should be limited in spectrum (**Table 2**).[1,6,12,14,15,86,121,122] Choices include:

Third-generation cephalosporins
Fluoroquinolones
Penicillins with gram-negative coverage but no antipseudomonal activity
Carbapenems with gram-negative coverage but no antipseudomonal activity

For patients with late-onset pneumonia, or risk factors for multidrug-resistant bacteria, initial therapy should include combination therapy targeted at non–lactose-fermenting gram-negative bacilli. Potential therapies include antipseudomonal beta-lactam agents, such as cefepime, piperacillin/tazobactam, or meropenem; plus an aminoglycoside or antipseudomonal fluoroquinolone, such as ciprofloxacin. Additionally, the patient requires coverage for possible MRSA pneumonia with vancomycin or linezolid. Antibiotic spectrum may then be adjusted based on culture results. However, recent data suggest evolving resistance of MRSA to both vancomycin and linezolid, based on increasing mean inhibitory concentration to these agents,[100,101] a problem that will have a significant impact on the future treatment of HAP.

OUTCOMES

HAP has a significant impact both medically and economically. Specifically, ICU patients with VAP experience longer ICU and hospital lengths of stay, cost more to treat, and have higher mortality rates than other patients.[4,5,7] In their evaluation of 127 episodes of VAP at a single institution, Warren and colleagues[3] cited increased costs of almost $50,000 per episode of VAP. Perhaps more importantly, VAP in this study was associated with an overall mortality of 32%, versus 11% in patients who did not have VAP.

These daunting statistics give urgency to the ongoing efforts to help hospitals and health care providers decrease the impact of HAP. Successful strategies focus on the implementation of evidence-based treatment guidelines, VAP-prevention bundles, and staff education initiatives.[107,121–124] Hospital authorities can decrease mortality rates through the use of treatment guidelines for nosocomial pneumonia that focus on early empiric therapy targeting organisms and sensitivities known to be prevalent at their institution.[98]

VAP-bundles are collections of educational materials, guidelines, and tools such as checklists that help clinicians deliver best-practice to every patient every time. The role of VAP-prevention bundles is also important to ensure all patients receive therapy known

Table 2
Causative organisms and empiric treatment

Infection	Causative Organisms	Empiric Therapy
Hospital acquired		
Early onset; no risk factors for multidrug-resistant organisms	*H influenzae; S pneumoniae*; MSSA; gram-negative bacilli or *Enterobacteraciae* (*Klebsiella, E Coli, Serratia*); anaerobes; *Legionella*	Ceftriaxone 1 g IV every 24 h or moxifloxacin 400 mg IV PO every 24 h
Late onset; risk factors for multidrug-resistant organisms	Above organisms and *P aeruginosa*; MRSA	Piperacillin/tazobactam 4.5 g IV every 6 h (3.375 g if not *Pseudomonas*), or cefepime 1 g IV every 8 h, or ciprofloxacin 400 g IV every 8 h plus clindamycin 600 g IV every 8 h
Ventilator associated		
Early onset (<5 d)	*S pneumoniae; H influenzae*; MSSA; *Enterobacteraciae*	Ceftriaxone 1 g IV every 24 h or moxifloxacin 400 mg IV/PO every 24 h
Late onset (≥5 d)	Enteric gram negative organisms; *Enterobacteraciae; P aeruginosa*; MRSA; *Acinetobacter* spp	Piperacillin/tazobactam 4.5 g IV every 6 h with or without aminoglycoside, or ciprofloxacin 400 mg IV every 12 h with or without aminoglycosid, or cefepime 1 g IV every 8 h with or without aminoglycoside; plus vancomycin 15 mg/kg IV every 12 h, or linezolid 600 mg IV every 12 h
Immunocompromised	*Legionella*; fungal	Azithromycin 500 mg IV every 24 h, fluconazole 200 mg IV every 24 h

Abbreviations: IV, intravenously; MSSA, methicillin-sensitive *Staphyloccous aureus*; PO, by mouth.

to be effective. Key components of these bundles include directives for semirecumbent positioning, continuous suction of subglottic secretions, appropriate provider hand hygiene, and care of ventilator circuits. Implementation of a VAP bundle alone did not decrease VAP rates from greater than the National Nosocomial Infections Surveillance System 90th percentile.[123] However, when this was combined with an auditing program providing weekly staff feedback, the rate decreased to the 25th percentile. Staff education sessions highlighting VAP risk factors and prevention strategies can help increase staff compliance with the VAP bundle[124] by showing practitioners the impact of the disease and how their actions can help improve outcomes.

In summary, HAP represents a significant problem in the United States and worldwide. An understanding of the pathophysiology and local microbiology of the disease is a critical factor in prevention, diagnosis, and treatment. Prompt and effective antibiotic therapy is necessary to ensure adequate treatment. Evidence-based practice guidelines and education programs can help decrease both the medical and economic impact of nosocomial pneumonia.

REFERENCES

1. American Thoracic Society. Guidelines for the management of adult with hospital-acquired, ventilator-associated and healthcare-associated pneumonia. Am J Respir Crit Care Med 2005;171:388–416.
2. Centers for Disease Control and Prevention (CDC). Guidelines for preventing health-care-associated pneumonia, 2003. MMWR Recomm Rep 2004;53:1–36.
3. Warren DK, Shukla SJ, Oslen MA, et al. Outcome and attributable cost of ventilator-associated pneumonia among intensive care unit patients in a suburban medical center. Crit Care Med 2003;31:1312–7.
4. Safdar N, Cameron D, Collard HR, et al. Clinical and economic consequences of ventilator-associated pneumonia: a systematic review. Crit Care Med 2005;33:2184–93.
5. Sopena N, Sabrià M, et al. Multicenter study of hospital-acquired pneumonia in non-ICU patients. Chest 2005;127:213–9.
6. Rello J. Bench to bedside review: therapeutic options and issues in the management of ventilator-associated bacterial pneumonia. Crit Care 2005;9:259–65.
7. Rello J, Ollendorf DA, Oster G, et al. Epidemiology and outcomes of ventilator-associated pneumonia in a large US database. Chest 2002;122:2115–21.
8. Berger MM, Eggimann P, Heyland DK, et al. Reduction of nosocomial pneumonia after major burns by trace element supplementation: aggregation of two randomized trials. Crit Care 2006;10:R153–60.
9. von Dossow V, Rotard K, Redlich U, et al. Circulating immune parameters predicting the progression from hospital-acquired pneumonia to septic shock in surgical patients. Crit Care 2005;9:R662–9.
10. Metheny NA, Clouse RE, Chang Y, et al. Tracheobronchial aspiration in critically ill tube-fed patients: frequency, outcomes and risk factors. Crit Care Med 2006;34:1007–15.
11. Hunter JP. Ventilator-associated pneumonia. Postgrad Med J 2006;82:172–8.
12. Metheny NA. Preventing respiratory complications of tube feedings: evidence-based practice. Am J Crit Care 2006;15:360–9.
13. Drakulovic MB, Torres A, Bauer TT, et al. Supine body position as a risk factor for nosocomial pneumonia in mechanically ventilated patients: a randomized trial. Lancet 1999;354:1851–8.
14. Howard LSGE, Sillis M, Pasteur MC, et al. Microbiological profile of community-acquired pneumonia in adults over the last 20 years. J Infect 2005;50:107–13.
15. Chastre J. Antimicrobial treatment of hospital-acquired pneumonia. Infect Dis Clin North Am 2003;17:727–37.
16. Park DR. The microbiology of ventilator-associated pneumonia. Respir Care 2005;50:742–65.
17. Dennesen PJ, van der Ven AJ, Kessels AG, et al. Resolution of infectious parameters after antimicrobial therapy in patients with ventilator associated pneumonia. Am J Respir Crit Care Med 2001;163:1371–5.
18. Sandiumenge A, Diaz E, Bodi M, et al. Therapy of ventilator-associated pneumonia: a patient-based approached based on the ten rules of the "Tarragona Strategy. Intensive Care Med 2003;29:876–83.

19. Rupp ME, Fey PD. Extended-spectrum beta-lactamase (ESBL)-producing Enterobacteriea: considerations for diagnosis, prevention and drug treatment. Drugs 2003;63:353–65.
20. Colodner R. Extended-spectrum beta-lactamases: a challenge for clinical microbiologists and infection control specialists. Am J Infect Control 2005;33: 104–7.
21. Zavaski AP, Barth AL, Fernandes AF, et al. Reappraisal of *Pseudomonas aeruginosa* hospital-acquired pneumonia in the era of metallo-β-lactamase-mediated multidrug resistance: a prospective, observational study. Crit Care 2006;10: R114–20.
22. Combes A, Luyt C, Fagon J, et al. Early predictors for infection recurrence and death in patients with ventilator-associated pneumonia. Crit Care Med 2007;35: 146–54.
23. Scott P, Deye G, Srinivasan A, et al. An outbreak of multidrug-resistant *Acinetobacter baumannii-caloaceticus* complex infection in the US military health care system associated with military operations in Iraq. Clin Infect Dis. 2007;44: 1577–84.
24. Maragakis LL, Perl TM. *Acinetobacter baumannii*: epidemiology, antimicrobial resistance and treatment options. Clin Infect Dis 2008;46:1254–63.
25. Bonomo RA, Szabo D. Mechanisms of multidrug resistance in Acinetobacter species and *Pseudomonas aeruginosa*. Clin Infect Dis 2006;43(suppl 2):49–56.
26. Garnacho-Montero J, Ortiz-Leyba C, Fernandez-Hinojosa E, et al. *Acinetobacter baumannii* ventilator-associated pneumonia: epidemiological and clinical findings. Intensive Care Med 2005;31:649–55.
27. Goldman L, Caldera DL, Nussbaum SR, et al. Multifactorial index of cardiac risk in noncardiac surgical procedures. N Engl J Med 1977;297:845–50.
28. Brooks-Brunn JA. Validation of a predictive model for postoperative pulmonary complications. Heart Lung 1998;27:151–8.
29. Castillo R, Haas A. Chest physical therapy: comparative efficacy of preoperative and postoperative in the elderly. Arch Phys Med Rehabil 1985;66:376–9.
30. Epstein SK, Faling LJ, Daly BD, et al. Predicting complications after pulmonary resection: preoperative exercise testing versus a multifactorial cardiopulmonary risk index. Chest 1993;104:694–700.
31. Arozullah AM, Daley J, Henderson WG, et al. Multifactorial risk index for predicting postoperative respiratory failure in men after major noncardiac surgery: the National Veterans Administration Surgical Quality Improvement Program. Ann Surg 2000;232:242–53.
32. Johnson RM, Arozullah AM, Neumayer L, et al. Multivariable predictors of postoperative respiratory failure after general and vascular surgery: results from the Patient Safety in Surgery Study. J Am Coll Surg 2007;204:1188–98.
33. Qaseem A, Snow V, Fitteman N, et al. Risk assessment for and strategies to reduce perioperative pulmonary complications for patients undergoing noncardiothoracic surgery: a guideline from the American College of Physicians. Ann Intern Med 2006;144:575–80.
34. Bluman LG, Masca L, Newman N, et al. Preoperative smoking habits and postoperative pulmonary complications. Chest 1998;113:883–9.
35. Moller AM, Maaloe R, Pedersen T. Postoperative intensive care admittance: the role of tobacco smoking. Acta Anaesthesiol Scand 2001;45:345–8.
36. Nakagawa M, Tanaka H, Tsukuma H, et al. Relationship between the duration of the preoperative smoke-free period and the incidence of postoperative pulmonary complications after pulmonary surgery. Chest 2001;120:705–10.

37. Warner MA, Offord KP, Warner ME, et al. Role of preoperative cessation of smoking and other factors in postoperative pulmonary complications: a blinded prospective study of coronary artery bypass patients. Mayo Clin Proc 1989;64:609–16.
38. Rodgers A, Walker N, Schug S, et al. Reduction of postoperative mortality and morbidity with epidural or spinal anaesthesia: results from an overview of randomized trials. BMJ 2000;321:1493–504.
39. Khan MA, Hussain SF. Pre-operative pulmonary evaluation. J Ayub Med Coll Abbottabad 2005;17:82–6.
40. Ferrer M, Torsten TB, Torres A, et al. Effect of nasogastric tube size on gastroesophageal reflux and microaspiration in intubated patients. Ann Intern Med 1999;130:991–4.
41. Holzapfel L, Chevert S, Madinier G, et al. Influence of long-term oro- or nasotracheal intubation on nosocomial maxillary sinusitis and pneumonia: results of a prospective, randomized clinical trial. Crit Care Med 1993;(8):1132–8.
42. Magne N, Marcy PY, Foa C, et al. Comparison between nasogastric tube feeding and percutaneous fluoroscopic gastrostomy tube feeding in advanced head and neck cancer patients. Eur Arch Otorhinolaryngol 2001;258:89–92.
43. Dodek P, Keenan S, Cook D, et al. Evidence-based clinical practice guideline for the prevention of ventilator-associated pneumonia. Ann Intern Med 2004;141: 305–13.
44. van Nieuwenhoven CA, Vandenbroucke-Graul SC, van Tiel FH, et al. Feasibility and effects of the semirecumbent position to prevent ventilator-associated pneumonia: a randomized study. Crit Care Med 2006;34:396–402.
45. de Jonge E, Schultz MJ, Spanjaard L, et al. Effects of selective decontamination of digestive tract on mortality and acquisition of resistant bacteria in intensive care: a randomized controlled trial. Lancet 2003;362:1011–6.
46. Ross A, Crumpler J. The impact of an evidence-based practice education program on the role of oral care in the prevention of ventilator-associated pneumonia. Intensive Crit Care Nurs 2007;23:132–6.
47. Segers P, Speekenbrink RGH, Ubbink DT, et al. Prevention of nosocomial infection in cardiac surgery by decontamination of the nasopharynx and oropharynx with chlorhexidine gluconate: a randomized controlled trial. JAMA 2006;296:2460–6.
48. Chlebicki MP, Safdar N. Topical chlorhexidine for prevention of ventilator-associated pneumonia: a meta-analysis. Crit Care Med 2007;35:595–602.
49. Kollef MH. Role of selective digestive tract decontamination on mortality and respiratory tract infections: a meta-analysis. Chest 1994;105:1101–8.
50. Cook D, Heyland D, Griffith D, et al. Risk factors for clinically important upper gastrointestinal bleeding in patients requiring mechanical ventilation; Canadian Critical Care Trials Group. Crit Care Med 1999;27:2812–7.
51. Cook D, Griffith LE, Walter SD, et al. The attributable mortality and length of intensive care unit stay of clinically important gastrointestinal bleeding in critically ill patients. Crit Care 2001;5:368–75.
52. Cook D, Guyhatt G, Marshall J, et al. A comparison of sucralfate and ranitidine for the prevention of upper gastrointestinal bleeding in patients requiring mechanical ventilation. N Engl J Med 1998;338:791–7.
53. Ramirez P, Ferrer M, Torres A. Prevention measures for ventilator-associated pneumonia: a new focus on the endotracheal tube. Curr Opin Infect Dis 2007; 20:190–7.
54. Holzapfel L, Chastang C, Demingeon G, et al. A randomized study assessing the systematic search for maxillary sinusitis in nasotracheally mechanically

ventilated patients. Influence of nosocomial maxillary sinusitis on the occurrence of ventilator-associated pneumonia. Am J Respir Crit Care Med 1999;159: 695–701.

55. Salord F, Gaussorgues P, Marti-Flich J, et al. Nosocomial maxillary sinusitis during mechanical ventilation: a prospective comparison of orotracheal versus the nasotracheal route for intubation. Intensive Care Med 1990;16:390–3.

56. Kollef MH, Skubas NJ, Sundt TM. A randomized clinical trial of continuous aspiration of subglottic secretions in cardiac surgery patients. Chest 1999;116: 1339–46.

57. Lorente L, Lecuona M, Jiménez A, et al. Influence of an endotracheal tube with polyurethane cuff and subglottic secretion drainage on pneumonia. Am J Respir Crit Care Med 2007;176:1079–83.

58. Dezfulian C, Shojania K, Collard HR, et al. Subglottic secretion drainage for preventing ventilator-associated pneumonia: a meta-analysis. Am J Med 2005;118: 11–8.

59. Niël-Weise BS, Snoeren RIMM, van den Broed DJ. Policies for endotracheal suctioning of patients receiving mechanical ventilation: a systematic review of randomized controlled trials. Infect Control Hosp Epidemiol 2007;28:178–84.

60. Combes P, Fauvage B, Oleyer C. Nosocomial pneumonia in mechanically ventilated patients, a prospective randomized evaluation of the stericath closed suctioning system. Intensive Care Med 2000;26:878–82.

61. Lorente M, Lecuona M, Martin MM, et al. Ventilator-associated pneumonia using a closed versus open tracheal suction system. Crit Care Med 2005;33:115–9.

62. Topeli A, Harmanci A, Cetinkaya Y, et al. Comparison of the effect of closed versus open endotracheal suction systems on the development of ventilator-associated pneumonia. J Hosp Infect 2004;58:14–9.

63. Gastmeier P, Geffers C. Prevention of ventilator-associated pneumonia: Analysis of studies published since 2004. J Hosp Infect 2007;67:1–8.

64. Kollef MH, Shapiro SD, Fraser VJ, et al. Mechanical ventilation with and without 7-day circuit changes, a randomized controlled trial. Ann Intern Med 1995;123: 168–74.

65. Dreyfuss D, Djedaini K, Weber P, et al. Prospective study of nosocomial pneumonia and of patient and circuit colonization during mechanical ventilation with circuit changes every 48 hours versus no change. Am Rev Respir Dis 1991;143:738–43.

66. Long MN, Wickstrom G, Grimes A, et al. Prospective, randomized study of ventilator-associated pneumonia in patients with one versus three ventilator circuit changes per week. Infect Control Hosp Epidemiol 1996;17:14–9.

67. Safdar N, Crnich CJ, Redlich U. The pathogenesis of ventilator-associated pneumonia: its relevance to developing effective strategies for prevention. Respir Care 2005;50:725–39.

68. Dreyfuss D, Djedaini K, Gros I, et al. Mechanical ventilation with heated humidifiers or heat and moisture exchangers: effects on patient colonization and incidence of nosocomial pneumonia. Am J Respir Crit Care Med 1995; 151:986–92.

69. Lacherade JC, Auburtin M, Cerf C, et al. Impact of humidification systems of ventilator-associated pneumonia. Am J Respir Crit Care Med 2005;172:1276–82.

70. Boots R, George N, Faoagali J, et al. Double-heater-wire circuits and head- and moisture exchanger and the risk of ventilator-associated pneumonia. Crit Care Med 2006;34:687–93.

71. Kress JP, As Pohlman, O'Connor MF, et al. Daily interruption of sedative infusions in critically ill patients undergoing mechanical ventilation. N Engl J Med 2000; 342:1461–77.
72. Schweickert WD, Gehlbach BK, Pohlman AS, et al. Daily interruption of sedative infusions and complications of critical illness in mechanically ventilated patients. Crit Care Med 2004;32:1272–6.
73. Marelich GP, Murin S, Battistella F, et al. Protocol weaning of mechanical ventilation in medical and surgical patients by respiratory care practitioners and nurses: effect on weaning time and incidence of ventilator-associated pneumonia. Chest 2000;118:459–67.
74. Girard TD, Kress JP, Fuchs BD, et al. Efficacy and safety of a paired sedation and ventilator weaning protocol for mechanically ventilated patients in intensive care (awakening and breathing controlled trial): a randomized controlled trial. Lancet 2008;371:126–34.
75. Smetana GW, Lawrence VA, Cornell JE. Preoperative pulmonary risk stratification for noncardiothoracic surgery: a systematic review for the American College of Physicians. Ann Intern Med 2006;144:581–95.
76. Freitas ERFS, Soares BGO, Cardoso JR, et al. Incentive spirometry for preventing pulmonary complications after coronary artery bypass graft [Review]. The Cochrane Collaboration 2007;1–18.
77. Criteria for defining nosocomial pneumonia. NHSN 2005;1:1–9.
78. Andrews CP, Coalson JJ, Smith JD, et al. Diagnosis of nosocomial bacterial pneumonia in acute, diffuse lung injury. Chest 1981;80:248–54.
79. Bell RC, Coalson JJ, Smith JD, et al. Multiple organ system failure and infection in adult respiratory distress syndrome. Ann Intern Med 1983;99:293–8.
80. Niederman MS. The clinical diagnosis of ventilator-associated pneumonia. Respir Care 2005;50:788–96.
81. Pugin J, Auckenthaler R, Mill N, et al. Diagnosis of ventilator-associated pneumonia by batcteriologic analysis of bronchoscopic and non-bronchoscopic "blind" bronchoalveolar lavage. Am Rev Respir Dis 1991;143:1121–9.
82. Luyt CE, Chastre J, Fagon JY, et al. Value of the clinical pulmonary infection score for the identification and management of ventilator-associated pneumonia. Intensive Care Med 2004;30:844–52.
83. Fagon J. Hospital acquired pneumonia: diagnostic strategies: lessons from clinical trials. Infect Dis Clin North Am 2003;17:717–26.
84. Singh N, Rogers P, Atwood C, et al. Short-course empiric antibiotic therapy for patients with pulmonary infiltrates in the intensive-care unit: a proposed solution for indiscriminate antibiotic use. Am J Respir Crit Care Med 2000;162:505–11.
85. Mueller EW, Croce MA, Boucher BA, et al. Repeat bronchoalveolar lavage to guide antibiotic duration for ventilator-associated pneumonia. J Trauma 2007; 63:1329–37.
86. Lode H, Raffenberg M, Erbes R, et al. Nosocomial pneumonia: epidemiology, pathogenesis, diagnosis, treatment and prevention. Curr Opin Infect Dis 2000; 13:377–84.
87. Heyland DK, Cook DJ, Marshall J, et al. The clinical utility of invasive diagnostic techniques in the setting of ventilator-associated pneumonia. Chest 1999;115:1076–84.
88. Timsit JF, Cheval C, Gachot B, et al. Usefulness of a strategy based on bronchoscopy with direct examination of bronchoalveolar lavage fluid in the initial antibiotic therapy of suspected ventilator-associated pneumonia. Intensive Care Med 2001;27:640–7.

89. Ruiz M, Torres A, Ewig S, et al. Noninvasive versus invasive microbial investigation in ventilator-associated pneumonia: evaluation of outcome. Am J Respir Crit Care Med 2000;162:119–25.

90. The Canadian Critical Care Trials Group. A randomized trial of diagnostic techniques for ventilator-associated pneumonia. N Engl J Med 2006;355:2619–30.

91. Fagon JY, Chastre J, Wolff M, et al. Invasive and non-invasive strategies for management of suspected ventilator-associated pneumonia: a randomized controlled trial. Ann Intern Med 2000;132:621–30.

92. Croce MA, Fabian TC, Schurr MJ, et al. Using bronchoalveolar lavage to distinguish nosocomial pneumonia from systemic inflammatory response syndrome: a prospective analysis. J Trauma 1995;39:1134–9.

93. Croce MA, Fabian TC, Waddle-Smith L, et al. Utility of Gram's stain and efficacy of quantitative culture for posttraumatic pneumonia: a prospective study. Ann Surg 1998;227:743–51.

94. Shorr AF, Sherner JH, Jackson WL, et al. Invasive approaches to the diagnosis of ventilator-associated pneumonia: a meta-analysis. Crit Care Med 2005;33:46–53.

95. Ioanas M, Ferrer M, Cavalcanti M, et al. Causes and predictors of non-response to treatment of intensive care unit-acquired pneumonia. Crit Care Med 2004;32:938–45.

96. Mueller EW, Hanes SD, Croce MA, et al. Effect from multiple episodes of inadequate empiric antibiotic therapy for ventilator-associated pneumonia on morbidity and mortality among critically ill trauma patients. J Trauma 2005;58:94–101.

97. Garcia JCP, Filho OFF, Grion CMC, et al. Impact of the implementation of a therapeutic guideline on the treatment of nosocomial pneumonia acquired in the intensive care unit of a university hospital. J Bras Pneumol 2007;33:175–84.

98. Kashuba ADM, Nafziger AN, Drusano GL, et al. Optimizing aminoglycoside therapy for nosocomial pneumonia caused by gram-negative bacteria. Antimicrobial Agents Chemother 1999;43:623–9.

99. Steinkraus G, White R, Friedrich L. Vancomycin MIC creep in non-vancomycin-intermediate *Staphylococcus aureus* (VISA), vancomycin-susceptible clinical methicillin-resistant *S. aureus* (MRSA) blood isolates from 2001–05. J Am Cult 2007;60:788–94.

100. Wang G, Hindler JF, Ward KW, et al. Increased vancomycin MICs for *Staphylococcus aureus* clinical isolates from a university hospital during a 5-year period. J Clin Microbiol 2006;44:3883–6.

101. Adler J. The use of daptomycin for *Staphylococcus aureus* infections in critical care medicine. Crit Care Clin 2008;24:349–63.

102. French GL. Bactericidal agents in the treatment of MRSA infections- the potential role of daptomycin. J Antimicrob Chemother 2006;58:1107–17.

103. Shorr AF, Combes A, Kollef MH, et al. Methicillin-resistant *Staphylococcus aureus* prolongs intensive care unit stay in ventilator-associated pneumonia, despite initially appropriate antibiotic therapy. Crit Care Med 2006;34:700–6.

104. Michalopoulos A, Fotakis D, Virtzili S, et al. Aerosolized colistin as adjunctive treatment of ventilator-associated pneumonia due to multidrug-resistant gram negative bacteria: a prospective study. Respir Med 2008;102:407–12.

105. Rios FG, Luna CM, Maskin B, et al. Ventilator-associated pneumonia due to colistin susceptible-only microorganisms. Eur Respir J 2007;30:307–13.

106. Linden PK, Paterson DL. Parenteral and inhaled colistin for treatment of ventilator-associated pneumonia. Clin Infect Dis 2006;43(Suppl 2):89–94.

107. Pieracci FM, Barie PS. Strategies in the prevention and management of ventilator-associated pneumonia. The American Surgeon 2007;73:419–32.

108. Lynch JP. Combination antibiotic therapy is appropriate for nosocomial pneumonia in the intensive care unit. Semin Respir Infect 1993;8:268–84.
109. Arbo MD, Snydman DR. Monotherapy is appropriate for nosocomial pneumonia in the intensive care unit. Semin Respir Infect 1993;8:259–67.
110. Croce MA, Fabian TC, Stewart RM, et al. Empiric monotherapy versus combination therapy of nosocomial pneumonia in trauma patients. J Trauma 1993;35:303–9.
111. Ibrahim EH, Ward S, Sherman G, et al. Experience with a clinical guideline for the treatment of ventilator-associated pneumonia. Crit Care Med 2001;29:1109–15.
112. Heyland DK, Dodek P, Muscedere J, et al. Randomized trial of combination versus monotherapy for the empiric treatment of suspected ventilator-associated pneumonia. Crit Care Med 2008;36:737–44.
113. Garnacho-Montero J, Sa-Borges M, Sole-Violan J, et al. Optimal management therapy for *Pseudomonas aeruginosa* ventilator-associated pneumonia: an observational, multicenter study comparing monotherapy with combination antibiotic therapy. Crit Care Med 2007;35:1888–95.
114. Chastre J, Wolff M, Fagon J, et al. Comparison of 8 vs. 15 days of antibiotic therapy for ventilator-associated pneumonia in adults. JAMA 2003;290:2588–98.
115. Trouillet JL, Chastre J, Vuagnat A, et al. Ventilator-associated pneumonia caused by potentially drug-resistant bacteria. Am J Respir Crit Care Med 1998;157:531–9.
116. Harris AD, McGregor JC, Johnson JA, et al. Risk factors for colonization with extended spectrum beta-lactamase-producing bacteria and intensive care unit admission. Emerging Infect Dis 2007;13:1144–9.
117. Alvarez-Lerma F, Alvarez B, Luque P, et al. Empiric broad-spectrum antibiotic therapy of nosocomial pneumonia in the intensive care unit: a prospective, observational study. Crit Care 2006;10:R78–88.
118. Rello J, Vidaur L, Sandiumenge A, et al. De-escalation therapy in ventilator-associated pneumonia. Crit Care Med 2004;32:2183–90.
119. Giantsou E, Liratzopoulos N, Efraimidou E, et al. De-escalation therapy rates are significantly higher by bronchalveolar lavage than by tracheal aspiration. Intensive Care Med 2007;33:1533–40.
120. Salahuddin N, Zafar A, Sukhyani L, et al. Reducing ventilator-associated pneumonia rates through a staff education programme. J Hosp Infect 2004;57:223–7.
121. The Johns Hopkins Hospital Antibiotic Management Program, Treatment Recommendations for Adult Inpatients, 2007.
122. Cocanour CS, Peninger M, Domonoske BD, et al. Decreasing ventilator-associated pneumonia in a trauma ICU. J Trauma 2006;61:122–30.
123. Tolentino-DelosReyes AF, Ruppert SD, Shiao SPK. Evidence-based practice: use of the ventilator bundle to prevent ventilator-associated pneumonia. Am J Crit Care 2007;16:20–7.
124. Holzapfel L, Chevert S, Madinier G, et al. Influence of long-term oro- or nasotracheal intubation on nosocomial maxillary sinusitis and pneumonia: results of a prospective, randomized clinical trial. Crit Care Med 1993;21:1132–8.

Catheter-Related Bloodstream Infection

Matthew R. Goede, MD[a], Craig M. Coopersmith, MD[b],*

KEYWORDS

- Central venous catheter • Infection
- Catheter-related bloodstream infection
- Intensive care unit • Bacteremia • Morbidity

Central venous catheters (CVCs) play an essential role in patient care, both in the inpatient and outpatient setting. CVCs can be used to measure central venous pressure, deliver parenteral nutrition, and administer medications that cannot be given safely by a peripheral catheter. The use of CVCs carries a risk of the development of catheter-related bloodstream infection (CR-BSI), however, which can be associated with significant morbidity and mortality. Although a subset of CR-BSIs have historically been believed to be preventable, recent evidence suggests that most, if not all, episodes of CR-BSI are actually preventable. This has recently resulted in CR-BSI being listed as a "never" complication by the Centers for Medicare and Medicaid Services.[1] Based on this designation, hospitals will no longer receive payment when Medicare patients develop CR-BSI, and it is expected that many private insurers also will rapidly adopt this policy. Between its designation as a "never" complication by the federal government and the institution of mandatory public reporting for CR-BSI rates by many states, this complication is rapidly developing a markedly increased public profile.

EPIDEMIOLOGY AND RISK FACTORS

The number of CR-BSIs has been estimated to be 250,000 per year.[2] CR-BSIs have recently been demonstrated to increase length of stay in the ICU by an average of 2.4 days and increase total hospital length of stay by 7.5 days.[3] Its effect on mortality is more controversial. Unadjusted mortality rates have ranged from 16% to 25%; however, this is complicated by the fact that patients with CVCs are likely to be sicker than a typical hospitalized patient.[4] Recent studies examining adjusted mortality that control for confounders have demonstrated mortality rates ranging from 0% to 17%, with

[a] Surgical Critical Care, Barnes-Jewish Hospital/Washington University School of Medicine, St. Louis, MO, USA
[b] Department of Surgery, Washington University School of Medicine, 660 South Euclid Avenue, Campus Box 8109, St. Louis, MO 63110, USA
* Corresponding author.
E-mail address: coopersmithc@wustl.edu (C.M. Coopersmith).

Surg Clin N Am 89 (2009) 463–474
doi:10.1016/j.suc.2008.09.003
0039-6109/08/$ – see front matter © 2009 Elsevier Inc. All rights reserved.

surgical.theclinics.com

rates in hospitalized patients noted to be as high as 23%.[5,6] The precise economic cost of a CR-BSI can be difficult to quantify, in light of the fact that patients with CVCs tend to have multiple coexisting medical problems. Estimates have varied greater than 10-fold in studies that have been published over the past decade, ranging from $4888 to $56,167,[7,8] although most studies have come up with estimates in the middle of this range.

Risk factors for CR-BSI include length of CVC duration; patient location (outpatient, inpatient floor, ICU); type of catheter; number of lumens; number of manipulations per day; emergent placement; use of catheter for parenteral nutrition; presence of needleless connectors (this increases risk); and whether or not best care practices are followed. CVCs in an ICU setting have a higher infection rate than those in the hospital ward or outpatient setting. According to the 2006 National Healthcare Safety Network report, medical and surgical wards had an incidence rate of 1.5 CR-BSI per 1000 catheter days compared with 2.4 per 1000 catheter days for medical and surgical ICUs.[9] The risk of infection also varies depending on type of ICU. Cardiothoracic ICUs have the lowest incidence at 1.6 per 1000 catheter days and burn ICUs have the highest rate of 6.8 per 1000 catheter days.[9] This difference in CR-BSI rates between different types of ICUs may be explained by differing disease processes, severity of illness, and potentially duration of CVC placement. Of note, with continued close scrutiny paid to CR-BSI rates, the incidence of this complication has decreased nearly twofold in under a decade.[9,10]

Nontunneled catheters are the most commonly inserted CVCs. Because of their prevalence and lack of an infection-suppressing cuff or tunnel, they have historically accounted for approximately 90% of CR-BSIs.[11] Several randomized trials have demonstrated that the risk of infection increases with the number of lumens in the catheter.[12] Except in specific clinical situations (ie, long-term parenteral nutrition), however, it may be difficult to predict the number of lumens that are needed, especially in critically ill patients. Because changing a catheter over a guidewire has significant implications for the sterility of the new catheter, most practitioners use multilumen catheters in the inpatient setting.

PREVENTION

Because of recent regulations suggesting that most if not all CR-BSIs are preventable, a large portion of this article focuses on evidenced-based practices that have been demonstrated to be effective at lowering or eliminating these infections.

Preventing CR-BSIs requires a multipronged strategy ranging from educational to technologic interventions. Attention must also be paid to prevention before a CVC is placed, when it is placed, and every day a catheter remains in place. Although the strategies listed next are applicable to all CVCs, they are focused on short-term access. It should be noted that subcutaneous cuffs and catheter tunneling are effective mechanical methods for preventing extraluminal infection, although both of these mechanisms increase the complexity and invasiveness of the insertion and removal of the catheter, and are not practical for temporary access.

Hand Hygiene

The first step in preventing CR-BSIs is the same as the first step in preventing infection in the operating room: strict adherence to aseptic techniques. This begins with hand hygiene. Although this should be obvious, many health care providers see a bedside procedure as somehow being "different" than even a minor operation, and do not feel the need to wash their hands before placing a CVC, despite the fact that the catheter can reasonably be expected to be in the central circulation in close proximity to the heart for a week or more, and there is little question that lack of hand hygiene can result in the spread of resistant infections.[13] Additionally, even if the person inserting a CVC knows that hand hygiene is appropriate, there is extensive literature to support the fact that health care workers repeatedly fail to wash their hands or use alcohol foam. The incidence of this failure has not changed appreciably over the past 30 years despite repeated admonitions from hospital administrators, the lay press, and infection control specialists.[14,15] Unfortunately, the literature also supports the observation that physicians perform appropriate hand hygiene less frequently than other health care workers, with estimates ranging from one third to one half the time. Of note, alcohol foam is generally as effective as washing hands with soap and water, and there is evidence that hand hygiene usage improves in physicians if alcohol foam is readily available.[16]

Skin Antisepsis

Similar to the operating room, thorough skin antisepsis before a procedure is an effective route of preventing infection days later. The use of 2% chlorhexidine (but not 0.5% chlorhexidine) has been shown to result in decreased CR-BSI compared with either 10% povidone iodine or 70% alcohol in a prospective randomized trial of 668 patients.[17,18] This is also supported by a meta-analysis comparing chlorhexidine with povidone iodine, which revealed a risk reduction of nearly 50%.[19] An economic analysis showed that even though chlorhexidine costs more on a per unit basis, the decreased incidence of CR-BSI (with its associated morbidity and potential mortality) leads to $113 in savings for each CVC placed.[20] It should also be noted that daily baths with 2% chlorhexidine washcloths as opposed to soap and water have been shown to decrease the rate of CR-BSI in a two-arm crossover study of 836 patients in a medical ICU.[21]

Full Barrier Precautions

When placing a CVC, the patient's room needs to be treated similar to an operating room. This means there should be full-sized sterile drapes on the patient and a mask, cap, sterile gown, and gloves on the person placing the CVC (full barrier precautions). An outpatient study of 343 patients demonstrated a sixfold decrease in the rate of CR-BSI when full barrier precautions were used as opposed to when sterile gloves and a small drape alone were used.[22] Additionally, a twofold decrease in CR-BSI rates was demonstrated in ICU patients undergoing pulmonary artery catheterization who had full barrier precautions compared with those with less stringent precautions.[23] An economic analysis also showed that even though full barrier precautions cost approximately $40 per CVC insertion, the decreased incidence of CR-BSI leads to $252 savings for each CVC placed.[24]

Anatomic Site of Insertion

In general, the subclavian vein is preferred to either the internal jugular or femoral vein for CVC insertion. Although this is not based on prospective, randomized trials, most studies examining this issue have demonstrated a twofold to threefold increase in CR-BSI when either of the latter approaches is used. This has led expert opinion to support placement of CVCs in the subclavian vein,[2] although the person performing the insertion should have appropriate expertise because of the increased risk of a pneumothorax when using this insertion site. Potential reasons to use a site other than the subclavian vein include significant coagulopathy, obvious site infection, inaccessibility, or a need for chronic dialysis, because subclavian stenosis and thrombosis may preclude subsequent use of this site. It should be noted that there is a greater than 10-fold increase in thrombotic complications when using the femoral vein to place a CVC,[25] and this site should generally only be used in life-threatening emergencies or when vascular access above the diaphragm is not technically feasible. The role of peripherally inserted central catheters (PICC) is unclear. Some studies have demonstrated that PICC lines may decrease CR-BSI. Some experts, however, believe that infection rates are similar between PICC lines and CVCs placed in the subclavian vein, but less attention may be placed to infection risks in PICC lines, leading to catheters being left in place (with resultant infection risk) longer than might a CVC.

Catheter Care After Insertion

A study comparing changing gauze dressings every other day to transparent dressings changed every 5 days demonstrated no difference in CR-BSI rate in pulmonary artery catheters.[26] Either strategy is equally acceptable, although if bleeding occurs, gauze dressings are preferred (and grossly soiled dressings should be changed immediately). Sustained-release chlorhexidine dressings have not been demonstrated to decrease CR-BSI rates but have been associated with a nearly twofold decrease in exit site colonization in a recent meta-analysis,[27] so their usefulness is currently unclear. Catheter care teams have been demonstrated to decrease infection rates in multiple trials, including one randomized trial,[28] although not all studies support this finding.[29] A recent meta-analysis demonstrates that administration sets do not need to be changed more frequently than every 96 hours, although administration sets containing blood or lipids need to be changed every 24 hours.[30] There is no role for antibiotic flush solution in routine adult CVCs. Vancomycin lock solution has been demonstrated to have use in highly selected groups including high-risk neonates with PICC lines and oncology patients with long-term tunneled catheters.[31,32] A recent meta-analysis suggests that antibiotic lock solutions may also prevent CR-BSI in hemodialysis catheters.[33] There is no benefit to prophylactic antibiotics in preventing CR-BSI in adults, and they should not be used. A recent meta-analysis of prophylactic antibiotics in neonates demonstrated reduced rates of documented or suspected bacteremia.[34] This was not associated with improved mortality, however, and because of this and concerns about selection of resistant organisms and lack of data on long-term neurodevelopmental outcome, the use of prophylactic antibiotics in neonates is not currently recommended.[34]

Educational Programs

Multiple studies have shown a significant reduction of CR-BSI when an educational program is initiated.[35,36] Successful educational programs stressing "best practice" can be targeted at either those placing CVCs or those responsible for maintaining them.

Comprehensive Prevention Programs

Comprehensive prevention programs have also been demonstrated to dramatically decrease CR-BSI rates.[37,38] These programs include an educational component but also stress specific bedside patterns that may reduce infections. One key component of this is asking whether a CVC is needed on a daily basis. Because the incidence of CR-BSI is proportional to line age, CVCs should be removed as soon as practicable. Although the logic behind this recommendation is clear, it requires a system to ensure that the health care team specifically assesses the need for a CVC each day. Of note, although CVCs should be removed as soon as possible, there is no benefit to routine replacement of CVCs, because studies examining scheduled replacement of catheters every 3 to 7 days have not been associated with a decrease in CR-BSI rates.[39,40] There is also no benefit to routine guidewire exchange of CVCs.[41]

Another important component of a comprehensive prevention program is empowering the bedside nurse to stop a CVC insertion if breaks in sterile technique are identified. Although it is understood that a scrub nurse is empowered to identify breaks in sterile technique in the operating room, the concept of a bedside nurse doing the equivalent is a cultural change for many institutions. Many experts believe, however, that this is one of the most important components of a prevention program because policies regarding antisepsis are only as good as their implementation.

A multifaceted prevention program from Johns Hopkins University was described in 2004 that virtually eliminated CR-BSI in the ICU.[37] The elements of this prevention program included (1) an educational program, (2) asking health care workers daily about the continued need for a CVC, (3) empowering the bedside nurse to stop a CVC insertion if guidelines were not followed correctly, (4) having a CVC insertion cart to ensure all elements of insertion were kept in one common location, and (5) a CVC checklist performed by the bedside nurse. This study decreased the rate of CR-BSI to 0.54 per 1000 catheter days over the course of 16 months.

Pronovost and colleagues[38] then demonstrated that this program could be successful on a large scale. A total of 103 ICUs in Michigan used a modified prevention program that included hand hygiene, full barrier precautions, 2% chlorhexidine as a skin preparation, avoidance of femoral catheters, and removing unnecessary CVCs. The program decreased CR-BSI rates statewide from 7.7 per 1000 catheter days to 1.4 per 1000 catheter days over the course of 18 months. Importantly, although the program was aimed at ICUs, it was not directed toward a specific ICU or hospital type, and included academic and community hospitals of all sizes with all types of ICUs.

Antiseptic- or Antibiotic-Coated Catheters

No area of infection control for the prevention of CR-BSIs has been the subject of as much study or seems to evoke as much passion as the use of antiseptic- or antimicrobial-impregnated catheters. There are currently two commonly used types of catheters: chlorhexidine–silver sulfadiazine (antiseptic impregnated) and minocycline-rifampin (antibiotic impregnated). There have been over 20 randomized, prospective trials evaluating the benefits of these catheters,[42] and a recent meta-analysis suggests that they are effective in preventing CR-BSIs.[43] Most of these studies demonstrate either decreased CR-BSI rates or decreased catheter colonization, and there is no evidence that these catheters increase the selection of resistant organisms. An economic analysis also showed that even though impregnated catheters cost more than uncoated CVCs, the decreased incidence of CR-BSI leads to $196 savings for each CVC placed.[44]

When to use these catheters is less clear. The Centers for Disease Control and Prevention recommends using an impregnated catheter when (1) a CVC is expected to be in place greater than 5 days; (2) the institution has a comprehensive strategy to prevent CR-BSIs in place, which includes full barrier precaution, 2% chlorhexidine preparation, and an educational program aimed at preventing infections; and (3) CR-BSIs are higher than goal rates set by an institution "based upon bench mark rates."[2] Although this sounds simple in theory, it is frequently not clear in advance whether a CVC needs to be in place for greater than 5 days. Similarly, it is not clear what the goal rate for CR-BSI should be in light of the fact that the federal government has indicated this is a "never" complication, suggesting it is preventable 100% of the time. National Healthcare Safety Network data indicate, however, that even though rates are decreasing, CR-BSI still occurs in most hospitals in the country. Additionally, the usefulness of impregnated catheters in an ICU whose CR-BSI rates are below the national average but are not zero is currently unclear.[45]

What type of catheter to use is also unclear. A meta-analysis of 11 studies comparing chlorhexidine–silver sulfadiazine CVCs with uncoated catheters demonstrates an odds ratio of 0.56 favoring the antiseptic-coated catheters.[46] A single prospective randomized trial comparing antiseptic-impregnated catheters with minocycline-rifampin–impregnated catheters demonstrated a marked reduction in CR-BSI in the latter (0.3% for the minocycline-rifampin catheters versus 3.4% for the chlorhexidine–silver sulfadiazine catheters).[47] It should be noted, however, that this study used a first-generation chlorhexidine–silver sulfadiazine catheter, and a newer version with both internal and external coating is now available. An additional type of catheter coated with silver-platinum-carbon has also recently been described. Its benefit versus uncoated catheters has not been clearly documented,[48] however, and it has been demonstrated to be associated with increased catheter colonization compared with minocycline-rifampin catheters,[49] so its use cannot be recommended at the current time.

DIAGNOSIS

The diagnosis of CR-BSI can be challenging. Physical examination is typically unrevealing, and the diagnosis generally relies on culture data. Positive culture data may be difficult to interpret, however, because clinicians must make the distinction between CR-BSI and catheter colonization. Further, distinctions must be made between CR-BSI and secondary bacteremia, with bloodstream infection resulting from a source other than a CVC (pneumonia, intra-abdominal infection, and so forth).

The first component necessary to the diagnosis of CR-BSI is clinical suspicion. The typical clinical sign that initiates a work-up for CR-BSI is a new fever, not obviously related to a distant infection. Although fever is the most sensitive sign of CR-BSI, it does not have appropriate specificity to make the diagnosis. As in any patient with suspected infection, a history and physical examination should always be performed. The history is generally unrevealing, however, except for the presence or absence of risk factors outlined previously, although it certainly may give clues as to whether another possible source of fever needs to be considered.

Physical examination is also generally unrevealing. Occasionally, it can reveal erythema, induration, or purulence from either the exit site or along the course of the catheter. Although these signs are highly suggestive of a CR-BSI, they are rarely present, however, and the absence of findings on physical examination does not lessen clinical suspicion for the presence of infection. Rarely, a patient with CR-BSI develops endocarditis. In patients with infection and a new murmur on physical examination or a prosthetic heart valve, serial blood cultures should be obtained. If these are positive, this strongly suggests the presence of endocarditis, necessitating a longer course of antibiotic treatment. This should be investigated using an echocardiogram. Although a transthoracic echocardiogram is technically easier, a study of 103 patients with *Staphylococcus aureus* bacteremia (both CR-BSI and non–catheter-related) demonstrated only a 32% sensitivity for transthoracic echocardiogram and 100% sensitivity for transesophageal echocardiogram.[50]

There is no gold standard for how to use blood cultures to assess for CR-BSI. The authors' ICU performs two simultaneous peripheral blood cultures. Another method is to send a simultaneous peripheral blood culture with one drawn through the CVC. A quantitative colony count that is 5- to 10-fold higher in the culture drawn through the CVC is predictive of CR-BSI in tunneled catheters.[51] This method has lower sensitivity, however, in nontunneled short-term CVCs. If paired cultures are drawn, it is likely that a CR-BSI is present if the catheter culture becomes positive greater than 2 hours before the peripheral culture. The "time to positivity" method has been demonstrated to be 81% sensitive and 92% specific for the diagnosis of CR-BSI.[52] The latter two techniques, however, put an additional burden on an institution's microbiology laboratory (quantitative cultures and time of positive culture, respectively) that many are unable to meet. When removing a CVC, some institutions send the catheter tip for quantitative culture. Two techniques for doing so include the sonication method and roll-plating. Of these, sonication better evaluates intra-luminal and extraluminal colonization, whereas roll-plating mostly evaluates extraluminal infection. It should be emphasized that neither a positive catheter tip culture nor a single positive blood culture drawn through a CVC is indicative of CR-BSI. Rather, these are consistent with catheter colonization, which is not equivalent to bacteremia and does not have the same treatment implications. It is this confusion between catheter colonization and infection that is the rationale for why the authors' ICU does not send either catheter tips or cultures drawn through a CVC. It should be noted that if a patient defervesces after a CVC is removed, this is indirect evidence that a catheter infection may have been present even if peripheral blood cultures are negative.

MICROBIOLOGY

CR-BSIs predominantly come from microorganisms that colonize either catheter hubs or the skin surrounding the insertion site.[53] Extraluminal colonization occurs from migration of organisms from the skin along the subcutaneous tract. Intraluminal colonization occurs from contamination by injection ports or hubs.

There are several microorganisms that cause CR-BSI. The most common are coagulase-negative staphylococci and *S aureus*, gram-negative bacilli, and *Candida albicans*.[54] The microbiology of CR-BSI is important not only for determining appropriate antibiotic therapy but also in the ultimate outcome from the disease. For instance, *S aureus* bacteremia has been demonstrated to have a mortality rate of 8.2%, whereas mortality from coagulase-negative staphylococci is greater than 10-fold lower (0.7%).[54] A special concern with *S aureus* is associated venous thrombosis. A recent study demonstrated that a total of 71% of patients with *S aureus* bacteremia from internal jugular, brachial, or subclavian veins had thrombosis on ultrasonography.[55] Importantly, death or recurrent bacteremia occurred in 32% of these patients. As such, patients with CR-BSI from *S aureus* should undergo ultrasonography even if physical examination is normal.

TREATMENT

The primary treatment of a CR-BSI is to remove the infected catheter. Although adjunctive antibiotic therapy is important, catheter removal represents source control, and there are very few instances (detailed next) where an infected catheter can be left in situ. In the case of nontunneled CVCs, catheter removal is easily accomplished after establishing appropriate access elsewhere. It should be realized that in patients who have a febrile illness in which their CVC is removed for presumed CR-BSI, most have sterile cultures.[56]

Although rare, there are times when the treating physician can consider leaving an infected CVC in place. Patients with coagulase-negative staphylococci may be candidates for catheter salvage if (1) they do not have persistent bacteremia, (2) they do not have evidence of tunnel infection, and (3) they do not have evidence of metastatic complications or severe sepsis.[54] There is evidence to suggest that patients recover faster with a higher cure rate if the CVC is removed, however, rather than attempting to salvage the catheter. In patients with tunneled catheters that are risky to remove or replace, antibiotic lock therapy may be used by filling the CVC with a solution containing concentrated antibiotics for a number of hours. Higher antibiotic concentrations must be used because of biofilm formation in these infections. Antibiotic lock solution for tunneled catheters has been demonstrated to result in a catheter salvage rate of 83%, which compares favorably with a salvage rate of 67% in patients treated without this therapy.[54]

As in other suspected infections, broad-spectrum antibiotics should be initiated when CR-BSI is suspected on clinical grounds. Antibiotics should be started before culture and sensitivity results are obtained, because waiting until these are known leaves the patient without antimicrobial therapy and likely increases their mortality if the patient is bacteremic. Once culture and sensitivity results are known, antimicrobial therapy should be narrowed as much as practicable effectively to treat only the causative organism. Generally, a single antimicrobial agent suffices but double coverage can be considered in *Pseudomonas aeruginosa* infections, in neutropenic patients, or in patients with *S aureus* bacteremia when the catheter cannot be safely removed.[54,57]

There is little level I evidence on length of treatment for CR-BSI, so recommendations are generally based on expert opinion and nonrandomized trials. In general, uncomplicated bacterial or fungal CR-BSIs should be treated for a 10- to 14-day course. Infections with coagulase-negative staphylococci can be treated for 5 to 7 days. Complicated infections with tunneled catheters that cannot be safely removed should be treated for at least 2 to 4 weeks. Patients with endocarditis require at least 6 weeks of therapy. Once a CVC has been removed and therapy initiated, it is appropriate to check follow-up blood cultures to verify the infection is being cleared. Patients with persistent fever, signs of sepsis, or risk factors for distant cardiac infection should have serial blood cultures drawn until these are negative. Patients who do not respond to antibiotic therapy after the suspected catheter has been removed for 3 days need to be evaluated further for possible other sources of infection including the possibility of secondary infections, such as endocarditis, septic thrombophlebitis, or osteomyelitis. Consultation with an infectious disease specialist may also be indicated. It should be noted that in addition to increased risk of thrombotic complications, *S aureus* infections also have an increased incidence of other secondary infections.

SUMMARY

CR-BSIs are a common complication of central venous catheterization, resulting in substantial morbidity. A large percentage of them are preventable, leading the Centers for Medicare and Medicaid Services recently to define this as a "never" complication. CR-BSIs can be prevented by use of appropriate hand hygiene, 2% chlorhexidine as a skin preparation, full barrier precautions, avoidance of femoral catheters, empowering the bedside nurse to halt a CVC insertion if sterile technique is not followed, removing unneeded catheters as soon as possible, and comprehensive educational programs. If all of these are unsuccessful, antiseptic- or antibiotic-impregnated catheters are an effective tool to prevent infections. The diagnosis of CR-BSI is made largely based on culture results, and broad-spectrum antibiotics should be initiated as soon as an infection is suspected. Antimicrobial therapy can subsequently be narrowed once the causative organism is known. Except in rare circumstances, patients with CR-BSI need to have their infected CVC removed.

REFERENCES

1. Medicare program: changes to the hospital inpatient prospective payment systems and fiscal year 2008 rates. Fed Regist 2007;72:47379–428.
2. O'Grady NP, Alexander M, Dellinger EP, et al. Guidelines for the prevention of intravascular catheter-related infections. Centers for Disease Control and Prevention. MMWR Recomm Rep 2002;51:1–29.
3. Warren DK, Quadir WW, Hollenbeak CS, et al. Attributable cost of catheter-associated bloodstream infections among intensive care patients in a nonteaching hospital. Crit Care Med 2006;34:2084–9.
4. Higuera F, Rosenthal VD, Duarte P, et al. The effect of process control on the incidence of central venous catheter-associated bloodstream infections and mortality in intensive care units in Mexico. Crit Care Med 2005;33:2022–7.
5. Digiovine B, Chenoweth C, Watts C, et al. The attributable mortality and costs of primary nosocomial bloodstream infections in the intensive care unit. Am J Respir Crit Care Med 1999;160:976–81.
6. Diekema DJ, Beekmann SE, Chapin KC, et al. Epidemiology and outcome of nosocomial and community-onset bloodstream infection. J Clin Microbiol 2003; 41:3655–60.
7. Rosenthal VD, Guzman S, Orellano PW. Nosocomial infections in medical-surgical intensive care units in Argentina: attributable mortality and length of stay. Am J Infect Control 2003;31:291–5.
8. Dimick JB, Pelz RK, Consunji R, et al. Increased resource use associated with catheter-related bloodstream infection in the surgical intensive care unit. Arch Surg 2001;136:229–34.
9. Edwards JR, Peterson KD, Andrus ML, et al. National Healthcare Safety Network (NHSN) Report, data summary for 2006, issued June 2007. Am J Infect Control 2007;35:290–301.
10. National Nosocomial Infections Surveillance (NNIS) System report, data summary from January 1990–May 1999, issued June 1999. Am J Infect Control 1999;27:520–32.
11. Pearson ML. Guideline for prevention of intravascular device-related infections. Hospital Infection Control Practices Advisory Committee. Infect Control Hosp Epidemiol 1996;17:438–73.
12. Farkas JC, Liu N, Bleriot JP, et al. Single- versus triple-lumen central catheter-related sepsis: a prospective randomized study in a critically ill population. Am J Med 1992;93:277–82.
13. Goldmann D. System failure versus personal accountability: the case for clean hands. N Engl J Med 2006;355:121–3.
14. Albert RK, Condie F. Hand-washing patterns in medical intensive-care units. N Engl J Med 1981;304:1465–6.
15. Jenner EA, Fletcher BC, Watson P, et al. Discrepancy between self-reported and observed hand hygiene behaviour in healthcare professionals. J Hosp Infect 2006;63:418–22.
16. Maury E, Alzieu M, Baudel JL, et al. Availability of an alcohol solution can improve hand disinfection compliance in an intensive care unit. Am J Respir Crit Care Med 2000;162:324–7.
17. Maki DG, Ringer M, Alvarado CJ. Prospective randomised trial of povidone-iodine, alcohol, and chlorhexidine for prevention of infection associated with central venous and arterial catheters. Lancet 1991;338:339–43.
18. Humar A, Ostromecki A, Direnfeld J, et al. Prospective randomized trial of 10% povidone-iodine versus 0.5% tincture of chlorhexidine as cutaneous antisepsis

for prevention of central venous catheter infection. Clin Infect Dis 2000;31: 1001–7.

19. Chaiyakunapruk N, Veenstra DL, Lipsky BA, et al. Chlorhexidine compared with povidone-iodine solution for vascular catheter-site care: a meta-analysis. Ann Intern Med 2002;136:792–801.
20. Chaiyakunapruk N, Veenstra DL, Lipsky BA, et al. Vascular catheter site care: the clinical and economic benefits of chlorhexidine gluconate compared with povidone iodine. Clin Infect Dis 2003;37:764–71.
21. Bleasdale SC, Trick WE, Gonzalez IM, et al. Effectiveness of chlorhexidine bathing to reduce catheter-associated bloodstream infections in medical intensive care unit patients. Arch Intern Med 2007;167:2073–9.
22. Raad II, Hohn DC, Gilbreath BJ, et al. Prevention of central venous catheter-related infections by using maximal sterile barrier precautions during insertion. Infect Control Hosp Epidemiol 1994;15:231–8.
23. Mermel LA, McCormick RD, Springman SR, et al. The pathogenesis and epidemiology of catheter-related infection with pulmonary artery Swan-Ganz catheters: a prospective study utilizing molecular subtyping. Am J Med 1991;91: 197S–205S.
24. Hu KK, Veenstra DL, Lipsky BA, et al. Use of maximal sterile barriers during central venous catheter insertion: clinical and economic outcomes. Clin Infect Dis 2004;39:1441–5.
25. Merrer J, De Jonghe B, Golliot F, et al. Complications of femoral and subclavian venous catheterization in critically ill patients: a randomized controlled trial. JAMA 2001;286:700–7.
26. Maki DG, Stolz SS, Wheeler S, et al. A prospective, randomized trial of gauze and two polyurethane dressings for site care of pulmonary artery catheters: implications for catheter management. Crit Care Med 1994;22:1729–37.
27. Ho KM, Litton E. Use of chlorhexidine-impregnated dressing to prevent vascular and epidural catheter colonization and infection: a meta-analysis. J Antimicrob Chemother 2006;58:281–7.
28. Sherertz R. Look before you leap: discontinuation of an infusion therapy team. Infect Control Hosp Epidemiol 1999;20:99–100.
29. bi-Said D, Raad I, Umphrey J, et al. Infusion therapy team and dressing changes of central venous catheters. Infect Control Hosp Epidemiol 1999;20:101–5.
30. Gillies D, O'Riordan L, Wallen M, et al, Optimal timing for intravenous administration set replacement Cochrane Database Syst Rev 2005;CD003588.
31. Garland JS, Alex CP, Henrickson KJ, et al. A vancomycin-heparin lock solution for prevention of nosocomial bloodstream infection in critically ill neonates with peripherally inserted central venous catheters: a prospective, randomized trial. Pediatrics 2005;116:e198–205.
32. van DW, van Woensel JB. Prophylactic antibiotics for preventing early central venous catheter gram positive infections in oncology patients Cochrane Database Syst Rev 2007;CD003295.
33. Jaffer Y, Selby NM, Taal MW. Meta-analysis of hemodialysis catheter locking solutions in the prevention of catheter-related infection. Am J Kidney Dis 2008;51:233–41.
34. Jardine LA, Inglis GD, Davies MW, et al. Prophylactic systemic antibiotics to reduce morbidity and mortality in neonates with central venous catheters. Cochrane Database Syst Rev 2008;CD006179.
35. Coopersmith CM, Rebmann TL, Zack JE, et al. Effect of an education program on decreasing catheter-related bloodstream infections in the surgical intensive care unit. Crit Care Med 2002;30:59–64.

36. Eggimann P, Harbarth S, Constantin MN, et al. Impact of a prevention strategy targeted at vascular-access care on incidence of infections acquired in intensive care. Lancet 2000;355:1864–8.
37. Berenholtz SM, Pronovost PJ, Lipsett PA, et al. Eliminating catheter-related bloodstream infections in the intensive care unit. Crit Care Med 2004;32:2014–20.
38. Pronovost P, Needham D, Berenholtz S, et al. An intervention to decrease catheter-related bloodstream infections in the ICU. N Engl J Med 2006;355: 2725–32.
39. Eyer S, Brummitt C, Crossley K, et al. Catheter-related sepsis: prospective, randomized study of three methods of long-term catheter maintenance. Crit Care Med 1990;18:1073–9.
40. Cobb DK, High KP, Sawyer RG, et al. A controlled trial of scheduled replacement of central venous and pulmonary-artery catheters. N Engl J Med 1992;327: 1062–8.
41. Cook D, Randolph A, Kernerman P, et al. Central venous catheter replacement strategies: a systematic review of the literature. Crit Care Med 1997;25: 1417–24.
42. Crnich CJ, Maki DG. Are antimicrobial-impregnated catheters effective? When does repetition reach the point of exhaustion? Clin Infect Dis 2005;41:681–5.
43. Hockenhull JC, Dwan K, Boland A, et al. The clinical effectiveness and cost-effectiveness of central venous catheters treated with anti-infective agents in preventing bloodstream infections: a systematic review and economic evaluation. Health Technol Assess 2008;12:1–154.
44. Veenstra DL, Saint S, Sullivan SD. Cost-effectiveness of antiseptic-impregnated central venous catheters for the prevention of catheter-related bloodstream infection. JAMA 1999;282:554–60.
45. Schuerer DJ, Zack JE, Thomas J, et al. Effect of chlorhexidine/silver sulfadiazine-impregnated central venous catheters in an intensive care unit with a low blood stream infection rate after implementation of an educational program: a before-after trial. Surg Infect (Larchmt) 2007;8:445–54.
46. Veenstra DL, Saint S, Saha S, et al. Efficacy of antiseptic-impregnated central venous catheters in preventing catheter-related bloodstream infection: a meta-analysis. JAMA 1999;281:261–7.
47. Darouiche RO, Raad II, Heard SO, et al. A comparison of two antimicrobial-impregnated central venous catheters. Catheter Study Group. N Engl J Med 1999; 340:1–8.
48. Kalfon P, de VC, Samba D, et al. Comparison of silver-impregnated with standard multi-lumen central venous catheters in critically ill patients. Crit Care Med 2007; 35:1032–9.
49. Fraenkel D, Rickard C, Thomas P, et al. A prospective, randomized trial of rifampicin-minocycline-coated and silver-platinum-carbon-impregnated central venous catheters. Crit Care Med 2006;34:668–75.
50. Fowler VG Jr, Li J, Corey GR, et al. Role of echocardiography in evaluation of patients with Staphylococcus aureus bacteremia: experience in 103 patients. J Am Coll Cardiol 1997;30:1072–8.
51. Fan ST, Teoh-Chan CH, Lau KF. Evaluation of central venous catheter sepsis by differential quantitative blood culture. Eur J Clin Microbiol Infect Dis 1989;8: 142–4.
52. Raad I, Hanna HA, Alakech B, et al. Differential time to positivity: a useful method for diagnosing catheter-related bloodstream infections. Ann Intern Med 2004; 140:18–25.

53. Mermel LA, Eggimann P, Harbarth S, et al. Prevention of intravascular catheter-related infections Impact of a prevention strategy targeted at vascular-access care on incidence of infections acquired in intensive care. Lancet 2000;355:1864–8.

54. Mermel LA, Farr BM, Sherertz RJ, et al. Guidelines for the management of intravascular catheter-related infections. Clin Infect Dis 2001;32:1249–72.

55. Crowley AL, Peterson GE, Benjamin DK Jr, et al. Venous thrombosis in patients with short- and long-term central venous catheter-associated *Staphylococcus aureus* bacteremia. Crit Care Med 2008;36:385–90.

56. Rello J, Coll P, Prats G. Evaluation of culture techniques for diagnosis of catheter-related sepsis in critically ill patients. Eur J Clin Microbiol Infect Dis 1992;11: 1192–3.

57. Leibovici L, Paul M, Poznanski O, et al. Monotherapy versus beta-lactam-aminoglycoside combination treatment for gram-negative bacteremia: a prospective, observational study. Antimicrob Agents Chemother 1997;41:1127–33.

Nosocomial Urinary Tract Infection

Michael F. Ksycki, DO, Nicholas Namias, MD, MBA*

KEYWORDS

- Nosocomial infection • Urinary tract infection
- Urinary catheter

Nosocomial urinary tract infection is a major cause of morbidity in hospitalized patients in general, and in postoperative surgical patients in particular. The major predisposing factor to the development of a urinary tract infection is the presence of a urinary catheter. The risk of infection increases with the duration of catheterization. It has been estimated that the risk of urinary tract infection increases by 5% to 10% per catheter day after the second day of catheterization.[1,2]

RISK FACTORS

A recent analysis of data from the National Surgical Infection Prevention Project revealed that 86% of patients undergoing major operations had indwelling urinary catheters in the perioperative period, with half of the patients remaining catheterized for more than 2 days. As expected, catheterization for more than 2 days was a significant risk factor for urinary tract infection (9.4% versus 4.5%; $P = .004$). Prolonged catheterization was also associated with a decreased likelihood for discharge to home, and with increased 30-day mortality.[3] Previously, duration of catheterization had not been linked to mortality.[4] The National Health Safety Network, a project of the Centers for Disease Control and Prevention, also investigated catheter use and catheter-related urinary tract infection as part of its surveillance activities. In 2006, it reported a catheter use index in surgically oriented intensive care units (ICUs). This index, a ratio of urinary catheter days to patient days, ranged from 0.69 to 0.91. In these same ICUs, there were 4.0 to 7.5 catheter-associated urinary tract infections per 1000 urinary catheter days.[5] Thus, perioperative catheterization is near ubiquitous, is a major risk factor for nosocomial urinary tract infection, and is linked to, if not directly causative of, a decreased likelihood of discharge to home and an increased 30-day mortality.

MICROBIOLOGY AND DIAGNOSIS

The most common causative agents of catheter-related urinary tract infection are the patients' own colonic flora. Additional organisms are usually not found until duration of

Miller School of Medicine, University of Miami, PO Box 016960 (D-40), Miami, FL 33101, USA
* Corresponding author.
E-mail address: nnamias@miami.edu (N. Namias).

Surg Clin N Am 89 (2009) 475–481
doi:10.1016/j.suc.2008.09.012
0039-6109/08/$ – see front matter © 2009 Elsevier Inc. All rights reserved.

catheterization exceeds 30 days.[6] The most common organisms causing these infections with short-term catheterizations are *Escherichia coli*, enterococci, *Pseudomonas*, *Klebsiella*, *Enterobacter*, *Staphylococcus epidermidis*, *Staphylococcus aureus*, and *Serratia*. Exogenous sources can also lead to catheter-related urinary tract infection, commonly with staphylococci, *Serratia marcescens*, *Burkholderia cepacia*, and *Stenotrophomonas maltophilia*.[7]

Wagenlehner and colleagues[8] recently analyzed their 12-year experience with urinary tract infections in hospitalized urology patients in one German hospital. *E coli* initially accounted for approximately one third of the urinary tract infections. This increased over the 12 years to approximately 40%, primarily displacing infections due to *Pseudomonas aeruginosa*. Other gram negatives accounted for another one third of the infections, and gram positives caused the remaining one third. Increasing resistance of *E coli* to the commonly used trimethoprim/sulfamethoxazole was noted, highlighting the importance of culture and sensitivity data not only in treating the individual patient, but also for planning effective empiric treatment strategies. The investigators did not include fungal urinary tract infections as part of their study.

Urinary cultures have been the standard means for diagnosing urinary tract infections. The standard cutoff has been the growth of 10^5 or more organisms per milliliter of urine. This number was originally based on studies of symptomatic patients with cystitis, and not hospitalized patients with infections related to indwelling urinary catheter. Nonetheless, this remains the number used to diagnose the presence of urinary tract infection in surgical patients, and in reporting the incidence of such infections to regulatory agencies.

In more critically ill surgical patients, candiduria remains a vexing clinical problem. It typically occurs in patients who have a multitude of reasons to manifest sepsis. Sobel and Lundstrom[9] reviewed the development of candiduria in 2001 and pointed out that 10% to 15% of nosocomial urinary tract infections are now caused by *Candida* sp, with the highest prevalence being in patients housed in ICUs, and those with leukemia or who had undergone bone marrow transplant. Diabetes predisposes to the development of candiduria in multiple ways. In women, diabetes promotes colonization of the vulvovestibular area with *Candida*. Glycosuria, if present, enhances urinary fungal growth. Diabetes also impairs host defenses, particularly phagocytosis. Finally, the development of a neurogenic bladder allows for urinary stasis and increases the likelihood that the urinary tract will be instrumented. Fungal urinary tract infections are also promoted in diabetics and nondiabetics alike by antibiotic therapy, which leads to fungal overgrowth in the colon and perineal area due to suppression of normal bacterial flora; the fungal organisms can then ascend the Foley catheter into the urinary system. Bukhary[10] in 2008 also identified similar risk factors in a review of 37 years of English-language literature on the topic of candiduria. This review indicated that the risk factors for candiduria were indwelling urinary catheters, use of antibiotics, advanced age, underlying anatomic urologic abnormality, previous surgery, and the presence of diabetes.

Sobel and Lundstrom[9] indicated that *Candida albicans* is the most common fungal species causing urinary fungal infections, with *Candida glabrata* being the second most common fungal pathogen. More than one candidal species are found simultaneously in 10% of cases. Bukhary[10] cited multiple reviews of the epidemiology of candiduria, and confirmed that with only one exception the overwhelming majority of candiduria is due to *C albicans*. *C glabrata* accounts for 12% to 18% of cases, *Candida tropicalis* for 8% to 22%, and all remaining species for less than 5% in almost all studies. Urinary tract infections due to noncandidal fungal organisms are very uncommon in surgical patients, and are usually encountered as part of a disseminated mycotic disease in highly immunosuppressed patients.[9]

The diagnosis of a urinary tract infection due to *Candida* is difficult because *Candida* in the urine can represent contamination, colonization of the drainage device, or a true infection. Small numbers of yeast from a colonized catheter, collection device, or the vulva may multiply rapidly in the collected urine, producing high colony counts that do not necessarily indicate infection. Further, although the presence of pyuria usually supports the diagnosis of infection, the mere presence of an indwelling catheter can lead to pyuria, as can a coexisting bacterial urinary tract infection. Thus, clinical judgment must be used in making the diagnosis, particularly in asymptomatic patients. Notably, asymptomatic candiduria rarely, if ever, leads to candidemia.[9]

PREVENTION

European and Asian guidelines have been developed based on a comprehensive review and meta-analysis of data on prevention and treatment of urinary catheter–associated infections. Not surprisingly, the principal findings are that minimization of duration of catheterization and maintenance of a closed system are the best means of avoiding infection.[6]

These 2008 European and Asian guidelines for the prevention of catheter-associated urinary tract infections are listed below. The letters in parentheses indicate the grade of the guideline recommendation. An "A" recommendation is based on clinical studies of good quality and consistency, including at least one randomized trial; a "B" recommendation is based on well-conducted clinical studies, but without randomized clinical trials; and a "C" recommendation is one developed by the expert panel in the absence of directly applicable clinical studies of good quality.

The catheter system should remain closed (A).
The duration of catheterization should be minimal (A).
Topical antiseptics or antibiotics applied to the catheter, urethra, or meatus are not recommended (A).
Benefits from prophylactic antibiotics and antiseptic substances have never been established; therefore, they are not recommended (A).
Removal of the indwelling catheter after a nonurological operation before midnight may be beneficial (B).
Long-term indwelling catheters should be changed in intervals adapted to the individual patient, but must be changed before blockage is likely to occur (B); however, there is no evidence for the exact intervals of changing catheters.
Chronic antibiotic suppressive therapy is generally not recommended (A).

Adherence to these basic recommendations could significantly decrease the risk of catheter-associated urinary tract infections. In a 10-year study of infection control and surveillance practices emphasizing some of these principles, there was a decrease of 70% over time in the risk of urinary tract infections in an ICU population.[11]

Nonetheless, prolonged use of urinary catheters is necessary in certain surgical patients. In such cases, clinicians cannot use the best tool for preventing catheter-associated infections—early removal of the devices. Therefore, there has been interest in the use of catheters that might be less prone to allowing an infection. One key way in which catheters predispose to urinary tract infection is by serving as a site for bacterial pathogens to create a biofilm. The organisms associated with catheter-associated urinary tract infection grow in a glycocalyx, protected from the antibiotics concentrated in the urine. This biofilm gradually thickens and can encapsulate all surfaces of the catheter. Within this dense biofilm, the bacteria create their own microenvironment, become metabolically inactive as compared with planktonic bacteria, and thereby become resistant to antibiotics because of the lack of metabolic activity.[12]

Attempts have been made to reduce catheter-associated urinary tract infection through use of advanced catheters designed to inhibit biofilm formation. The primary technology for this is the use of antibiotic- or antiseptic-coated catheters. There have been two systematic reviews of silver alloy and nitrofurazone-impregnated urinary catheters in recent years.[13,14] The difficulty in evaluating the utility of these products is stressed in one of these reviews,[14] which included trials that were deemed to be of variable levels of quality. The combined data available on all 13,319 participants suggested that antimicrobial urinary catheters prevented or delayed the onset of catheter-associated bacteriuria compared with control catheters. However, the magnitude of this effect varied, and was systematically overestimated in many studies because of dropouts and exclusions. The effects of these catheters on morbidity, including bloodstream infection, remained unknown.[15]

Thus, although these devises seem promising, the analysis of the literature by Tenke and colleagues[6] described in the European and Asian guidelines suggests that the role of these devices is limited at the present time, with the indications for their use remaining to be established. Recommendations and their level of evidence included:

Antibiotic-impregnated catheters may decrease the frequency of asymptomatic bacteriuria within 1 week. There is, however, no evidence they decrease symptomatic infection. Therefore, they cannot be recommended routinely (B).
Silver alloy catheters significantly reduce the incidence of asymptomatic bacteriuria, but only for less than 1 week. There was some evidence of reduced risk for symptomatic urinary tract infection. Therefore, such catheters may be useful in some settings (B).

Research into urinary catheter design continues because of the clear need to reduce the incidence of catheter-associated urinary tract infections. The newest technology involves use of protamine sulfate and chlorhexidine to prevent or delay biofilm formation. These catheters proved less likely to become colonized in vivo than silver-coated or uncoated catheters, but their clinical efficacy, as with the older types of impregnated catheters, has yet to be proven.[15]

TREATMENT

Treatment of nosocomial urinary tract infections needs to be considered separately for patients with asymptomatic bacteriuria and for those with symptomatic urinary tract infection. In general, asymptomatic bacteriuria in catheterized patients should not be treated. Removal of the catheter allows resolution of bacteriuria in one third to one half of cases.[6] The European and Asian guidelines[1] recommend treatment of asymptomatic bacteriuria in the following circumstances:

For patients undergoing urological surgery or implantation of prostheses (A)
When treatment may be part of a plan to control nosocomial infection due to a particularly virulent organism prevailing in a treatment unit (B)
For patients who have a high risk of serious infectious complications (eg, patients who are immunosuppressed) (C)
For infections caused by strains causing a high incidence of bacteremia (eg, S marcescens) (B)

Treatment of symptomatic urinary tract infection is usually more straightforward. Clinical symptoms and signs, such as frequency, dysuria, or suprapubic pain directly attributable to an infection, are an indication for treatment.

The most common symptom attributed to a urinary tract infection in hospitalized patients is usually fever. Bacteriuria may or may not be the source of a fever or another nonspecific indicator of infection, such as leukocytosis. It has been suggested that if the patient has a low-grade fever, is clinically stable, and has no other indication for antibiotics, observation, rather than immediate antimicrobial therapy, can be entertained. In these patients, it may also be useful to replace the catheter with a new one to eliminate the burden of the existing biofilm.[7]

If the patient is systemically ill, empiric antibiotics should be started, based on knowledge of the local bacterial ecology, and then tailored based on definitive culture and susceptibility results. There are no adequate clinical studies to guide the duration of therapy; clinical judgment and patient response should be used to determine the duration of the antibiotic course.[7] The choice of antibiotic may be complicated by the development of resistant bacteria. In particular, there is greater resistance of E coli, other Enterobacteriaceae, and P aeruginosa in catheterized patients compared with noncatheterized patients.[16] In the absence of an indwelling catheter, as with community-acquired urinary tract infections, resistance has not generally been an important issue because antibiotics typically used for community-acquired infections, such as amoxicillin, cephalexin, trimethoprim/sulfamethoxazole, ciprofloxacin, and levofloxacin, are highly concentrated in the urine, from nearly 100 up to several hundred times.[17] However, in patients with nosocomial urinary tract infections, who may have indwelling urinary catheters and highly resistant pathogens, the perception that bacterial susceptibilities are unimportant may not necessarily be accurate. Thus, clinical judgment and the patient's response to therapy dictate the degree to which susceptibility data are used to direct treatment of symptomatic urinary tract infections in hospitalized patients.

Some of these same considerations apply to the dilemma as to whether or not to treat the patient with candiduria. In the past, when the only option for treatment was amphotericin B, patients were rarely treated. The development of fluconazole and other less toxic antifungal agents has greatly increased the likelihood that clinicians will treat patients with candiduria. As with other asymptomatic urinary tract infections, however, asymptomatic candiduria needs no pharmacologic therapy, and can usually be treated by removal of Foley catheters or replacement of the catheter to reduce the biofilm burden. Pharmacologic therapy with an antifungal agent should generally be limited to patients with symptomatic candiduria after confirmation of the infection from a second urine sample.[18]

Unfortunately, the critically ill patient is the one most likely to have candiduria, and the one least likely to be able to complain of symptoms. Furthermore, this is the patient most likely to suffer a poor outcome if a necessary treatment is withheld. Thus, it is somewhat difficult to define which of these patients should be treated. Suggested indications for the treatment of candiduria include low birth weight infants and patients who have undergone renal transplantation, have neutropenia, or who have a planned invasive urologic procedure. If asymptomatic candiduria progresses to symptomatic cystitis, it ought to be treated as well.[9]

Fluconazole is the antifungal agent most commonly given to eradicate candiduria. Oral fluconazole is both convenient and effective, and should be used if it is feasible to give the patient an oral or enteral agent. Because fluconazole concentrates in the urine to more than 100 μg/mL after a 400-mg dose, even C glabrata, which is relatively resistant to fluconazole with a minimal inhibitory concentration of 8 to 16 μg/mL, can be successfully treated with fluconazole. Candiduria frequently recurs 2 weeks after successful treatment with fluconazole if the underlying patient conditions conducive to the development of candiduria have not been eliminated. In the presence of renal failure, when a drug cannot be effectively delivered into the urinary tract, amphotericin B bladder irrigations can be used to treat a lower urinary tract infection due to *Candida*.[9]

SUMMARY

Nosocomial urinary tract infections are a common complication in surgical patients. The use of urinary catheters is the major risk factor for the development of these infections. Discontinuation of catheterization within 2 days is key to avoiding nosocomial urinary tract infections. Patients with asymptomatic bacteriuria can generally be treated initially with catheter removal or catheter exchange, and do not necessarily need antimicrobial therapy. Symptomatic patients should receive antibiotic therapy. Resistance of urinary pathogens to common antibiotics is not usually an issue because of the concentration of most antibiotics in the urine. However, it is uncertain if different empiric antimicrobial regimens are needed when highly resistant bacteria are involved in nosocomial urinary tract infections. The treatment of patients with candiduria generally follows the same principles. Patients with asymptomatic candiduria usually can be treated with catheter removal or exchange, and do not need specific antifungal therapy. However, selected high-risk patients as well as those with symptomatic fungal urinary tract infections should receive antifungal therapy, generally using fluconazole.

REFERENCES

1. Schaeffer AJ. Catheter-associated bacteriuria. Urol Clin North Am 1986;13(4): 735–47.
2. Stamm WE. Guidelines for prevention of catheter-associated urinary tract infections. Ann Intern Med 1975;82(3):386–90.
3. Wald HL, Ma A, Bratzler DW, et al. Indwelling urinary catheter use in the postoperative period: analysis of the national surgical infection prevention project data. Arch Surg 2008;143(6):551–7.
4. Clec'h C, Schwebel C, Francais A, et al. Does catheter-associated urinary tract infection increase mortality in critically ill patients? Infect Control Hosp Epidemiol 2007;28(12):1367–73.
5. Edwards JR, Peterson KD, Andrus ML, et al. National Healthcare Safety Network (NHSN) Report, data summary for 2006, issued June 2007. Am J Infect Control 2007;35(5):290–301.
6. Tenke P, Kovacs B, Bjerklund Johansen TE, et al. European and Asian guidelines on management and prevention of catheter-associated urinary tract infections. Int J Antimicrob Agents 2008;31(Suppl 1):S68–78.
7. Sedor J, Mulholland SG. Hospital-acquired urinary tract infections associated with the indwelling catheter. Urol Clin North Am 1999;26(4):821–8.
8. Wagenlehner FM, Niemetz AH, Weidner W, et al. Spectrum and antibiotic resistance of uropathogens from hospitalised patients with urinary tract infections: 1994–2005. Int J Antimicrob Agents 2008;31(Suppl 1):S25–34.
9. Sobel JD, Lundstrom T. Management of candiduria. Curr Urol Rep 2001;2(4): 321–5.
10. Bukhary ZA. Candiduria: a review of clinical significance and management. Saudi J Kidney Dis Transpl 2008;19(3):350–60.

11. Vanhems P, Baratin D, Voirin N, et al. Reduction of urinary tract infections acquired in an intensive care unit during a 10-year surveillance program. Eur J Epidemiol 2008;23:641–5.
12. Ha US, Cho YH. Catheter-associated urinary tract infections: new aspects of novel urinary catheters. Int J Antimicrob Agents 2006;28(6):485–90.
13. Drekonja DM, Kuskowski MA, Wilt TJ, et al. Antimicrobial urinary catheters: a systematic review. Expert Rev Med Devices 2008;5(4):495–506.
14. Johnson JR, Kuskowski MA, Wilt TJ, et al. Systematic review: antimicrobial urinary catheters to prevent catheter-associated urinary tract infection in hospitalized patients. Ann Intern Med 2006;144(2):116–26.
15. Darouiche RO, Mansouri MD, Gawande PV, et al. Efficacy of combination of chlorhexidine and protamine sulphate against device-associated pathogens. J Antimicrob Chemother 2008;61(3):651–7.
16. Ko MC, Liu CK, Woung LC, et al. Species and antimicrobial resistance of uropathogens isolated from patients with urinary catheter. Tohoku J Exp Med 2008; 214(4):311–9.
17. Gupta K, Hooton TM, Stamm WE, et al. Increasing antimicrobial resistance and the management of uncomplicated community-acquired urinary tract infections. Ann Intern Med 2001;135(1):41–50.
18. Sobel JD, Kauffman CA, McKinsey D, et al. Candiduria: a randomized, double-blind study of treatment with fluconazole and placebo. The National Institute of Allergy and Infectious Diseases (NIAID) mycoses study group. Clin Infect Dis 2000;30(1):19–24.

Clostridium difficile Colitis

Philip A. Efron, MD, John E. Mazuski, MD, PhD*

KEYWORDS

• *Clostridium difficile* • Colitis • Diarrhea • Infection

Clostridium difficile is an anaerobic, gram-positive, spore-forming bacillus capable of producing significant diarrhea or colitis in the hospitalized patient, particularly one previously exposed to antibiotics. Even though no microbial pathogen is identified in most patients with antibiotic-associated diarrhea, *C difficile* accounts for 15% to 25% of such cases and is the most common pathogen associated with infectious diarrhea in hospitalized patients.[1] *C difficile*–associated disease (CDAD) is common in the surgical population because of the frequent use of prophylactic and therapeutic antimicrobial agents. Although uncommon, a *C difficile* infection can progress to fulminant colitis that requires surgical intervention.[2–5] In recent years, *C difficile* infections have been increasing in incidence and severity. This may be caused by the emergence of a more pathogenic strain of *C difficile*, the BI/NAP1/027 strain, which has been implicated in several outbreaks of CDAD in North America and Europe.[2–5]

CDAD is associated with significant morbidity, some mortality, and significant health care costs. Although it may only be a marker of patient illness, the all-cause death rate of patients infected with *C difficile* was reported to be about 10% greater than the overall hospital death rate of 3.4%.[6] In the United States, each case of CDAD was found to be associated with additional costs of more than $3600 in 1998, and total costs of CDAD may have exceeded $1 billion dollars that year.[7] Because of the frequency of CDAD in the surgical population and the possible need for surgical therapy in those patients, the surgeon should have a good understanding of this disease, including its pathogenesis, clinical features, diagnosis, and medical and surgical treatment.

PATHOGENESIS

In the absence of exposure to the health care setting, acquisition of *C difficile* is uncommon. Less than 5% of the healthy adult population is colonized with this bacterium.[8] A total of 20% to 30% of hospitalized patients become colonized with *C difficile*, although most of these patients remain asymptomatic.[9–11] Because of its

Department of Surgery, Washington University School of Medicine, Campus Box 8109, 660 South Euclid Avenue, St. Louis, MO 63110, USA
* Corresponding author.
E-mail address: mazuskij@wudosis.wustl.edu (J.E. Mazuski).

Surg Clin N Am 89 (2009) 483–500
doi:10.1016/j.suc.2008.09.014   surgical.theclinics.com
0039-6109/08/$ – see front matter © 2009 Elsevier Inc. All rights reserved.

ability to form resistant spores, *C difficile* is not easily eradicated from the hospital environment with standard cleansing procedures.[9,12] Medical staff may transmit the spores after contact with an infected patient; the most common sites of contamination include fingernails, fingertips, palms, and the undersides of rings.[13]

Colonic proliferation of *C difficile* is thought to occur when the bacterial environment has been altered by current or previous exposure to an antibiotic.[14–16] The association of any specific antibiotic with CDAD may be related to the capacity of that agent to suppress commensal bacterial growth, the concentration that the drug reaches in the colonic lumen, and the resistance of *C difficile* to the antibiotic.[2,15,17,18] *C difficile* infection can also occur in the absence of exposure to antibiotics; in many such cases, CDAD is associated with the use of antineoplastic medications.[15]

Only *C difficile* strains that produce exotoxins, specifically toxins A and B, are pathogenic. Toxin B is approximately 10 times more potent than toxin A.[19–22] Since 2000, a *C difficile* strain known as "BI/NAP1/027" has progressively emerged. This strain produces increased amounts of toxins A and B. A deletion in this strain's *tcdC* gene, which is a negative regulator of toxin production, causes production of both toxins A and B to increase by 16- to 23-fold.[2,23,24] This strain is also more resistant to fluoroquinolones, has hypersporulation capacity, and produces an additional binary toxin.[25] The hypersporulation capacity potentially accounts for the enhanced transmission of this strain in hospitals as compared with previous strains.

The BI/NAP1/027 strain has now spread throughout the United States, Canada, and Europe.[26] It is associated with an increased severity of disease; patients infected with this strain more frequently have pseudomembranous colitis.[27–29] In the United States, the incidence of *C difficile* infection has more than doubled and *C difficile*–related mortality has quadrupled since the emergence of the BI/NAP1/027 strain.[30–32] There is no evidence, however, that this strain is any more resistant to standard medical therapy than are other *C difficile* strains.[5,33–35]

RISK FACTORS

Major risk factors for CDAD include antibiotic exposure, hospitalization, and advanced age.[1] Previous antibiotic exposure was reported to increase the risk for the development of *C difficile* diarrhea sixfold.[17] Although a single dose of antibiotics can lead to *C difficile* colonization and proliferation, prolonged antibiotic exposure further increases the risk of a *C difficile* infection.[36,37]

Almost any antibiotic can predispose a patient to a *C difficile* infection. Historically, such drugs as clindamycin, cephalosporins, and certain penicillins were the ones most commonly associated with CDAD.[15,17,18] More recently, fluoroquinolones have been implicated as a cause of this infection.[3,33,38,39] There is some controversy regarding the role of specific antibiotics in the current outbreak of the BI/NAP1/027 strain. A prospective study of 12 hospitals in Quebec, Canada found exposure to fluoroquinolones or cephalosporins to be risk factors for CDAD because of this strain.[33] Fluoroquinolone use was also cited as a risk factor for BI/NAP1/027 CDAD outbreaks in various geographic areas in the United States.[38] In a subsequent review of the 2001 to 2004 outbreak of BI/NAP1/027 in Quebec, Canada, however, it was concluded that there was no direct link between the outbreak and specific antibiotics. Instead, the CDAD outbreak was thought to be secondary to poor infection control.[24]

Exposure to the health care setting also increases the risk of acquiring CDAD. The spores are more prevalent in hospital and long-term care facilities, and colonization is greater among patients in those locales, thereby facilitating transmission.[9,40,41] Within the hospital setting, patients housed in an intensive care unit and those having a prolonged hospital stay are more likely to become infected with *C difficile*.[17,42]

Age is also a significant risk factor for the development of CDAD. Patients older than 65 years have a 20-fold greater chance of developing a *C difficile* infection compared with younger patients.[33,39,43,44] Immunosuppressed patients are also at greater risk.[44] Weaker risk factors include the severity of the underlying disease and treatment with nonsurgical gastrointestinal procedures.[17,42] It has been suggested by some that antiulcer medications, by allowing increased survival of *C difficile* spores, play a role in the spread of this disease; however, this hypothesis has been questioned by others.[17,42]

CLINICAL PRESENTATION

Patients with a *C difficile* infection usually present with diarrhea several days after receiving an antibiotic, although symptoms may occur as long as 2 months after antibiotic treatment.[45] Symptomatic patients with mild to moderate disease usually have less than 10 watery bowel movements per day. Typically, stools have a characteristic odor, but stool characteristics can vary greatly. Clinically evident lower gastrointestinal bleeding is rare with CDAD.[45,46] More severe forms of the disease are associated with increased abdominal cramping and pain and signs of systemic inflammation, such as fever, leukocytosis, and hypoalbuminemia.[3,45]

Diarrhea may be absent in some patients with a *C difficile* infection. This may be caused by several factors, including a paralytic ileus secondary to a recent surgical procedure or the use of narcotics or other agents that impair bowel motility. Much more ominously, it may signal the progression of the infection to its most fulminant form.[3,45,47]

Patients with fulminant CDAD may initially present with nonspecific clinical symptoms and signs, such as nausea, vomiting, dehydration, lethargy, and tachycardia. These patients frequently go on to develop septic shock with concomitant organ dysfunction, such as renal failure.[3,45,47] The disease may also progress to toxic megacolon or, rarely, colonic perforation. Systemic symptoms are caused by toxin-induced inflammatory mediators and not bacteremia, which is reported extremely rarely in association with CDAD.[48] None of the features of *C difficile* infection are highly specific, and other infectious and noninfectious causes need to be considered in such patients. The possibility of CDAD should be considered, however, in critically ill patients with signs of septic shock and an obscure source of infection because the most fulminant form of CDAD may occur in the absence of diarrhea.[1]

DIAGNOSIS

Several laboratory tests are available to diagnose *C difficile* infections. When the patient has clinically evident disease, however, the physician should not wait for a positive test before instituting treatment.[22] Culture of the stool for *C difficile* is a sensitive test; however, not all *C difficile* strains produce toxin and the test may be positive for a nontoxigenic strain.[15,49–51] It may require 48 hours for a culture to become positive. This test is not used routinely in the United States except for epidemiologic studies and antibiotic susceptibility testing.[52]

Most other tests rely on identification of *C difficile* toxins in the stool. The cytotoxicity assay for *C difficile* toxins is considered the gold standard; it is sensitive to less than 10 pg of toxin. This test is very specific, but may be falsely negative if there has been toxin degradation because of improper stool sample storage. Because of the sensitivity of the test, it is not usually necessary to test multiple stool samples. The results of this test are usually not available for several days, however, and even more time is needed when the test is performed in combination with stool culture.[1,15,49,50,53,54]

Many clinical laboratories use ELISA/enzyme immunoassays or immunochromatography to detect toxin A or toxin B. These tests are relatively specific but less sensitive; they have been reported to have false-negative rates up to 40%. These tests, however, allow for results to be available within hours.[49–51,55–58] Commercially available tests that test only for toxin A can miss small numbers of infections because of strains that produce only toxin B; these strains have been responsible for some epidemics.[59]

There are also tests for microbial proteins other than the C difficile toxins. An ELISA/enzyme immunoassay for glutamate dehydrogenase, an enzyme constitutively produced by C difficile, has been used. As with C difficile cultures, this test lacks specificity because it does not prove that a toxin-producing strain is present. In addition, other fecal microbes occasionally produce the enzyme. Nonetheless, it is a fairly sensitive, inexpensive, and rapid test that can be used as a screening tool for further C difficile testing.[52,60] A latex agglutination test is another rapid test that identifies a protein common to C difficile organisms. Similarly, this assay does not differentiate between toxigenic and nontoxigenic strains.[15,49,51] Both the ELISA/enzyme immunoassays and latex agglutination assays also have an elevated false-negative rate compared with other tests and may require analysis of repeated samples in a symptomatic patient.[49,61]

Polymerase chain reaction analyses have been developed to detect C difficile and its toxins. These are exquisitely sensitive, because they are capable of detecting very small amounts of genetic material. Technical difficulties related to sample preparation and to performance of the assay prevent their widespread clinical use.[62]

Overall, no laboratory test is ideal. The use of a cell cytotoxicity assay or ELISA with stool culture can allow for sensitive and specific detection of a toxigenic organism, but requires prolonged time and is labor intensive.[63] In the United States, most laboratories currently use the ELISA/enzyme immunoassays tests because they are rapid, inexpensive, and technically simple. However, this may result in a higher false-negative rate compared with the use of stool culture as a screen followed by a toxin assay to determine pathogenicity.[64]

Direct endoscopic visualization of the colonic mucosa can be useful in making the diagnosis of CDAD. Greater than 95% of patients identified with pseudomembranes have a C difficile infection.[14] Many patients with C difficile colitis, however, do not have pseudomembranes; nonspecific colitis may be the only endoscopic finding in such patients. In addition, 20% to 33% of patients with pseudomembranes only have lesions proximal to the sigmoid colon; the diagnosis would be missed using flexible sigmoidoscopy as compared with full colonoscopy.[15,19,49,51,65,66] Overall, endoscopy for the diagnosis of a C difficile infection can have a 10% false-negative rate.[6] Because of concern for colonic perforation, this technique has generally been reserved for patients with severe disease and negative laboratory results in whom there is a need for rapid diagnosis.[15,19,49,51,65,66]

Although they are rarely required, radiographic studies can be useful for differentiating C difficile infection from other causes of colitis. CT can help determine the extent of the disease and the presence of pneumatosis or colonic perforation.[49,67,68] Intravenous or oral contrast is usually not required to make the diagnosis.[22] Typically, the scan demonstrates the nonspecific finding of a thickened colonic wall. Other signs may be found with CDAD, however, including pericolonic stranding; an "accordion sign" (high-attenuation oral contrast in the colonic lumen alternating with low-attention inflamed mucosa); a "double-halo sign target sign" (intravenous contrast displaying varying degrees of attenuation caused by submucosal inflammation and hyperemia); and ascites (caused by hypoalbuminenia).[49,67,68] Except for an ileus, small bowel findings are usually absent, although *C difficile* enteritis has been occasionally reported.[1,68,69]

MEDICAL THERAPY

The first step in treating any *C difficile* infection is to discontinue the causative antibiotic if at all possible (**Fig. 1**). If not, changing to antibiotics with less association with CDAD, such as macrolides, aminoglycosides, sulfamethoxazole, tetracyclines, or vancomycin, might be attempted. There are no controlled studies that demonstrate the benefit of this approach, however, and there remains disagreement about which antibiotics, if any, are safest for use in patients with *C difficile* infections.[24,25] Antiperistaltic agents should not be used in patients with CDAD. Opiates should be avoided or minimized to the extent possible.[70] Reduction of peristaltic activity by those agents allows toxins to accumulate in the gastrointestinal lumen and exacerbate the disease.[37]

Antimicrobial Treatment with Metronidazole and Vancomycin

Although other antimicrobial regimens are potentially available for the treatment of *C difficile* infection, the two most commonly used antibiotics are metronidazole and intraluminal vancomycin. Only intraluminal vancomycin has been approved by the Food and Drug Administration as a medical therapy for *C difficile*.[71] Both medications are highly active against *C difficile*. Significant resistance to either drug has not been demonstrated.[71–74] Metronidazole, however, is much less expensive than oral vancomycin.[71]

Empiric treatment is often instituted before the availability of *C difficile* laboratory results to avoid undue delay in therapy.[48] Typically, patients are treated for 10 to 14 days after discontinuation of an offending antimicrobial.[25] A response to medical treatment, such as improvement in the patient's leukocytosis, fever, abdominal pain, or diarrhea, should be apparent within 1 to 2 of days of therapy. Complete resolution of diarrhea may take up to a week. Anecdotal reports indicate that patients infected with the BI/NAP1/027 strain may require longer periods of time to show improvement in their clinical symptoms and signs.[25] Patients who do not demonstrate some improvement after several days or whose condition worsens should have their treatment escalated.[25] It is not recommended that stool be tested in patients who have completed their medical therapy and have resolution of their symptoms because patients may shed the organism or one of its toxins for several weeks after completion of treatment.[75–77]

Oral metronidazole is completely absorbed by the small intestine. After absorption, secretion of the drug into the colon can produce therapeutic fecal concentrations of the drug. Because of this secretion into the colon, fecal metronidazole levels can also be attained with parental administration.[78] Metronidazole reaches the colonic wall in about 1 to 2 hours, but it is not known how long it takes to be secreted out of the colon into the stool.[26] This process is apparently somewhat variable. Fecal metronidazole levels decrease significantly with resolution of diarrhea and are undetectable in the stool of asymptomatic patients colonized with *C difficile*.[78,79] Colonic inflammation with severe *C difficile* infections may also interfere with the delivery of metronidazole to the colonic lumen.[80]

Side effects of metronidazole include gastrointestinal intolerance and, with prolonged courses of therapy, polyneuropathy. This latter side effect should be taken

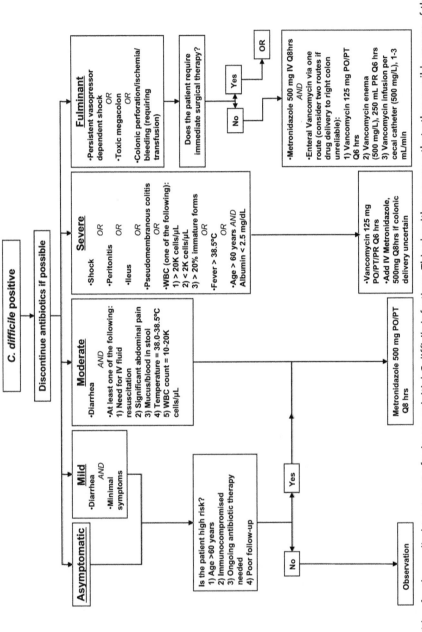

Fig. 1. Algorithm for the medical treatment of primary or initial *C difficile* infections. This algorithm assumes that other possible causes of the patient's signs and symptoms have been excluded. Treatment should be for 10–14 days, with consideration given to continuing treatment for 7 days after discontinuation of potentially causative antibiotics. Metronidazole therapy should be used with caution in pregnant patients.

into account if an antibiotic course greater than 14 days is anticipated.[26] Metronidazole probably does not have teratogenic properties, but should nonetheless be used with caution in pregnant or lactating women and in children younger than 10 years of age.[12,22] Allergic reactions to metronidazole are rare. Oral dosing is typically 250 mg four times per day or 500 mg three times per day.[25]

The use of supplemental agents along with metronidazole has not been shown to be beneficial. Combination therapy of metronidazole and oral rifampin demonstrated no advantage over metronidazole alone in the treatment of *C difficile* infections.[81]

Oral vancomycin is not absorbed from the gastrointestinal tract and can achieve very high colonic concentrations that do not vary with the degree of the patient's diarrhea.[78,79] In patients without an ileus, it takes less than 6 hours for the ingested drug to reach the ileocecal valve.[26] Oral vancomycin has relatively few side effects or allergic reactions.[26] Because of the expense of the oral formulation, it is a common practice to administer the intravenous form of vancomycin enterally in the hospital setting, especially in patients who receive medications through a gastric or intestinal tube.[71] This formulation has a noxious taste, however, and may not be well tolerated with oral administration.[71] Further, this option may not be available for outpatient treatment because many community pharmacies do not carry parenteral vancomycin. Typical dosing of oral vancomycin is 125 mg 4 times per day.[25,26]

Delivery of vancomycin to the colon may be an issue in patients with a nonfunctioning gastrointestinal tract. Under such circumstances, vancomycin can be instilled directly into the colon by an enema or through a catheter placed during colonoscopy. Carefully done trials of this type of treatment, however, are lacking; most of the supportive evidence comes from small series of patients. There is also the potential risk of iatrogenic perforation in patients with a friable colon caused by fulminant colitis.[48]

The available clinical data do not indicate any preference for one agent over the other. Earlier prospective studies demonstrated equivalency of metronidazole and oral vancomycin in the treatment of *C difficile* infection, with neither drug being superior in preventing relapse.[72,74,80,82–87] The numbers of subjects in these clinical trials were relatively small, however, making a type II error possible. In addition, the studies were typically not blinded and the patients were not stratified according to severity of disease.[26,71,80]

More recent prospective trials have suggested that cure rates are higher in patients with severe *C difficile* infections treated with oral vancomycin compared with oral metronidazole.[71,80,88] In one study, patients with severe *C difficile* infections were identified as those having pseudomembranous colitis or meeting two of the following criteria: age greater than 60 years, serum albumin less than 2.5 mg/mL, peripheral leukocyte count greater than 15,000 cells/mL, or a temperature greater than 38.3°C.[80] In a second study, patients with severe colitis were defined as those having 10 or more bowel movements per day, a peripheral leukocyte count greater than or equal to 20,000 cells/mL, or severe abdominal pain.[71,88] Two criticisms of these trials are that the scoring systems used for defining severe *C difficile* infection had not been previously validated, and that they reported intermediate end points, such as cessation of diarrhea or a negative toxin assay, as their end points.[26]

Nonetheless, these data suggest that oral vancomycin may be preferable for the treatment of patients with more severe disease even though neither drug has been proved superior for the treatment of infections caused by the BI/NAP1/027 strain.[26] In addition to the severity of the infection, the presence of an ileus, which limits delivery of oral agents to the colon, may influence the choice of therapy.[25] For patients with mild or moderate *C difficile* infections, there does not seem to be any advantage of oral vancomycin over oral metronidazole. It is still unclear whether patients with mild *C difficile* infections require any treatment other than discontinuation of the inciting antibiotic.[89]

Other Therapies

Other antimicrobial regimens may be of potential use for *C difficile* infection, although they have been little used in this regard. Antibiotics that have been studied include bacitracin, teicoplanin, and fusidic acid.[22] In some studies, bacitracin demonstrated efficacy equivalent to that of metronidazole and vancomycin for relief of symptoms secondary to *C difficile* infection.[90,91] Bacitracin was less effective, however, at eliminating *C difficile* from the stool. Teicoplanin and fusidic acid, neither of which are available in the United States, display efficacies similar to bacitracin.[90,91] Nitazoxanide, a thiazolide antiparasitic agent that blocks anaerobic metabolism, is a relatively new agent that has demonstrated potential for the treatment of *C difficile* infection.[34,92] Nitazoxanide and its metabolite, tizoxanide, inhibit growth of *C difficile* in vitro. Approximately two thirds of an oral dose is recovered in the stool.[92,93] Dosed orally at 500 mg twice a day, nitazoxanide seemed similar to oral metronidazole for the treatment of *C difficile* infections. It was also used successfully in an uncontrolled study to treat patients who had failed previous therapy with metronidazole.[92,93] Nitazoxanide is much more expensive, however, than oral metronidazole.

Agents other than antibiotics have also been studied with regard to their potential for treating *C difficile* infections.[34,92] Tolevamer is an anionic polymer binding agent. When used at a high dose (6 g per day) to treat mild to moderate *C difficile* infections, this agent demonstrated noninferiority to oral vancomycin.[94]

There has also been considerable interest in the use of probiotics as complements to antimicrobial therapy for CDAD, particularly with regard to their role in restoring a more normal colonic flora. Two randomized trials demonstrated increased efficacy with addition of *Saccharomyces boulardii* to specific antibiotic therapies.[95,96] Other probiotics seem to be less effective in this regard. A recent meta-analysis concluded that only *S boulardii* was an effective therapy for *C difficile* infection.[97] Even this evidence is disputed by some; Dendukuri and colleagues[98] believed that current data did not support the use of any probiotics for *C difficile* infection. Although usually considered harmless, both *S boulardii* and *Lactobacillus* therapy are capable of inducing fungemia and bacteremia, respectively.[99–102]

Experimental treatments being developed to treat *C difficile* infections include tinidazole; tiacumicin B complex (OPT-80); ramoplanin; rifalazil; and rifaximin.[103–108] The use of passive immunity for patients with CDAD is being studied, and efforts to develop a vaccine effective against *C difficile* are proceeding.[25]

Treatment of Recurrent C difficile Infections

Recurrent *C difficile* infections are most likely to develop in the first or second week after completion of therapy. Overall, 15% to 35% of patients infected with *C difficile* develop a recurrence. Recurrences, which occur even more commonly after a second episode of CDAD, are found in 33% to 65% of patients with two or more episodes of *C difficile* infections.[76,87,109–112] The early onset of recurrence may indicate that these are relapses rather than reinfections; the recurrence may result from re-establishment of the infection because of endogenous spores that remain in the patient's gastrointestinal tract after an initial course of therapy.[84,113] Recurrence may also be caused by a new infection following ingestion of spores from an exogenous source, particularly if the patient remains in an environment where such contamination is prevalent. Antimicrobial resistance has not been shown to play a role in recurrence. Rather, recurrence likely reflects inadequate host defenses against the infection.[114,115] The advanced age and pre-existing comorbidities characteristic of the patients who develop CDAD, and the frequent need for continuation of systemic antibiotics, are factors that may make a *C difficile* infection refractory to treatment.[114–116]

The development of a recurrent *C difficile* infection after successful treatment of a first episode does not necessitate any change in therapy. Secondary response rates are similar with use of either metronidazole or vancomycin. Although complications are more likely to develop with a second or subsequent episode of CDAD, the risk of such complications is also similar with use of either antibiotic.[75,84] High-quality data, however, regarding the optimal treatment of recurrent *C difficile* infections are lacking.[25] Combination therapy of vancomycin and rifampin has been shown to be somewhat efficacious, but this method is limited because of patient intolerance of high-dose rifampin, the numerous interactions of rifampin with other drugs, and emerging resistance to rifampin.[25,117] Cholestyramine, an anion-exchange binding resin that can bind the toxins, has not been demonstrated to be an effective treatment for recurrent *C difficile* infection. In addition, cholestryramine can bind to drugs used to treat *C difficile* infection, such as vancomycin.[25,118] Intravenous immunoglobulin has been used when no other therapeutic options are available. This therapy, however, seems to be of marginal efficacy, optimal dosing has not been determined, and these preparations are very expensive and in short supply.[25] The use of rifaximin following initial vancomycin therapy seemed promising at first, but resistance to rifaximin after treatment has now been documented.[119] The efficacy of probiotic therapy for recurrent *C difficile* infections, as with primary infections, continues to be debated, as are attempts to re-establish normal colonic therapy using stool infusion therapy.[25,95–102]

FULMINANT *C DIFFICILE* COLITIS

Fulminant colitis develops in approximately 3% to 8% of patients with *C difficile* infections, but accounts for most of the serious complications caused by this disease.[22,48] Mortality for fulminant *C difficile* infection ranges from 30% to 90%.[22] Predictors of mortality with fulminant *C difficile* colitis include a patient's American Society of Anesthesiology classification, a need for vasopressor therapy, and a low serum albumin level.[48] Fulminant *C difficile* colitis is associated with a prolonged hospital course in 40% of patients, and with relapse in 20% of patients following adequate medical therapy.[22]

Fulminant CDAD is more likely to develop in patients who have undergone recent surgery, chemotherapy, transplantation, immunosuppression, and those who have autoimmune diseases or HIV-AIDS. Antimicrobial exposure within 2 weeks of the onset of symptoms is also a risk factor for fulminant disease.[48] The emergence of the BI/NAP1/027 strain of *C difficile* has been associated with the development of more severe disease.

Hallmarks of fulminant disease include hypotension, hypoalbuminemia, and a pronounced leukocytosis.[22] Often, patients with fulminant colitis present with an acute surgical abdomen or unexplained shock.[48] Typically, patients with fulminant colitis have a marked leukocytosis. This leukocytosis usually precedes the development of hypotension and the need for vasopressor therapy; the diagnosis of CDAD should be considered in a patient with a marked elevation in the white blood cell count in an appropriate clinical setting.[22,48]

Diagnosis may be problematic in many patients with fulminant disease. About 20% of these patients do not have diarrhea because of an ileus or colonic atony. The clinical findings may be attributed to routine postoperative sequelae of patients who have undergone recent abdominal operations.[48] In the absence of diarrhea, patients may have negative assays for *C difficile* toxin in the stool, further complicating the diagnosis.[22,48] CT of the abdomen can suggest the diagnosis of fulminant *C difficile* infection in patients with otherwise obscure clinical findings. Colonoscopic findings of pseudomembranes or severe inflammation also suggest the disease and the need for aggressive therapy.[48,49,68] The results of these tests may trigger earlier surgical intervention, which may decrease the morbidity and mortality of a fulminant *C difficile* infection.[48]

Optimal treatment of fulminant *C difficile* has yet to be determined. No drug has been demonstrated to be superior to intraluminal vancomycin as a medical treatment for severe *C difficile* infections. Because gastrointestinal motility is compromised in many of these patients, however, delivery of the antibiotic to the colonic lumen cannot be guaranteed. To obtain significant colonic concentrations of the drug in the setting of an adynamic ileus, vancomycin can be delivered directly into the intestine through a tube positioned beyond the ligament of Treitz, or it can be administered rectally by an enema. Neither of these approaches, however, ensures that the drug reaches significant concentrations in the right colon. Direct instillation of vancomycin into the colon through a tube introduced colonscopically into the right colon has been used successfully to treat fulminant *C difficile* colitis.[120,121] Nonetheless, a controlled trial of this approach is lacking. Intravenous metronidazole is frequently used in the treatment of fulminant *C difficile* colitis, although there are no carefully designed trials of its use in this setting. A typical approach for the treatment of patients with fulminant disease is to administer intravenous metronidazole along with intraluminal vancomycin by the oral, enteral, or rectal route. A failure of such medical therapy in patients with fulminant disease is usually an indication for colectomy.[25,122]

SURGICAL THERAPY

Approximately 0.4% to 3.5% of patients with a *C difficile* infection undergo colectomy. Indications for surgical therapy include the rare colonic perforation caused by CDAD, toxic megacolon, and refractory disease associated with ongoing sepsis.[91] Risk factors for surgical therapy parallel risk factors for fulminant colitis, and include advanced age, malignancy, immunosuppression, renal failure, and the use of antiperistaltic agents.[22,91] Patients who have undergone a surgical procedure within the previous 8 weeks, particularly a cardiothoracic, vascular, or transplantation procedure, represent a significant proportion of the patients undergoing colectomy for *C difficile* infections.[6]

The primary surgical strategy is to resect the involved bowel and to create proximal fecal diversion.[48] Nonresectional therapy with only an ileostomy or cecostomy has been used for fulminant disease; however, this is associated with a higher mortality than is colectomy and fecal diversion.[48] Successful outcomes have been reported for patients undergoing only segmental colonic resections for fulminant *C difficile* infection.[6,48] Regardless multiple patient series indicate that survival is higher with subtotal colectomy than with segmental colectomy or colostomy with catheter placement.[123–129] The current recommendation is to perform subtotal colectomy in patients undergoing surgical treatment of fulminant *C difficile* infection, because the disease is likely to be pancolonic in most patients.

Although emergent colectomy can salvage patients with fulminant *C difficile* colitis, patients undergoing a surgical procedure still have about a 50% overall mortality.[6,48,122] The outcome is worse in patients who have colonic perforation or who have refractory shock requiring vasopressor therapy for blood pressure maintenance at the time of the surgical procedure. It is desirable to intervene before the development of these complications.[22,48,122] Unfortunately, it is not possible to predict which patients are likely to develop these problems. Ultimately, the need for and the timing of operative intervention for fulminant *C difficile* colitis is best determined by having an experienced surgeon carefully follow these patients and their response to medical therapy.

PREVENTION

Prevention of *C difficile* infections requires appropriate infection control practices and avoidance of unnecessary antibiotics.[37] Once a patient is infected with *C difficile*, strict isolation measures should be implemented to prevent further spread of the disease, because health care workers and patients can transmit the disease throughout an institution and to other institutions. Patients should optimally be housed in a single room or, if necessary, in a room shared with another patient with CDAD.[33,130] Health care workers should wear gowns and gloves when entering the room. Equipment used on the patient (ie, blood pressure cuffs and stethoscopes) should be used only for that particular patient or cleaned before use on another patient.[33,131] Rectal thermometers should be avoided.[37] Environmental cleaning should be performed with a sporacidal agent, such as bleach.[132] Alcohol is ineffective at eliminating *C difficile* spores; health care workers should wash their hands with soap or chlorhexidine and water when caring for these patients.[133] Implementation of these and other infection control measures, along with careful use of antibiotics, are the most important means of limiting the spread of *C difficile* infection within the hospital setting.[33]

SUMMARY

Clostridium difficile is a common cause of diarrhea and an occasional cause of colitis in the surgical population. The emergence of a new strain of this bacterium, the highly toxigenic BI/NAP1/027 strain, has not only increased outbreaks of *C difficile* infections but has also led to an increase in the morbidity and mortality of CDAD. Most patients with mild to moderate or severe *C difficile* infections can be treated medically; however, fulminant *C difficile*, which is frequently lethal, often requires early surgical intervention for optimal management. Containment of this nosocomial infection can only be achieved through careful infection control measures and appropriate antimicrobial-prescribing practices by physicians. It is vital that antibiotics have a clear indication for use, and that unnecessarily prolonged therapy be avoided.

REFERENCES

1. Bartlett JG, Gerding DN. Clinical recognition and diagnosis of *Clostridium difficile* infection. Clin Infect Dis 2008;46:S12–8.
2. McDonald LC, Kilgore GE, Thompson A, et al. An epidemic, toxin gene-variant strain of *Clostridium difficile*. N Engl J Med 2005;353(23):2433–41.
3. Sunenshine RH, McDonald LC. *Clostridium difficile*-associated disease: new challenges from an established pathogen. Cleve Clin J Med 2006;73:187–97.
4. Bartlett JG, Perl TM. The new *Clostridium difficile*: what does it mean? N Engl J Med 2005;353:2503–5.
5. Hubert B, Loo VG, Bourgault AM, et al. A portrait of the geographic dissemination of the *Clostridium difficile* colitis North American pulsed-field type 1 strain and the epidemiology of *C difficile*-associated disease in Quebec. Clin Infect Dis 2007;44:238–44.

6. Dallal RM, Harbrecht BG, Boujoukas AJ, et al. Fulminant *Clostridium difficile*: an underappreciated and increasing cause of death and complications. Ann Surg 2002;235:363–72.
7. Kyne L, Hamel MB, Polavaram R, et al. Health care costs and mortality associated with nosocomial diarrhea due to *Clostridium difficile*. Clin Infect Dis 2002; 24:346–53.
8. Viscidi R, Willey S, Bartlett JG. Isolation rates and toxigenic potential of *Clostridium difficile* isolates from various patient populations. Gastroenterology 1981;81:5–9.
9. McFarland LV, Mulligan ME, Kwok RYY, et al. Nosocomial acquisition of *Clostridium difficile* infection. N Engl J Med 1989;320:204–10.
10. Bender BS, Bennett R, Laughon BE, et al. Is *Clostridium difficile* endemic in chronic care facilities? Lancet 1986;2:11–3.
11. Johnson S, Clabots CR, Linn FV, et al. *Clostridium difficile* colonization and disease. Lancet 1990;336:97–100.
12. Mazuski JE, Longo WE. *Clostridium difficile* colitis. Problems in General Surgery 2002;19(1):121–32.
13. Fordtran JS. Colitis due to *Clostridium difficile* toxins: underdiagnosed, highly virulent, and nosocomial. Proc (Bayl Univ Med Cent) 2006;19:3–12.
14. Bartlett JG. *Clostridium difficile*: clinical considerations. Rev Infect Dis 1990; 12(Suppl 2):S243–51.
15. Reinke CM, Messick CR. Update on *Clostridium difficile*-induced colitis, part 1. Am J Hosp Pharm 1994;51:1771–81.
16. Wilson KH. The microecology of *Clostridium difficile*. Clin Infect Dis 1993; 16(Suppl 4):S214–8.
17. Bignardi GE. Risk factors for *Clostridium difficile* infection. J Hosp Infect 1998; 40:1–15.
18. Kelly CP, Pothoulakis C, LaMont JT. *Clostridium difficile* colitis. N Engl J Med 1994;330:257–62.
19. Kelly CP, LaMont TJ. *Clostridium difficile* infection. Annu Rev Med 1998;49:375–90.
20. Riegler M, Sedivy R, Pothoulakis C, et al. *Clostridium difficile* toxin B is more potent than toxin A in damaging human colonic epithelium in vitro. J Clin Invest 1995;95:2004–11.
21. Hurley BW, Nguyen CC. The spectrum of pseudomembranous enterocolitis and antibiotic-associated diarrhea. Arch Intern Med 2002;162:2177–84.
22. Adams SD, Mercer DW. Fulminant *Clostridium difficile* colitis. Curr Opin Crit Care 2007;13:450–5.
23. MacCannell DR, Louie TJ, Gregson DB, et al. Molecular analysis of *Clostridium difficile* PCR ribotype 027 isolates from Eastern and Western Canada. J Clin Microbiol 2006;44:2147–52.
24. Weiss K, Bergeron L, Bernatchez H, et al. *Clostridium difficile*-associated diarrhoea rates and global antibiotic consumption in five Quebec institutions from 2001 to 2004. Int J Antimicrob Agents 2007;30:309–14.
25. Gerding DN, Muto CA, Owens RC. Treatment of *Clostridium difficile* infection. Clin Infect Dis 2008;46:S32–42.
26. Pepin J. Vancomycin for the treatment of *Clostridium difficile* infection: for whom is this expensive bullet really magic? Clin Infect Dis 2008;46:1493–8.
27. Rupnik M, Avesani V, Janc M, et al. A novel toxinotyping scheme and correlation of toxinotypes with serogroups of *Clostridium difficile* isolates. J Clin Microbiol 1998;36:2240–7.

28. Geric B, Rupnik M, Gerding DN, et al. Distribution of *Clostridium difficile* variant toxinotypes and strains with binary toxin genes among clinical isolates in an American hospital. J Med Microbiol 2004;53:887–94.
29. Warny M, Pepin J, Fang A, et al. Toxin production by an emerging strain of *Clostridium difficile* associated with outbreaks of severe disease in North America and Europe. Lancet 2005;366:1079–84.
30. McDonald LC, Owings M, Jernigan DB. *Clostridium difficile* infection in patients discharged from US short-stay hospitals, 1996–2003. Emerg Infect Dis 2006;12: 409–15.
31. Redelings MD, Sorvillo F, Mascola L. Increase in *Clostridium difficile*-related mortality, United States, 1999–2004. Emerg Infect Dis 2007;13:1417–9.
32. Ricciardi R, Rothenberger DA, Madoff RD, et al. Increasing prevalence and severity of *Clostridium difficile* colitis in hospitalized patients in the United States. Arch Surg 2007;142:624–31.
33. Loo VG, Poirier L, Miller MA, et al. A predominantly clonal multi-institutional outbreak of *Clostridium difficile*-associated diarrhea with high morbidity and mortality. N Engl J Med 2005;353(23):2442–9.
34. Musher DM, Aslam S, Logan N, et al. Relatively poor outcome after treatment of *Clostridium difficile* colitis with metronidazole. Clin Infect Dis 2005;40: 1586–90.
35. Bourgault AM, Lamothe F, Loo VG, et al. In vitro susceptibility of *Clostridium difficile* clinical isolates from a multi-institutional outbreak in Quebec. Antimicrob Agents Chemother 2006;50:3473–5.
36. Privitera G, Scarpellini P, Ortisi G, et al. Prospective study of *Clostridium difficile* intestinal colonization and disease following single-dose antibiotic prophylaxis in surgery. Antimicrob Agents Chemother 1991;35:208–10.
37. Bartlett JG. Clinical practice: antibiotic-associated diarrhea. N Engl J Med 2002; 346:334–9.
38. Gaynes R, Rimland D, Killum E, et al. Outbreak of *Clostridium difficile* infection in a long-term care facility: association with gatifloxicin use. Clin Infect Dis 2004;38: 640–5.
39. Pepin J, Saheb N, Coulombe MA, et al. Emergence of fluoroquinilones as the predominant risk factor for *Clostridium difficile*-associated diarrhea: a cohort study during an epidemic in Quebec. Clin Infect Dis 2005;41:1254–60.
40. Bartlett JG. *Clostridium difficile*: history of its role as an enteric pathogen and the current state of knowledge about the organism. Clin Infect Dis 1994;18(Suppl 4): S265–72.
41. Simor AE, Bradley SF, Strausbaugh LJ, et al. *Clostridium difficile* in long-term-care facilities for the elderly. Infect Control Hosp Epidemiol 2002;23:696–703.
42. Chang VT, Nelson K. The role of physical proximity in nosocomial diarrhea. Clin Infect Dis 2000;31:717–22.
43. Aronsson B, Molly R, Nord CE. Diagnosis and epidemiology of *Clostridium difficile*-associated diarrhea in Sweden. The Swedish *C difficile* Study Group. J Antimicrob Chemother 1984;14(Suppl D):85–95.
44. Yolken RH, Bishop C, Townsend TR, et al. Infectious gastroenteritis in bone-marrow-transplant recipients. N Engl J Med 1982;306:1010–2.
45. Mogg GA, Keighley MR, Burdon DW, et al. Antibiotic-associated colitis: a review of 66 cases. Br J Surg 1979;66:738–42.
46. Bartlett JG, Taylor NS, Chang T, et al. Clinical and laboratory observations in *Clostridium difficile* colitis. Am J Clin Nutr 1980;33(11 Suppl):2521–6.

47. Tedesco FJ, Barton RW, Alpers DH. Clindamycin-associated colitis: a prospective study. Ann Intern Med 1974;81:429–33.
48. Longo WE, Mazuski JE, Virgo KS, et al. Outcome after colectomy for *Clostridium difficile* colitis. Dis Colon Rectum 2004;47(10):1620–6.
49. Fekety R. Guidelines for the diagnosis and management of *Clostridium difficile*-associated diarrhea and colitis. Am J Gastroenterol 1997;92:739–50.
50. Schue V, Green GA, Monteil H. Comparison of the ToxA test with cytotoxicity assay and culture for the detection of *Clostridium difficile*-associated diarrhoeal disease. J Med Microbiol 1994;41:316–8.
51. Mylonakis E, Ryan ET, Calderwood SB. *Clostridium difficile*-associated diarrhea. Arch Intern Med 2001;161:525–33.
52. Wilkins TD, Lyerly DM. *Clostridium difficile* testing: after 20 years, still challenging. J Clin Microbiol 2003;41:531–4.
53. Chang TW, Bartlett JG, Gorbach SL, et al. Clindamycin-induced enterocolitis in hamsters a as a model of pseudomembranous colitis in patients. Infect Immun 1978;20:526–9.
54. Borek AP, Aird DZ, Carroll KC. Frequency of sample submission for optimal utilization of the cell culture cytotoxicity assay for detection of *Clostridium difficile* toxin. J Clin Microbiol 2005;43:2994–5.
55. Whittier S, Shapiro DS, Kelly WF, et al. Evaluation of four commercially available enzyme immunoassays for laboratory diagnosis of *Clostridium difficile*-associated diseases. J Clin Microbiol 1993;31:2861–5.
56. Merz CS, Kramer C, Forman M, et al. Comparison of four commercially available rapid enzyme immunoassays with cytotoxin assay for detection of *Clostridium difficile* toxin(s) from stool specimens. J Clin Microbiol 1994;32:1142–7.
57. Delmee M, Van Broeck J, Simon A, et al. Laboratory diagnosis of *Clostridium difficile*-associated diarrhoea: a plea for culture. J Med Microbiol 2005;54:187–91.
58. George WL, Sutter VL, Citron D, et al. Selective and differential medium for isolation of *Clostridium difficile*. J Clin Microbiol 1979;9:214–9.
59. Shanholtzer CJ, Willard KE, Holter JJ, et al. Comparison of the Vidas *Clostridium difficile* toxin A immunoassay with *C difficile* culture and cytotoxin and latex tests. J Clin Microbiol 1992;30:1837–40.
60. Ticehurst JR, Aird DZ, Dam LM, et al. Effective detection of toxigenic *Clostridium difficile* by a two step algorithm including test for antigen and cytotoxin. J Clin Microbiol 2006;44:1145–9.
61. Manabe YC, Vinetz JM, Moore RD, et al. *Clostridium difficile* colitis: an efficient clinical approach to diagnosis. Ann Intern Med 1995;123:835–40.
62. Kato N, Ou CY, Kato H, et al. Detection of toxigenic *Clostridium difficile* in stool specimens by the polymerase chain reaction. J Infect Dis 1993;167:455–8.
63. National *Clostridium difficile* Standards Group: report to the Department of Health. J Hosp Infect 2004;56(Suppl 1):1–38.
64. Riley TV, Cooper M, Bell B, et al. Community-acquired *Clostridium difficile*-associated diarrhea. Clin Infect Dis 1995;20(Suppl 2):S263–5.
65. Tedesco FJ, Corless JK, Brownstein RE. Rectal sparing in antibiotic-associated pseudomembranous colitis: a prospective study. Gastroenterology 1982;83:1259–60.
66. Tedesco FJ. Antibiotic associated pseudomembranous colitis with negative proctosigmoidoscopy examination. Gastroenterology 1979;77:295–7.
67. Fisherman EK, Kavuru M, Jones B, et al. Pseudomembranous colitis: CT evaluation of 26 cases. Radiology 1991;180:57–60.

68. Kawamoto S, Horton KW, Fishman EK. Pseudomembranous colitis: spectrum of imaging findings with clinical and pathologic correlation. Radiographics 1999; 19:887–97.
69. Hayetian FD, Read TE, Brozovich M, et al. Ileal perforation secondary to *Clostridium* difficile enteritis: report of 2 cases. Arch Surg 2006;141(1):97–9.
70. Fekety R, Shah AB. Diagnosis and treatment of *Clostridium difficile* colitis. JAMA 1993;269:71–5.
71. Bartlett JG. The case for vancomycin as the preferred drug for treatment of *Clostridium difficile* infection. Clin Infect Dis 2008;46:1489–92.
72. Teasley DG, Gerding DN, Olson MM, et al. Prospective randomized trial of metronidazole vs. vancomycin fro *Clostridium difficile*-associated diarrhea and colitis. Lancet 1983;2:1043–6.
73. Fekety R, Silva J, Buggy B, et al. Treatment of antibiotic-associated colitis with vancomycin. J Antimicrob Chemother 1984;12(Suppl D):97–102.
74. Bartlett JG, Tedesco FJ, Shull S, et al. Symptomatic relapse after oral vancomycin therapy of antibiotic-associated pseudomembranous colitis. Gastroenterology 1980;78:431–4.
75. Gerding DN, Johnson S, Peterson LR, et al. *Clostridium difficile*-associated diarrhea and colitis. Infect Control Hosp Epidemiol 1995;16:459–77.
76. Fekety R, Silva J, Kauffman C, et al. Treatment of antibiotic-associated *Clostridium difficile* colitis with oral vancomycin: comparison of two dosage regimens. Am J Med 1989;86:15–9.
77. Poutanen SM, Simor AE. *Clostridium difficile*-associated diarrhea in adults. CMAJ 2004;171:51–8.
78. Bolton RP, Culshaw MA. Faecal metronidazole concentrations during oral and intravenous therapy for antibiotic associated colitis due to *Clostridium difficile*. Gut 1986;27:1169–72.
79. Johnson S, Hormann SR, Bettin KM, et al. Treatment of asymptomatic *Clostridium difficile* carriers (fecal excretors) with vancomycin or metronidazole: a randomized, placebo controlled trial. Ann Intern Med 1992;117:297–302.
80. Zar FA, Bakkanagari SR, Moorthi MKLST, et al. A comparison of vancomycin and metronidazole for the treatment of *Clostridium difficile*-associated diarrhea, stratified by disease severity. Clin Infect Dis 2007;45:302–7.
81. Lagrotteria D, Holmes S, Smieja M, et al. Prospective, randomized inpatient study of oral metronidazole versus oral metronidazole and rifampin for treatment of primary episode of *Clostridium difficile*-associated diarrhea. Clin Infect Dis 2006;3:547–52.
82. Pepin J, Valiquette L, Gagnon S, et al. Outcomes of *Clostridium difficile*-associated disease treated with metronidazole or vancomycin before and after the emergence of NAP1/027. Am J Gastroenterol 2007;102:2781–8.
83. Bartlett JG. Narrative review: the new epidemic of *Clostridium difficile*-associated enteric disease. Ann Intern Med 2006;145:758–64.
84. Pepin J, Routhier S, Gagnon S, et al. Management and outcomes of a first recurrence of *Clostridium difficile*-associated disease in Quebec, Canada. Clin Infect Dis 2006;42:758–64.
85. McFarland LV, Elmer GW, Surawicz CM. Breaking the cycle: treatment strategies for 163 cases of recurrent *Clostridium difficile* disease. Am J Gastroenterol 2002; 97:1769–75.
86. De Lalla F, Nicolin R, Rinaldi E, et al. Prospective study of oral teicoplanin versus oral vancomycin for therapy of pseudomembranous colitis and *Clostridium difficile*-associated diarrhea. Antimicrob Agents Chemother 1992;36:2192–6.

87. Wenisch C, Parschalk B, Hasenundl M, et al. Comparison of vancomycin, teicoplanin, metronidazole and fusidic acid for the treatment of *Clostridium difficile*-associated diarrhea. Clin Infect Dis 1996;22:813–8.

88. Louie T, Gerson M, Grimard D, et al. Results of a phase III trial comparing tolevamer, vancomycin and metronidazole for the treatment of *Clostridium difficile*-associated diarrhea (CDAD) [abstract K-4259]. In: Program and abstracts of the 47th Interscience Conference on Antimicrobial Agents and Chemotherapy (Washington, DC). Herndon (VA): ASM Press; 2007.

89. Nelson R. Antibiotic treatment for *Clostridium difficile*-associated diarrhea in adults. Cochrane Database Syst Rev 2007;3:CD004610.

90. Aslam S, Musher DM. An update on diagnosis, treatment and prevention of *Clostridium difficile*-associated disease. Gastroenterol Clin North Am 2006;35: 315–35.

91. Malnick SD, Zimhony O. Treatment of *Clostridium difficile*-associated diarrhea. Ann Pharmacother 2002;36:1767–75.

92. Musher DM, Logan N, Hamill RJ, et al. Nitazoxanide for the treatment of *Clostridium difficile* colitis. Clin Infect Dis 2006;43:421–7.

93. Musher DM, Logan N, Mehendiratta V, et al. *Clostridium difficile* colitis that fails conventional metronidazole therapy: response to nitazoxanide. J Antimicrob Chemother 2007;59:705–10.

94. Louie TJ, Peppe J, Watt CK, et al. Tolevamer, a novel nonantibiotic polymer, compared with vancomycin in the treatment of mild to moderately severe *Clostridium difficile*-associated diarrhea. Clin Infect Dis 2006;43:411–20.

95. McFarland LV, Surawicz CM, Greenberg RN, et al. A randomized placebo-controlled trial of *Saccharomyces boulardii* in combination with standard antibiotics for *Clostridium difficile* disease. JAMA 1994;271:1913–8.

96. Surawicz CM, McFarland LV, Greenberg RN, et al. The search for a better treatment for recurrent *Clostridium difficile* disease: use of high-dose vancomycin combined with Saccharomyces boulardii. Clin Infect Dis 2000;31:1012–7.

97. McFarland LV. Meta-analysis of probiotics for the prevention of antibiotic-associated diarrhea and the treatment of *Clostridium difficile* disease. Am J Gastroenterol 2006;101:812–22.

98. Dendukuri N, Costa V, McGregor M, et al. Probiotic therapy for the prevention and treatment of *Clostridium difficile*-associated diarrhea: a systematic review. CMAJ 2005;173:167–70.

99. Cassone M, Serra P, Mondello F, et al. Outbreak of *Saccharomyces cerevisiae* subtype *boulardii* infection fungemia in patients neighboring those treated with a probiotic preparation of the organism. J Clin Microbiol 2003;41:5340–3.

100. Enache-Angoulvant A, Hennequin C. Invasive *Saccharomyces* infection: a comprehensive review. Clin Infect Dis 2005;41:1559–68.

101. Lherm T, Monet C, Nougiere B, et al. Seven cases of fungemia with *Saccharomyces boulardii* in critically ill patients. Intensive Care Med 2002;28:797–801.

102. Salminen MK, Rautelin H, Tynkkynen S, et al. *Lactobacills* bacteremia, clinical significance, and patient outcome, with special focus on probiotic *L. rhamnosus* GG. Clin Infect Dis 2004;38:62–9.

103. Pelaez T, Alcala L, Alonso R, et al. In vitro activity of ramoplanin against *Clostridium difficile*, including strains with reduced susceptibility to vancomycin or with resistance to metronidazole. Antimicrob Agents Chemother 2004;48: 2280–2.

104. Ackermann G, Loffler B, Adler D, et al. In vitro activity of OPT-80 against *Clostridium difficile*. Antimicrob Agents Chemother 2004;48:2280–2.

105. Anton PM, O'Brien M, Kokkotou E, et al. Rifalazil treats and prevents relapse of *Clostridium difficile*-associated diarrhea in hamsters. Antimicrob Agents Chemother 2004;48:3975–9.
106. Citron DM, Tyrell KL, Warren YA, et al. In vitro activities of tinidazole and metronidazole against *Clostridium difficile, Prevotella bivia*, and *Bacteroides fragilis*. Anaerobe 2005;113:15–7.
107. Adachi JA, DuPont HL. Rifaximin: a novel nonabsorbed rifamycin for gastrointestinal disorders. Clin Infect Dis 2006;42:541–7.
108. Taylor DN, Bourgeois AL, Ericsson CD, et al. A randomized, double-blind, multicenter study of rifaximin compared with placebo and with ciprofloxacin in the treatment of travelers' diarrhea. Am J Trop Med Hyg 2006;74:1060–6.
109. Pepin J, Alary ME, Valiquette L, et al. Increasing risk of relapse after treatment of *Clostridium difficile* colitis in Quebec, Canada. Clin Infect Dis 2005;40:1591–7.
110. Barbut F, Richard A, Hamadi K, et al. Epidemiology of recurrences or reinfections of *Clostridium difficile*-associated diarrhea. J Clin Microbiol 2000;38:2386–8.
111. McFarland LV. Alternative treatments for *Clostridium difficile* disease: what really works? J Med Microbiol 2005;54:101–11.
112. McFarland LV, Surawicz CM, Rubin M, et al. *Clostridium difficile* disease: epidemiology and clinical characteristics. Infect Control Hosp Epidemiol 1999;20:43–50.
113. Aas J, Gessert CE, Bakken JS. Recurrent *Clostridium difficile* colitis: case series involving 18 patients treated with donor stool administered via nasogastric tube. Clin Infect Dis 2003;36:580–5.
114. Sanchez JL, Gerding DN, Olson MM, et al. Metronidazole susceptibility in *Clostridium difficile* isolates recovered from cases of *C difficile*-associated disease treatment failures and successes. Anaerobe 1999;5:201–4.
115. Kyne L, Warny M, Qamar A, et al. Association between antibody response to toxin A and protection against recurrent *Clostridium difficile* diarrhoea. Lancet 2001;357:189–93.
116. Nair S, Yadav D, Corpuz M, et al. *Clostridium difficile* colitis: factors influencing treatment failure and relapse – prospective evaluation. Am J Gastroenterol 1998;93:1873–6.
117. Buggy BP, Fekety R, Silva J Jr. Therapy of relapsing *Clostridium difficile*-associated diarrhea and colitis with the combination of vancomycin and rifampin. J Clin Gastroenterol 1987;9:155–9.
118. Taylor NS, Bartlett JG. Binding of *Clostridium difficile* cytotoxin and vancomycin by anion-exchange resins. J Infect Dis 1980;141:92–7.
119. Johnson S, Schriever C, Galang M, et al. Interruption of recurrent *Clostridium difficile*-associated diarrhea episodes by serial therapy with vancomycin and rifaximin. Clin Infect Dis 2007;44:846–8.
120. Olson MM, Shanholtzer CJ, Lee JT, et al. Ten years of prospective *Clostridium difficile*-associated disease surveillance and treatment at the Minneapolis VA Medical Center, 1982–1991. Infect Control Hosp Epidemiol 1994;15:371–81.
121. Pasic M, Jost R, Carrel T, et al. Intracolonic vancomycin for pseudomembranous colitis. N Engl J Med 1993;329:583.
122. Lamontagne F, Labbe AC, Haeck O, et al. Impact of emergency colectomy on survival of patients with fulminant *Clostridium difficile* colitis during an epidemic caused by a hypervirulent strain. Ann Surg 2007;245:267–72.
123. Morris JB, Zollinger RM, Stellato TA. Role of surgery in antibiotic-induced pseudomembranous enterocolitis. Am J Surg 1990;160:535–9.

124. Drapkin MS, Worthington MG, Chang TW, et al. *Clostridium difficile* colitis mimicking acute peritonitis. Arch Surg 1985;120:1321–2.
125. Lipsett PA, Samantaray DL, Tam ML, et al. Pseudomembranous colitis: a surgical disease? Surgery 1994;116:491–6.
126. Synott K, Mealy K, Merry C, et al. Timing of surgery for fulminating pseudomembranous colitis. Br J Surg 1998;85:229–31.
127. Medich DS, Lee KK, Simmons RL, et al. Laparotomy for fulminant pseudomembranous colitis. Arch Surg 1992;127:847–53.
128. Bradbury AW, Barrett S. Surgical aspects of *Clostridium difficile* colitis. Br J Surg 1997;84:150–9.
129. Grundfest-Broniatowski S, Quader M, Alexander F, et al. *Clostridium difficile* colitis in the critically ill. Dis Colon Rectum 1996;39:619–23.
130. Samore MH, Venkataraman L, DeGirolami PC, et al. Clinical and molecular epidemiology of sporadic and clustered cases of nosocomial *Clostridium difficile* diarrhea. Am J Med 1996;100:32–40.
131. Garner JS. Guideline for isolation precautions in hospitals. Infect Control Hosp Epidemiol 1996;17:53–80 [Erratum, Infect Control Hosp Epidemiol 1996;17:214].
132. Sehulster L, Chinn RY. Guidelines for environmental infection control in health-care facilities: recommendations of CDC and the Healthcare Infection Control Practices Advisory Committee [HICPAC]. MMWR Recomm Rep 2003;55(RR-10):1–42.
133. Boyce JM, Pittet D. Guideline for hand hygiene in health-care settings: recommendations of the Healthcare Infection Control Practices Advisory Committee and the HICPAC/SHEA/APIC/IDSA Hand Hygiene Task Force. Infect Control Hosp Epidemiol 2002;23(Suppl):S3–40.

Preventing Bacterial Resistance in Surgical Patients

Heather L. Evans, MD, MS[a],*, Robert G. Sawyer, MD, FACS[b,c]

KEYWORDS

- Bacterial resistance • Health care–associated infections
- Multidrug-resistant organisms • Antibiotic cycling
- Infection control

Antimicrobial resistance is a major public health concern. Whether administering perioperative antibiotics to prevent surgical site infection or performing operative debridement to attain source control, surgeons are integral to the effort to contain the spread of resistant organisms. The rising acuity of hospitalized patients and the dramatic increase in community-acquired antibiotic-resistant infections highlight the need for judicious antimicrobial prescription balanced with early, aggressive intervention. This article demonstrates that comprehensive treatment and prevention of surgical infections mandates both an awareness of the changing epidemiology and a commitment to implementation of the multifaceted approach to treatment and control of antimicrobial resistance. A summary of the scope of the problem of resistant surgical infections is followed by a review of the current practices and controversies in infection treatment and infection control in surgical patients.

IMPACT OF RESISTANT ORGANISMS ON SURGICAL PRACTICE

The surgeon most commonly encounters infection either as a primary surgical disease, as in complicated skin and skin-structure infections or intra-abdominal infections, or as a health care–associated infection following injury or instrumentation. With the development of resistance to commonly used antibiotics, understanding the principles of adequate empiric antimicrobial treatment with subsequent

[a] Department of Surgery, University of Washington, Harborview Medical Center, Box 359796, 325 Ninth Avenue, Seattle, WA 98104–2499, USA
[b] Division of Acute Care Surgery, Department of Surgery, University of Virginia School of Medicine, Box 800709, Charlottesville, VA 22908–0709, USA
[c] Department of Public Health Sciences, University of Virginia School of Medicine, Charlottesville, VA 22908, USA
* Corresponding author. Department of Surgery, University of Washington, Box 359796, 325 Ninth Avenue, Seattle, WA 98104–2499.
E-mail address: hlevans@u.washington.edu (H.L. Evans).

Surg Clin N Am 89 (2009) 501–519
doi:10.1016/j.suc.2008.09.011
0039-6109/08/$ – see front matter © 2009 Elsevier Inc. All rights reserved.

surgical.theclinics.com

de-escalation, and appropriate perioperative prophylaxis, has become as important as knowing how to conduct an operation and achieve source control for the surgeon.

Complicated Skin and Skin-Structure Infections

The most comprehensive microbiologic data regarding complicated skin and skin-structure infections in hospitalized patients suggests that although resistance patterns do vary by geography, these infections are predominantly caused by gram-positive skin organisms, and overwhelmingly by *Staphylococcus aureus*.[1] In the United States, the proportion of methicillin-resistant *S aureus* (MRSA) isolates has steadily increased over time. By 2003, the incidence of MRSA in National Nosocomial Infection Surveillance reporting ICUs reached 59%.[2] Simultaneous with the increase in resistance among health care–associated infections was a disturbing and unexpected rise in community-acquired MRSA complicated skin and skin-structure infections, characterized by necrotizing features.[3–6] It is now estimated that 60% to 80% of community-acquired complicated skin and skin-structure infections are caused by community-acquired MRSA.[7,8]

Appropriate initial therapy for complicated skin and skin-structure infections includes the combined administration of empiric broad-spectrum antimicrobials and aggressive surgical debridement.[9] With the increasing prevalence of MRSA, there has been a dramatic increase in the empiric administration of vancomycin. Associated with this increased use has been an associated increase in the drug's minimum inhibitory concentration over the same time period, however, potentially compromising responses to this agent.[3,10] Particularly in the case of severe necrotizing infections with systemic illness, use of alternative agents, such as linezolid, daptomycin, and tigecycline, may be indicated in addition to supportive critical care and serial operative assessment and excision.[3,7,11] It is worthwhile to remember that complicated skin and skin-structure infections include a spectrum of disease from cellulitis to abscess to diabetic foot infection to necrotizing fasciitis. As such, these infections are frequently polymicrobial, harboring gram-negative and anaerobic organisms.[9,12] Increasing resistance of *Enterobacteriaceae* to fluoroquinolones and cephalosporins has been reported, influencing a shift in the initial antibiotic choice toward such alternative agents as aminoglycosides, carbapenems, and extended-spectrum penicillins with β-lactamase inhibitors.

Intra-Abdominal Infections

The term "intra-abdominal infection" comprises a constellation of diverse infections between the diaphragm and pelvis, and as such the epidemiology is somewhat unclear.[13] Ranging from spontaneous bacterial peritonitis in cirrhotic patients to simple appendicitis to multiple loculated abscesses following liver transplantation, intra-abdominal infections require a tailored approach depending on the etiology, microbiology, and timing of the pathology.[14,15] Primary peritonitis is predominantly a monomicrobial infection seen in patients with ascites or peritoneal dialysis, and is treated with antibiotics, not surgically. Secondary peritonitis is characterized by a breach in the gastrointestinal tract; the primary treatment is source control through surgical debridement, repair, or excision of involved organs. Tertiary peritonitis is distinguished from secondary peritonitis as either recurrent or persistent intra-abdominal infection in the setting of failure of initial operative source control, inadequate empiric antibiotic coverage, or deleterious host factors.[16] Most commonly presenting in critically ill patients, tertiary peritonitis is usually diagnosed in the setting of persistent systemic illness after operative intervention and continued antibiotic therapy. Major risk factors include malnutrition, a high Acute Physiology and Chronic Health Evaluation

II score, the presence of organisms resistant to antimicrobial therapy, and organ system failure; the mortality associated with this disease is as high as 60%.[16] The characteristic microbiology of tertiary peritonitis tends toward that of other health care–associated infections including coagulase-negative *Staphylococcus*; *Candida* species; *Pseudomonas aeruginosa*; and multidrug-resistant organisms, such as vancomycin-resistant *Enterococcus*.[17–19] As such, tertiary peritonitis may be more difficult to treat, and antimicrobials should be adjusted according to available culture and drug sensitivity results.[20–24]

Patients who have ongoing signs of peritonitis or systemic illness beyond 5 to 7 days of antibiotic treatment warrant aggressive diagnostic investigation to determine whether additional surgical intervention is necessary to address an ongoing uncontrolled source of infection or antimicrobial treatment failure. Perhaps the most important factor in the treatment of intra-abdominal infections, in conjunction with timely appropriate operative intervention, is selecting the right initial antimicrobial therapy. Failure to do so is associated with development of tertiary peritonitis, more lengthy hospitalizations, use of longer courses of antibiotic therapy, and higher mortality.[20,21,23,24] It is also worthwhile to consider that delays in administration of antibiotic therapy may impart further risk to patients, as evidenced by higher mortality with every hour delayed in initiation of antibiotic therapy in the setting of septic shock.[25]

Surgical Site Infections

It is estimated that 1 in 10 surgical patients develop a health care–associated infection.[26] Of the 1.7 million health care–associated infections documented in the United States in 2002, 22% were surgical site infections (SSI).[27] Surgical wounds are at risk for infection from organisms that reside on the skin and within the operative field exposed in the course of the intervention. The microbiology of SSI is largely dependent on the kind of operation performed (eg, with higher likelihood of gram-negative infection in gastrointestinal tract surgery). Even so, gram-positive organisms that colonize the skin, such as *S aureus*, coagulase-negative *Staphylococcus*, and *Enterococcus* species, predominate, and the isolates from SSI cultures have remained fairly consistent over time, as have the drugs used to provide perioperative prophylaxis.[12,28]

Recent evidence calls into question the adequacy of traditional prophylactic regimens. First, administration of antibiotics beyond as little as 24 hours after surgery has been shown to promote higher rates of vancomycin-resistant *Enterococcus*, cephalosporin-resistant *Enterobacteriaceae*, and MRSA.[29–32] The Surgical Infection Prevention recommendations currently include direction to discontinue antibiotics within 24 hours of operation.[33] Interestingly, a subsequent retrospective analysis of the Medicare population by the same workgroup revealed that although 99% of patients received timely antibiotics before surgery, only 40% had appropriate discontinuation of antibiotics.[34] Second, the rising prevalence of MRSA colonization is associated with increasing rates of MRSA SSI[12,28] and increasing incidence of infected vascular grafts associated with limb loss and fatal outcomes as a result of MRSA graft infections.[35,36] Targeted preoperative screening of those patients at high risk for MRSA colonization has been suggested as a possible way to identify patients who may benefit from vancomycin prophylaxis.[37] Because of the risk of MRSA mediastinitis, which carries significant morbidity and mortality, preoperative decolonization through nasal mupirocin application has been advocated in cardiac surgery, and it is likely to be adopted by other fields, despite inconsistent evidence of its effectiveness.[38–40] Third, although second-generation cephalosporins have been a mainstay for preventing SSI in elective colon surgery, a randomized controlled trial comparing cefotetan with ertapenem prophylaxis revealed higher rates of SSI and organisms resistant to cefotetan in the cefotetan group.[41] As resistance to commonly used antibiotics increases, surgeons must continually weigh the benefit of preventing resistant SSI with promotion of more difficult-to-treat multidrug-resistant organisms.

Outcomes From Multidrug-Resistant Organism Infections

A thorough summary of the extent of the problem of multidrug-resistant infection and the available evidence as to how best to prevent and treat multidrug-resistant organisms is beyond the scope of this article.[42] It is essential to acknowledge, however, that although multidrug-resistant infections may have similar clinical manifestations to infections caused by susceptible organisms, outcomes are uniformly worse. Resistant gram-negative rod infections are associated with prolonged hospitalizations, higher health care cost, and increased mortality.[43,44] These findings have also been reported when resistant gram-positive organisms contribute to intra-abdominal infection[18,45] and in vancomycin-resistant enterococcal bacteremia.[46] Two meta-analyses of MRSA bacteremia conclude that methicillin resistance is independently predictive of death, perhaps because of a lethal combination of the decreased effectiveness of vancomycin, delay in selection of appropriate antibiotic coverage, and the enhanced virulence of the organisms.[47,48] Interestingly, it has also been observed that during outbreaks of these infections, outcomes improve, likely because of heightened awareness of the problem and more rapid initiation of therapy. Even SSI is associated with higher mortality when caused by MRSA. One study reported a more than 12-fold increase in the 90-day postoperative mortality rate when patients with a MRSA SSI were compared with patients who did not develop SSI, and a more than threefold increase when these patients were compared with patients with a methicillin-sensitive S aureus SSI.[49]

PREVENTING RESISTANCE
Centers for Disease Control and Prevention Campaign to Prevent Antimicrobial Resistance in Health Care Settings

Antibiotic resistance has been recognized for nearly 60 years, but by 2002 the proportion of bacteria resistant to at least one antibiotic causing hospital-acquired infection was estimated to be 70%. With the acknowledgment that this was associated with increased lengths of hospitalization and more costly and potentially problematic treatments, and that the development of antibiotic resistance was largely a result of overuse of antibiotics and uncontrolled transmission between patients, the Centers for Disease Control and Prevention (CDC) developed an integrated campaign from existing evidence-based guidelines to address these problems in health care facilities.[50]

The campaign outlined a 12-step approach to prevent antimicrobial resistance with four main strategies: (1) prevent infection, (2) diagnose and treat infection effectively, (3) use antimicrobials wisely, and (4) prevent transmission (**Fig. 1**). Through creation of a campaign-specific Web site, the CDC disseminated education tools for providers and patients in a variety of media and encouraged implementation of the program.[51] Notably, five steps are devoted to redirecting prescribing patterns of antibiotics. Subsequent studies reported varying degrees of acceptance of the 12-steps, but demonstrated that the program afforded structure and external support for educating providers on appropriate antimicrobial prescribing practices and changing local culture.[52,53]

Specialty societies endorsed respective programs targeted at specific providers, with the Surgical Infection Society publishing a joint position paper with the CDC summarizing the evidence supporting implementation in surgical patients and calling on

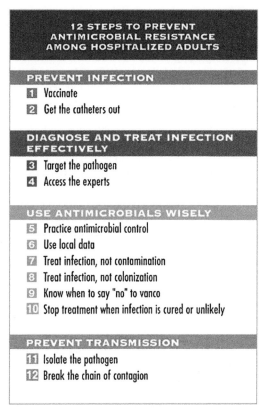

Fig. 1. Centers for Disease Control and Prevention campaign to prevent antimicrobial resistance pocket card, 2002.

surgeons to become involved in policy development.[54] Particularly important developments highlighted in that publication were new CDC guidelines for the prevention of intravascular catheter-related infections and guidelines on hand hygiene.[55,56] The former publication was produced by a multidisciplinary group of experts in critical care, surgery, infectious disease, and other fields as an updated review and evaluation of the level of evidence for issues regarding insertion, maintenance, and discontinuation of intravascular catheters. Areas of emphasis that represented change since the last guidelines included education and training in the proper insertion and maintenance of catheters, using full barrier methods during central venous catheter insertion or change, preference for 2% chlorhexidine skin preparation, and avoidance of routine central venous catheter insertion. For the first time, antiseptic or antibiotic impregnated central venous catheters were also recommended for use if rates of catheter-related bloodstream infections were high at the institution despite adherence to the previous recommendations. In regard to the 12-step campaign, central venous catheters appeared prominently in steps 2 and 10, in which providers were called to remove catheters as soon as they were not required, avoid culturing catheter tips, and to treat documented bacteremia and not catheter tip colonization.

The hand hygiene document, produced jointly by the Healthcare Infection Control Practices Advisory Committee and the hand hygiene task force comprised of representatives from the Healthcare Infection Control Practices Advisory Committee and three major infectious disease societies, begins with a comprehensive historical review of the scientific data supporting hand washing since 1829.[55,57–59] What follows is a systematic analysis of skin microbiology and physiology, pathogen transmission, and the efficacy of cleansing using various evaluative methods, cleansing products, and regimens. Several studies cited demonstrate a temporal relationship between improved hand hygiene compliance and decreased incidence of multidrug-resistant organisms, although these analyses may be confounded, as in other infection-control studies, by the presence of multiple concurrent infection-control measure implementations.[57–59] The practice of hand hygiene by health care workers is examined in terms of compliance, barriers to adoption, and possible areas for promotion. The essential conclusion is that nothing short of multimodal, hospital-wide adoption of system change promoting institutional safety results in longstanding effectiveness.[60] The authors admit that this is beyond the scope of infection-control practitioners. Yet, the innovative group at the University of Geneva Hospitals has partnered with experts in human factors engineering, cognitive behavioral science, and marketing to develop a new program for hand hygiene using a novel user-centered design that can be applied worldwide.[61] The result is an original, interactive model that transforms the invisible transmission of organisms to a systematic task-based and contact-driven experience that is intended to evoke ownership and commitment to the hand hygiene process each time contact is made through understanding of the implications of organism transmission. Through defining two zones of work (the health care zone and the patient zone) and two critical sites within the patient zone (clean sites and body fluid sites) the creators of the model have designed a system where the health care worker is reminded, merely by the act of moving between sites or zones, to wash their hands at five moments in care: (1) before patient contact, (2) before an aseptic task, (3) after body fluid exposure risk, (4) after patient contact, and (5) after contact with patient surroundings. Furthermore, the systematic nature of the model allows for ease of standardization of behavior, facilitating education and increasing patient safety through cleaner care. The estimate that health care workers should be washing their hands as often as every 2 minutes during intensive care seems like an unattainable goal, but this model provides a framework for improvement, monitoring, and behavioral change.

In 2007, the CDC published a review of multidrug-resistant organism infection diagnosis and management.[42] This document contains a comprehensive assessment of current recommendations, including a new emphasis on the importance of administrative support in the success of infection-control initiatives. Examples of this include increased staffing levels, and installation of sufficient and appropriately placed hand hygiene equipment and resources to encourage lasting culture change and adherence to recommended precautions and policies.[57] Additional emphasis was placed on education and training efforts to facilitate understanding of rationale for behavior changes and encourage a culture that supports lasting compliance.[60] The recognition that sustained acceptance of infection-control practices requires ongoing human resources, team building, and reinforcement signals a profound shift from the punitive to the inspired.

The authors also acknowledge that despite the tremendous volume of evidence in the literature, a universally accepted set of infection-control measures, including when to use contact precautions over standard precautions, cannot be agreed on because of the quality and inconsistency of the data; local circumstances need to direct facilities as to best practices.[42] Further, the position that active surveillance cultures (screening cultures performed on admission to a hospital unit to identify MRSA carriers) should not be mandated is elaborated in a joint publication by the Society for

Healthcare Epidemiology of America and the Association for Professionals in Infection Control and Epidemiology,[62] and supported by additional data that such a practice has no impact on decreasing either the rate of MRSA colonization or subsequent infection.[63,64] The routine use of decolonization regimens to rid patients of MRSA colonization is discouraged because of the potential for developing mupirocin-resistant S aureus strains;[65,66] rather this practice is probably best reserved for outbreak situations or decolonization of a health care worker when linked to transmission,[10] particularly when decolonization involves topical and systemic antibiotic regimens. Subsequent to this CDC review, there have been several reports of decontamination of ICU patients through whole-body skin cleansing with chlorhexidine gluconate, effecting reduced rates of bloodstream infection caused by vancomycin-resistant enterococcus, MRSA, and Acinetobacter.[67–70] This practice is appealing because it provides an additional means of reducing the reservoir of resistant skin pathogens with little risk of inducing further bacterial resistance.

STEWARDSHIP: THE ROLE OF ANTIMICROBIAL RESTRICTION PROGRAMS

Antibiotic stewardship refers to an integrated effort to manage the administration of antimicrobials to ensure the best treatment selection for individual patients while attempting to prevent the development of resistance.[71] Comprehensive antibiotic management strategies may use a variety of methods to limit antibiotic use in volume, duration, and spectrum, and means to monitor compliance with clinical practice guidelines, policies, and protocols. Formulary restriction, selective reporting of culture susceptibilities, decision support tools, and antibiotic cycling are among the means by which antimicrobial use is directed.

Antibiotic Formulary Restriction

Formulary restriction was developed as an external control over clinician prescribing when antimicrobial resistance continued to increase in the face of noncompliance with clinical practice guidelines. Restrictions may be at various levels, from a closed formulary, where only a defined selection of antibiotics are available; to one where additional antibiotics are available with prior approval from infectious disease specialists; to one in which providers may use any antibiotic as long as predefined criteria are met. Initial restriction policies, characterized by individualized education of a practitioner by an expert in infectious disease, without the authority to stop the dispensing of the drug, sufficed to change prescribing practices in most cases, effectively reducing use of targeted antimicrobials.[72,73] Subsequent studies in which restricted antibiotics were only released after approval by infectious disease and pharmacy consultants revealed improvement in antibiotic sensitivities and significant cost savings through use of less expensive unrestricted antibiotics.[74,75] It is likely that the cost savings and prescribing pattern changes were effected through a combination of personal education and the desire to avoid having to interact with a consultant by simply ordering a less restricted drug. But because the "antibiotic police" have established a presence in many institutions, practitioners have devised means for subverting the established rules and obtaining access to restricted antimicrobial drugs.[76,77] These reports signal a larger problem common to infection-control measures: policies that involve changing behaviors without addressing a change in culture and incorporating provider contribution at the time of enacting the policy may result in dissent rather than cooperation. Carling and colleagues[78] reported that the ultimate success of their stewardship effort depended on a high degree of provider acceptance, attributed to having non–infectious disease personnel involved in the effort. Successful stewardship requires multidisciplinary cooperation, systems-based change, and support from hospital leadership.[79,80]

Although formulary restriction has been in practice for over 30 years and has been shown repeatedly to reduce hospital expenditures, it does not seem to have had significant enduring impact on the ongoing development of resistance. The one area in which formulary restriction seems to be particularly effective in manipulating antibiotic resistance is in the setting of outbreak, in conjunction with other infection-control methods.[81] With the rise of extended-spectrum β-lactamase–producing gram-negative organisms, many hospitals have demonstrated effective reduction in the isolation of these bacteria through restricting use of cephalosporins and encouraging use of β-lactamase inhibitors, such as piperacillin-tazobactam or imipenem-cilastatin.[82–85] Reduction in vancomycin-resistant enterococci and *Clostridium difficile* infections has also been seen in some cases.[81,86–88] The downside to systematic formulary changes such as these is the potential for inducing resistance to the replacement class,[84,89] a phenomenon described as "squeezing the balloon."[90] There is at least one population-based analysis that concluded that restricted formularies were associated with a higher rate of antimicrobial resistance, which may represent the end result of this reactionary method of manipulating prescribing patterns.[91]

Selective Reporting of Bacterial Susceptibilities: Helpful or Harmful?

Use of culture data to direct antimicrobial therapy is one of the cornerstones of the CDC program to prevent antimicrobial resistance, both to target the pathogen and to de-escalate therapy from broad-spectrum empiric drugs. Culture data reporting, however, is another means to enact infection-control. The task of testing culture susceptibilities is based on the organisms isolated and the institutional environment in which the culture is obtained. These criteria are systematically outlined by the Clinical and Laboratory Standards Institute through a hierarchy of testing measures, whereby the most common drugs to which an organisms is usually sensitive are tested first, with additional testing of more broad-spectrum, costly antimicrobials reserved for resistance to multiple agents in the first group or through special request by the ordering physician.[92] Based on the conclusion that reporting results for every antimicrobial agent tested without censoring inappropriate results may encourage inappropriate antimicrobial use, selective reporting of susceptibilities has been recommended for some time and is currently listed among the guidelines for antimicrobial stewardship.[93,94] This practice is frequently defended by citing a case report of increased use of rifampicin when microbiology culture reporting began routinely including rifampicin susceptibility information in a single institution.[95] In reality, the impact of susceptibility reporting on prescribing behavior is controversial. Some studies have suggested a significant influence,[96,97] whereas others have shown that there is little correlation between susceptibility reporting and appropriate therapy initiation, concluding that providers may be overwhelmed with information, unable accurately to interpret the report as provided, or unwilling to alter antimicrobial therapy for fear of relapse.[98,99]

Interestingly, the studies on which these recommendations are based are largely derived from community-based populations with urinary tract infections, rather than the complex, critically ill hospitalized patients to whom these measures are often directed. An alternative view is that clinicians at the point of care should have access to the best available information optimally to interpret a complex clinical situation, of which microbiologic laboratories and infection-control monitors may not be aware. Although broader-spectrum, more costly agents may not be the first-line treatment for a specific infection, integration of all available clinical information may direct clinicians to choose such therapies. Considerations, such as other concurrent infections or the best empiric therapy for the potential source sepsis, and patient factors, such as allergies and concomitant organ failure, may all be important. Full laboratory reporting may contribute to better understanding of culture data and implementation of antibiotic therapy,[100] although improved outcomes also depend on active communication and collaboration between the primary clinician, pharmacists, the microbiology laboratory, and infectious disease experts.[101,102]

Integrated Decision Support Tools

Through the implementation of clinical information systems into the hospital environment comes new opportunity to integrate education, medical decision making, delivery of care, and monitoring of outcomes. On the simplest level, connection to the Internet at the point of care provides unprecedented access to the medical literature and practice guidelines. Hospital-based policies and educational initiatives can be promoted and integrated into provider workflows. Physician order entry allows real-time computerized feedback on treatment choices. Some institutions with this capability have adopted computerized educational interventions to maintain formulary restrictions, such as prompting justification for ordering a specific antibiotic, or choosing from a set of approved indications.[103–105] As with other restrictive policies, prescribers may seek to circumvent the process by selecting an approved indication when the drug is to be used for other purposes.[103] Other major barriers to integrating technology-based methods include prior experience with earlier, dysfunctional medical information systems; potential interference with the doctor-patient relationship; a threat to the clinician's autonomy; and the potential for increasing workload because of excessive electronic reminders.[106]

With expert decision support systems, computer algorithms can amalgamate patient-specific culture and laboratory data with the local antibiogram and prescribing policies to suggest tailor-made treatment regimens. Continuous tracking of antibiotic usage, susceptibilities, and patient outcomes allow unprecedented analysis of the impact of care. These are not new developments in some institutions; the group at the Latter-Day Saints hospital in Salt Lake City, Utah, has been using and refining a locally developed rules-based system since 1988.[107,108] Using a before-and-after comparison design, they have demonstrated a significant decrease in antibiotic expenditures despite an overall increase in the number of antibiotics administered, and a stable pattern of antimicrobial resistance despite an open formulary and increased severity of illness. More recently, an interventional cluster randomized trial of a novel computerized decision support system for empiric antibiotic treatment was conducted in three countries.[109] The system was shown to outperform clinicians by more frequently recommending appropriate empiric therapy, including withholding therapy when indicated. Clinicians did not consistently follow the recommendations of the system, however, decreasing the effectiveness of the intervention.

ANTIBIOTIC CYCLING

The scheduled periodic withdrawal and reintroduction of different antibiotic classes within a clinical environment is known as "antibiotic rotation" or "cycling." This regimen of empiric antibiotic administration is designed to address selective antibiotic pressure, the preferential selection of resistant microbes through inappropriate antibiotic use. Resistant bacterial strains are assumed to have a growth disadvantage when homogenous antibiotic pressure is withdrawn, so in the absence of cross-resistance, exposure to the new class of antibiotics should eliminate resistance selected during the previous cycle.

In the setting of increasing gram-negative resistance to aminoglycosides in the 1980s, the association between a change in antibiotic usage and alteration of antibiotic sensitivities was recognized in the initial reports of antibiotic restriction in the ICU.[110–113] It was determined that resistance to gentamicin dropped substantially when its use was restricted and amikacin was used in its place. In 1991, Gerding and colleagues[114] observed that gradual increase of gentamicin use after formulary restriction was not associated with increase in resistance to any of the aminoglycosides in use. Kollef and colleagues[115] then demonstrated a reduction in the incidence of nosocomial pneumonia when quinolones were used instead of third-generation cephalosporins in the empiric treatment of suspected gram-negative infection following cardiac surgery. After a second antibiotic class switch to cefepime, the efficacy of the cycling regimen was demonstrated by a reduction in the isolation of organisms not covered by the administered empiric antibiotic (inadequate treatment) and a reduction in mortality among the most severely ill patients.[116]

Other investigators have designed cycling regimens using predominant resistance patterns in the units of study as the basis for the drug choices. Gruson and colleagues[117] detailed a comprehensive effort to control rising quinolone and cephalosporin resistance in a medical ICU through a combined cycling and antibiotic restriction schedule devised each month, based on the previous month's antibiotic use and microbial resistance pattern. Although the drugs chosen for the rotation schedule were again targeting gram-negative organisms, the incidence of MRSA pneumonia decreased during the study period. This report was also the first specifically to detail improved drug sensitivities for several commonly resistant gram-negative organisms responsible for ventilator associated pneumonia following the institution of cycling. Similarly, Allegranzi and colleagues[89] cycled empiric antibiotics based on resistance patterns and found decreased resistance to a variety of drugs in *S aureus*, coagulase-negative staphylococcus, and *P aeruginosa* isolates from blood, sputum, urine, and surgical sites.

Despite the encouraging results from these early studies of single antibiotic class cycling, mathematical models suggest that the temporal cycling of antibiotics is inferior to mixing, a strategy whereby multiple antibiotic classes are used simultaneously in the environment to increase antibiotic heterogeneity.[118–120] Out of concern for sustained antibiotic pressure with a single class of antibiotics over a 3-month period, Raymond and colleagues[121] at the University of Virginia designed a study that combined antibiotic mixing and rotation, with two antibiotic classes used in the environment simultaneously (to be distinguished from double-coverage or two-drug antibiotic therapy in an individual patient) for the empiric treatment of suspected intra-abdominal infection and sepsis of unknown origin, or pneumonia. Using a before-and-after design, the investigators found a decrease in the incidence of all infections, infections caused by resistant gram-negative organisms, and in-hospital mortality during the rotation period. At the same time, there was a reduction in hospital-acquired and resistant hospital-acquired infection rates on the non-ICU wards where ICU patients in the rotation study were transferred, suggesting that the influence of antibiotic rotation on resistance patterns in one unit may be sustained after the patients are transferred to a new location.[122] Antibiotic rotation was independently predictive of survival when subjected to logistic regression analysis, but the study was criticized in that infection-control measures that were introduced during the first study period may have confounded the analysis.[123,124] To control for these factors, the dual-antibiotic rotation was subsequently discontinued and compared with consecutive periods of undirected and then single-cycled empiric antibiotic use.[125] Further analysis of the nature of the resistance in gram-negative isolates revealed greater heterogeneity of organisms and increased multiple drug class resistance during the single-antibiotic rotation.[126] It was also determined, however, that compliance with the rotation schedule was significantly worse in the single-antibiotic rotation period. More antibiotic classes were used per quarter in the single-antibiotic rotation than in the dual-antibiotic rotation, leading to the conclusion that increased antibiotic heterogeneity may not confer protection against resistance. Additional support for this conclusion is found in a recent prospective crossover study comparing a mixing strategy with a cycling strategy, where greater resistance to cephalosporins and carbapenemems was observed during the mixing period.[127]

An alternative explanation is that prolonged exposure to a group of antibiotics without removal of that antibiotic class is associated with increased resistance. This was the conclusion reached when an outbreak of multidrug-resistant *P aeruginosa* occurred in the medical ICU at the University of Virginia during the conduction of a CDC-sponsored multicenter trial of antibiotic cycling.[128] In contrast, in the more heterogenous ICU population studied by Warren and colleagues[129] at Barnes-Jewish Hospital in St. Louis, no significant change in *Enterobacteriaceae* and *P aeruginosa* susceptibilities was observed with antibiotic cycling, despite a longer ICU length of stay and a hospital-wide increase in resistant gram-negative bacilli. Hedrick and colleagues[128] noted that the higher baseline rate of fluoroquinolone use and the larger proportion of patients with chronic obstructive pulmonary disease, and thereby increased prior antibiotic exposure, in their cohort may have contributed to these differences in outcomes. Additionally, other studies of single-agent cycling that involve monthly switching of antibiotic classes have shown improved susceptibility profiles for *P aeruginosa*, among other gram-negative isolates, and high rates of appropriate empiric antibiotic therapy.[130,131]

Investigators at the University of Virginia have recently published results from the only study to date of empiric gram-positive antibiotic rotation.[132] Designed to reduce the incidence of vancomycin-resistant enterococcus in the ICU through quarterly cycling of linezolid and vancomycin, the study demonstrated a surprising, dramatic decrease in ICU-acquired MRSA infections, despite stable rates of MRSA infection in non-ICU patients during the same period. The low rate of vancomycin-resistant enterococcus infection remained stable, and the minimum inhibitory concentration for vancomycin was maintained at less than or equal to 1 μg/mL throughout the 6-year study. No linezolid-resistant strains were noted in the ICU, but there were two isolates from infections on the non-ICU ward that displayed intermediate sensitivity to linezolid (minimum inhibitory concentration, 4 μg/mL).

SUMMARY

The prevention of infections with antimicrobial-resistant pathogens in surgical patients begins with the recognition of their prevalence (common) and importance (costly and deadly). Although hospitals remain the epicenter of these infections, it is important to remember that resistant bacteria are becoming more common among outpatients, particularly with the increasing isolation of community-acquired *S aureus*. The approach to preventing these infections must be multifaceted and multidisciplinary. Some interventions that can help in this area include more precise antimicrobial use, hand hygiene procedures, meticulous surgical technique, and the identification and prompt treatment of patients actively infected with these organisms. In reality, different interventions certainly have different levels of importance between different populations, when one considers the wide array of patients treated throughout health care systems today. It is only through the cooperation between surgeons and multiple other health care professionals, including nurses, administrators, epidemiologists, other ancillary personnel, and different governmental bodies, that optimal outcome can be achieved.

REFERENCES

1. Moet GJ, Jones RN, Biedenbach DJ, et al. Contemporary causes of skin and soft tissue infections in North America, Latin America, and Europe: report from the SENTRY Antimicrobial Surveillance Program (1998–2004). Diagn Microbiol Infect Dis 2007;57:7–13.
2. National Nosocomial Infections Surveillance System. National Nosocomial Infections Surveillance (NNIS) System Report, data summary from January 1992 through June 2004, issued October 2004. Am J Infect Control 2004;32:470–85.
3. Awad SS, Elhabash SI, Lee L, et al. Increasing incidence of methicillin-resistant Staphylococcus aureus skin and soft-tissue infections: reconsideration of empiric antimicrobial therapy. Am J Surg 2007;194:606–10.
4. Lee TC, Carrick MM, Scott BG, et al. Incidence and clinical characteristics of methicillin-resistant Staphylococcus aureus necrotizing fasciitis in a large urban hospital. Am J Surg 2007;194:809–12.
5. Miller LG, Perdreau-Remington F, Rieg G, et al. Necrotizing fasciitis caused by community-associated methicillin-resistant Staphylococcus aureus in Los Angeles. N Engl J Med 2005;352:1445–53.
6. Young DM, Harris HW, Charlebois ED, et al. An epidemic of methicillin-resistant Staphylococcus aureus soft tissue infections among medically underserved patients. Arch Surg 2004;139:947–51.
7. Daum RS. Clinical practice: skin and soft-tissue infections caused by methicillin-resistant Staphylococcus aureus. N Engl J Med 2007;357:380–90.
8. Moran GJ, Krishnadasan A, Gorwitz RJ, et al. Methicillin-resistant S. aureus infections among patients in the emergency department. N Engl J Med 2006; 355:666–74.
9. Stevens DL, Bisno AL, Chambers HF, et al. Practice guidelines for the diagnosis and management of skin and soft-tissue infections. Clin Infect Dis 2005;41:1373–406.
10. Wang JT, Chang SC, Ko WJ, et al. A hospital-acquired outbreak of methicillin-resistant Staphylococcus aureus infection initiated by a surgeon carrier. J Hosp Infect 2001;47:104–9.
11. Solomkin JS, Bjornson HS, Cainzos M, et al. A consensus statement on empiric therapy for suspected gram-positive infections in surgical patients. Am J Surg 2004;187:134–5.
12. Jones ME, Karlowsky JA, Draghi DC, et al. Epidemiology and antibiotic susceptibility of bacteria causing skin and soft tissue infections in the USA and Europe: a guide to appropriate antimicrobial therapy. Int J Antimicrob Agents 2003;22: 406–19.
13. Farthmann EH, Schoffel U. Epidemiology and pathophysiology of intraabdominal infections (IAI). Infection 1998;26:329–34.
14. Evans HL, Raymond DP, Pelletier SJ, et al. Diagnosis of intra-abdominal infection in the critically ill patient. Curr Opin Crit Care 2001;7:117–21.
15. Solomkin JS, Mazuski JE, Baron EJ, et al. Guidelines for the selection of anti-infective agents for complicated intra-abdominal infections. Clin Infect Dis 2003; 37:997–1005.

16. Malangoni MA. Evaluation and management of tertiary peritonitis. Am Surg 2000;66:157–61.

17. Evans HL, Raymond DP, Pelletier SJ, et al. Tertiary peritonitis (recurrent diffuse or localized disease) is not an independent predictor of mortality in surgical patients with intraabdominal infection. Surg Infect (Larchmt) 2001;2:255–63.

18. Pelletier SJ, Raymond DP, Crabtree TD, et al. Outcome analysis of intraabdominal infection with resistant Gram-positive organisms. Surg Infect (Larchmt) 2002; 3:11–9.

19. Roehrborn A, Thomas L, Potreck O, et al. The microbiology of postoperative peritonitis. Clin Infect Dis 2001;33:1513–9.

20. Bare M, Castells X, Garcia A, et al. Importance of appropriateness of empiric antibiotic therapy on clinical outcomes in intra-abdominal infections. Int J Technol Assess Health Care 2006;22:242–8.

21. Krobot K, Yin D, Zhang Q, et al. Effect of inappropriate initial empiric antibiotic therapy on outcome of patients with community-acquired intra-abdominal infections requiring surgery. Eur J Clin Microbiol Infect Dis 2004;23:682–7.

22. Mazuski JE, Sawyer RG, Nathens AB, et al. The Surgical Infection Society guidelines on antimicrobial therapy for intra-abdominal infections: an executive summary. Surg Infect (Larchmt) 2002;3:161–73.

23. Sturkenboom MC, Goettsch WG, Picelli G, et al. Inappropriate initial treatment of secondary intra-abdominal infections leads to increased risk of clinical failure and costs. Br J Clin Pharmacol 2005;60:438–43.

24. Tellado JM, Sen SS, Caloto MT, et al. Consequences of inappropriate initial empiric parenteral antibiotic therapy among patients with community-acquired intra-abdominal infections in Spain. Scand J Infect Dis 2007;39:947–55.

25. Kumar A, Roberts D, Wood KE, et al. Duration of hypotension before initiation of effective antimicrobial therapy is the critical determinant of survival in human septic shock. Crit Care Med 2006;34:1589–96.

26. Vazquez-Aragon P, Lizan-Garcia M, Cascales-Sanchez P, et al. Nosocomial infection and related risk factors in a general surgery service: a prospective study. J Infect 2003;46:17–22.

27. Klevens RM, Edwards JR, Richards CL Jr, et al. Estimating health care-associated infections and deaths in U.S. hospitals, 2002. Public Health Rep 2007; 122:160–6.

28. Giacometti A, Cirioni O, Schimizzi AM, et al. Epidemiology and microbiology of surgical wound infections. J Clin Microbiol 2000;38:918–22.

29. Harbarth S, Samore MH, Lichtenberg D, et al. Prolonged antibiotic prophylaxis after cardiovascular surgery and its effect on surgical site infections and antimicrobial resistance. Circulation 2000;101:2916–21.

30. Kachroo S, Dao T, Zabaneh F, et al. Tolerance of vancomycin for surgical prophylaxis in patients undergoing cardiac surgery and incidence of vancomycin-resistant enterococcus colonization. Ann Pharmacother 2006;40:381–5.

31. Nelson CL, Green TG, Porter RA, et al. One day versus seven days of preventive antibiotic therapy in orthopedic surgery. Clin Orthop Relat Res 1983;176:258–63.

32. Terpstra S, Noordhoek GT, Voesten HG, et al. Rapid emergence of resistant coagulase-negative staphylococci on the skin after antibiotic prophylaxis. J Hosp Infect 1999;43:195–202.

33. Bratzler DW, Houck PM. Antimicrobial prophylaxis for surgery: an advisory statement from the National Surgical Infection Prevention Project. Clin Infect Dis 2004;38:1706–15.

34. Bratzler DW, Houck PM, Richards C, et al. Use of antimicrobial prophylaxis for major surgery: baseline results from the National Surgical Infection Prevention Project. Arch Surg 2005;140:174–82.

35. Nasim A, Thompson MM, Naylor AR, et al. The impact of MRSA on vascular surgery. Eur J Vasc Endovasc Surg 2001;22:211–4.

36. Taylor MD, Napolitano LM. Methicillin-resistant *Staphylococcus aureus* infections in vascular surgery: increasing prevalence. Surg Infect (Larchmt) 2004;5:180–7.

37. Muto CA, Jernigan JA, Ostrowsky BE, et al. SHEA guideline for preventing nosocomial transmission of multidrug-resistant strains of *Staphylococcus aureus* and enterococcus. Infect Control Hosp Epidemiol 2003;24:362–86.

38. Kluytmans JA, Mouton JW, VandenBergh MF, et al. Reduction of surgical-site infections in cardiothoracic surgery by elimination of nasal carriage of *Staphylococcus aureus*. Infect Control Hosp Epidemiol 1996;17:780–5.

39. Mekontso-Dessap A, Kirsch M, Brun-Buisson C, et al. Poststernotomy mediastinitis due to *Staphylococcus aureus*: comparison of methicillin-resistant and methicillin-susceptible cases. Clin Infect Dis 2001;32:877–83.

40. Perl TM, Cullen JJ, Wenzel RP, et al. Intranasal mupirocin to prevent postoperative *Staphylococcus aureus* infections. N Engl J Med 2002;346:1871–7.

41. Itani KM, Wilson SE, Awad SS, et al. Ertapenem versus cefotetan prophylaxis in elective colorectal surgery. N Engl J Med 2006;355:2640–51.

42. Siegel JD, Rhinehart E, Jackson M, et al. Management of multidrug-resistant organisms in health care settings, 2006. Am J Infect Control 2007;35:S165–93.

43. Evans HL, Lefrak SN, Lyman J, et al. Cost of gram-negative resistance. Crit Care Med 2007;35:89–95.

44. Raymond DP, Pelletier SJ, Crabtree TD, et al. Impact of antibiotic-resistant gram-negative bacilli infections on outcome in hospitalized patients. Crit Care Med 2003;31:1035–41.

45. Gleason TG, Crabtree TD, Pelletier SJ, et al. Prediction of poorer prognosis by infection with antibiotic-resistant gram-positive cocci than by infection with antibiotic-sensitive strains. Arch Surg 1999;134:1033–40.

46. Song X, Srinivasan A, Plaut D, et al. Effect of nosocomial vancomycin-resistant enterococcal bacteremia on mortality, length of stay, and costs. Infect Control Hosp Epidemiol 2003;24:251–6.

47. Cosgrove SE, Sakoulas G, Perencevich EN, et al. Comparison of mortality associated with methicillin-resistant and methicillin-susceptible *Staphylococcus aureus* bacteremia: a meta-analysis. Clin Infect Dis 2003;36:53–9.

48. Whitby M, McLaws ML, Berry G. Risk of death from methicillin-resistant *Staphylococcus aureus* bacteraemia: a meta-analysis. Med J Aust 2001;175:264–7.

49. Engemann JJ, Carmeli Y, Cosgrove SE, et al. Adverse clinical and economic outcomes attributable to methicillin resistance among patients with *Staphylococcus aureus* surgical site infection. Clin Infect Dis 2003;36:592–8.

50. Stephenson J. CDC campaign targets antimicrobial resistance in hospitals. JAMA 2002;287:2351–2.

51. Centers for Disease Control and Prevention. 12 steps to prevent antimicrobial resistance among hospitalized patients: campaign to prevent antimicrobial resistance. Available at: http://www.cdc.gov/drugresistance/healthcare/default.htm; 2002. Accessed August 28, 2008.

52. Brinsley K, Srinivasan A, Sinkowitz-Cochran R, et al. Implementation of the Campaign to prevent antimicrobial resistance in healthcare settings: 12 steps to prevent antimicrobial resistance among hospitalized adults–experiences from 3 institutions. Am J Infect Control 2005;33:53–4.

53. Cosgrove SE, Patel A, Song X, et al. Impact of different methods of feedback to clinicians after postprescription antimicrobial review based on the Centers For Disease Control and Prevention's 12 steps to prevent antimicrobial resistance among hospitalized adults. Infect Control Hosp Epidemiol 2007;28:641–6.

54. Raymond DP, Kuehnert MJ, Sawyer RG. Preventing antimicrobial-resistant bacterial infections in surgical patients. Surg Infect (Larchmt) 2002;3:375–85.

55. Boyce JM, Pittet D. Guideline for hand hygiene in health-care settings: recommendations of the Healthcare Infection Control Practices Advisory Committee and the HICPAC/SHEA/APIC/IDSA Hand Hygiene Task Force. Infect Control Hosp Epidemiol 2002;23:S3–40.

56. O'Grady NP, Alexander M, Dellinger EP, et al. Guidelines for the prevention of intravascular catheter-related infections. Infect Control Hosp Epidemiol 2002;23:759–69.

57. Pittet D, Hugonnet S, Harbarth S, et al. Effectiveness of a hospital-wide programme to improve compliance with hand hygiene. Infection Control Programme. Lancet 2000;356:1307–12.

58. Webster J, Faoagali JL, Cartwright D. Elimination of methicillin-resistant *Staphylococcus aureus* from a neonatal intensive care unit after hand washing with triclosan. J Paediatr Child Health 1994;30:59–64.

59. Zafar AB, Butler RC, Reese DJ, et al. Use of 0.3% triclosan (Bacti-Stat) to eradicate an outbreak of methicillin-resistant *Staphylococcus aureus* in a neonatal nursery. Am J Infect Control 1995;23:200–8.

60. Larson EL, Early E, Cloonan P, et al. An organizational climate intervention associated with increased handwashing and decreased nosocomial infections. Behav Med 2000;26:14–22.

61. Sax H, Allegranzi B, Uckay I, et al. My five moments for hand hygiene: a user-centred design approach to understand, train, monitor and report hand hygiene. J Hosp Infect 2007;67:9–21.

62. Weber SG, Huang SS, Oriola S, et al. Legislative mandates for use of active surveillance cultures to screen for methicillin-resistant *Staphylococcus aureus* and vancomycin-resistant enterococci: position statement from the Joint SHEA and APIC Task Force. Am J Infect Control 2007;35:73–85.

63. Harbarth S, Fankhauser C, Schrenzel J, et al. Universal screening for methicillin-resistant *Staphylococcus aureus* at hospital admission and nosocomial infection in surgical patients. JAMA 2008;299:1149–57.

64. McGinigle KL, Gourlay ML, Buchanan IB. The use of active surveillance cultures in adult intensive care units to reduce methicillin-resistant *Staphylococcus aureus*-related morbidity, mortality, and costs: a systematic review. Clin Infect Dis 2008;46:1717–25.

65. Miller MA, Dascal A, Portnoy J, et al. Development of mupirocin resistance among methicillin-resistant *Staphylococcus aureus* after widespread use of nasal mupirocin ointment. Infect Control Hosp Epidemiol 1996;17:811–3.

66. Walker ES, Vasquez JE, Dula R, et al. Mupirocin-resistant, methicillin-resistant *Staphylococcus aureus*: does mupirocin remain effective? Infect Control Hosp Epidemiol 2003;24:342–6.

67. Bleasdale SC, Trick WE, Gonzalez IM, et al. Effectiveness of chlorhexidine bathing to reduce catheter-associated bloodstream infections in medical intensive care unit patients. Arch Intern Med 2007;167:2073–9.

68. Borer A, Gilad J, Porat N, et al. Impact of 4% chlorhexidine whole-body washing on multidrug-resistant *Acinetobacter baumannii* skin colonisation among patients in a medical intensive care unit. J Hosp Infect 2007;67:149–55.

69. Evans HL, Chan J, Dellit TH, et al. Impact of 2% chlorhexidine whole body washing on nosocomial infections among trauma patients. Surg Infect (Larchmt) 2008;9:239–40 [abstract].

70. Vernon MO, Hayden MK, Trick WE, et al. Chlorhexidine gluconate to cleanse patients in a medical intensive care unit: the effectiveness of source control to reduce the bioburden of vancomycin-resistant enterococci. Arch Intern Med 2006;166:306–12.

71. MacDougall C, Polk RE. Antimicrobial stewardship programs in health care systems. Clin Microbiol Rev 2005;18:638–56.

72. Craig WA, Uman SJ, Shaw WR, et al. Hospital use of antimicrobial drugs: survey at 19 hospitals and results of antimicrobial control program. Ann Intern Med 1978;89:793–5.

73. McGowan JE Jr, Finland M. Usage of antibiotics in a general hospital: effect of requiring justification. J Infect Dis 1974;130:165–8.

74. Cannon JP, Silverman RM. A pharmacist-driven antimicrobial approval program at a Veterans Affairs hospital. Am J Health Syst Pharm 2003;60:1358–62.

75. White AC Jr, Atmar RL, Wilson J, et al. Effects of requiring prior authorization for selected antimicrobials: expenditures, susceptibilities, and clinical outcomes. Clin Infect Dis 1997;25:230–9.

76. LaRosa LA, Fishman NO, Lautenbach E, et al. Evaluation of antimicrobial therapy orders circumventing an antimicrobial stewardship program: investigating the strategy of stealth dosing. Infect Control Hosp Epidemiol 2007;28:551–6.

77. Linkin DR, Fishman NO, Landis JR, et al. Effect of communication errors during calls to an antimicrobial stewardship program. Infect Control Hosp Epidemiol 2007;28:1374–81.

78. Carling P, Fung T, Killion A, et al. Favorable impact of a multidisciplinary antibiotic management program conducted during 7 years. Infect Control Hosp Epidemiol 2003;24:699–706.

79. Goldmann DA, Weinstein RA, Wenzel RP, et al. Strategies to prevent and control the emergence and spread of antimicrobial-resistant microorganisms in hospitals: a challenge to hospital leadership. JAMA 1996;275:234–40.

80. Larson EL, Quiros D, Giblin T, et al. Relationship of antimicrobial control policies and hospital and infection control characteristics to antimicrobial resistance rates. Am J Crit Care 2007;16:110–20.

81. Quale J, Landman D, Saurina G, et al. Manipulation of a hospital antimicrobial formulary to control an outbreak of vancomycin-resistant enterococci. Clin Infect Dis 1996;23:1020–5.

82. Lan CK, Hsueh PR, Wong WW, et al. Association of antibiotic utilization measures and reduced incidence of infections with extended-spectrum beta-lactamase-producing organisms. J Microbiol Immunol Infect 2003;36:182–6.

83. Piroth L, Aube H, Doise JM, et al. Spread of extended-spectrum beta-lactamase-producing *Klebsiella pneumoniae*: are beta-lactamase inhibitors of therapeutic value? Clin Infect Dis 1998;27:76–80.

84. Rahal JJ, Urban C, Horn D, et al. Class restriction of cephalosporin use to control total cephalosporin resistance in nosocomial *Klebsiella*. JAMA 1998;280:1233–7.

85. Rice LB, Lakticova V, Helfand MS, et al. In vitro antienterococcal activity explains associations between exposures to antimicrobial agents and risk of colonization by multiresistant enterococci. J Infect Dis 2004;190:2162–6.

86. May AK, Melton SM, McGwin G, et al. Reduction of vancomycin-resistant enterococcal infections by limitation of broad-spectrum cephalosporin use in a trauma and burn intensive care unit. Shock 2000;14:259–64.

87. O'Connor KA, Kingston M, O'Donovan M, et al. Antibiotic prescribing policy and *Clostridium difficile* diarrhoea. QJM 2004;97:423–9.
88. Wilcox MH, Freeman J, Fawley W, et al. Long-term surveillance of cefotaxime and piperacillin-tazobactam prescribing and incidence of *Clostridium difficile* diarrhoea. J Antimicrob Chemother 2004;54:168–72.
89. Allegranzi B, Luzzati R, Luzzani A, et al. Impact of antibiotic changes in empirical therapy on antimicrobial resistance in intensive care unit-acquired infections. J Hosp Infect 2002;52:136–40.
90. Burke JP. Antibiotic resistance–squeezing the balloon? JAMA 1998;280:1270.
91. Zillich AJ, Sutherland JM, Wilson SJ, et al. Antimicrobial use control measures to prevent and control antimicrobial resistance in US hospitals. Infect Control Hosp Epidemiol 2006;27:1088–95.
92. Clinical and Laboratory Standards Institute. Performance standards for antimicrobial susceptibility testing: sixteenth informational supplement M100-S16; 2006.
93. Dellit TH, Owens RC, McGowan JE Jr, et al. Infectious Diseases Society of America and the Society for Healthcare Epidemiology of America guidelines for developing an institutional program to enhance antimicrobial stewardship. Clin Infect Dis 2007;44:159–77.
94. Sharp SE. Effective reporting of susceptibility test results. Diagn Microbiol Infect Dis 1993;16:251–4.
95. Steffee CH, Morrell RM, Wasilauskas BL. Clinical use of rifampicin during routine reporting of rifampicin susceptibilities: a lesson in selective reporting of antimicrobial susceptibility data. J Antimicrob Chemother 1997;40:595–8.
96. Langdale P, Millar MR. Influence of laboratory sensitivity reporting on antibiotic prescribing preferences of general practitioners in the Leeds area. J Clin Pathol 1986;39:233–4.
97. Tan TY, McNulty C, Charlett A, et al. Laboratory antibiotic susceptibility reporting and antibiotic prescribing in general practice. J Antimicrob Chemother 2003;51:379–84.
98. Barnes MP. Influence of laboratory reports on prescribing of antimicrobials for urinary tract infection. J Clin Pathol 1980;33:481–3.
99. Campo L, Mylotte JM. Use of microbiology reports by physicians in prescribing antimicrobial agents. Am J Med Sci 1988;296:392–8.
100. Cunney RJ, Smyth EG. The impact of laboratory reporting practice on antibiotic utilisation. Int J Antimicrob Agents 2000;14:13–9.
101. Morgan MS. Perceptions of a medical microbiology service: a survey of laboratory users. J Clin Pathol 1995;48:915–8.
102. Schentag JJ, Ballow CH, Fritz AL, et al. Changes in antimicrobial agent usage resulting from interactions among clinical pharmacy, the infectious disease division, and the microbiology laboratory. Diagn Microbiol Infect Dis 1993;16:255–64.
103. Calfee DP, Brooks J, Zirk NM, et al. A pseudo-outbreak of nosocomial infections associated with the introduction of an antibiotic management programme. J Hosp Infect 2003;55:26–32.
104. Richards MJ, Robertson MB, Dartnell JG, et al. Impact of a web-based antimicrobial approval system on broad-spectrum cephalosporin use at a teaching hospital. Med J Aust 2003;178:386–90.
105. Shojania KG, Yokoe D, Platt R, et al. Reducing vancomycin use utilizing a computer guideline: results of a randomized controlled trial. J Am Med Inform Assoc 1998;5:554–62.

106. Varonen H, Kortteisto T, Kaila M. What may help or hinder the implementation of computerized decision support systems (CDSSs): a focus group study with physicians. Fam Pract 2008;25:162–7.

107. Evans RS, Pestotnik SL, Classen DC, et al. A computer-assisted management program for antibiotics and other antiinfective agents. N Engl J Med 1998; 338:232–8.

108. Pestotnik SL, Classen DC, Evans RS, et al. Implementing antibiotic practice guidelines through computer-assisted decision support: clinical and financial outcomes. Ann Intern Med 1996;124:884–90.

109. Paul M, Andreassen S, Tacconelli E, et al. Improving empirical antibiotic treatment using TREAT, a computerized decision support system: cluster randomized trial. J Antimicrob Chemother 2006;58:1238–45.

110. Betts RF, Valenti WM, Chapman SW, et al. Five-year surveillance of aminoglycoside usage in a university hospital. Ann Intern Med 1984;100: 219–22.

111. Gerding DN, Larson TA. Aminoglycoside resistance in gram-negative bacilli during increased amikacin use. Comparison of experience in 14 United States hospitals with experience in the Minneapolis Veterans Administration Medical Center. Am J Med 1985;79:1–7.

112. Ruiz-Palacios GM, Ponce de Leon S, Sifuentes J, et al. Control of emergence of multi-resistant gram-negative bacilli by exclusive use of amikacin. Am J Med 1986;80:71–5.

113. Young EJ, Sewell CM, Koza MA, et al. Antibiotic resistance patterns during aminoglycoside restriction. Am J Med Sci 1985;290:223–7.

114. Gerding DN, Larson TA, Hughes RA, et al. Aminoglycoside resistance and aminoglycoside usage: ten years of experience in one hospital. Antimicrob Agents Chemother 1991;35:1284–90.

115. Kollef MH, Vlasnik J, Sharpless L, et al. Scheduled change of antibiotic classes: a strategy to decrease the incidence of ventilator-associated pneumonia. Am J Respir Crit Care Med 1997;156:1040–8.

116. Kollef MH, Ward S, Sherman G, et al. Inadequate treatment of nosocomial infections is associated with certain empiric antibiotic choices. Crit Care Med 2000; 28:3456–64.

117. Gruson D, Hilbert G, Vargas F, et al. Rotation and restricted use of antibiotics in a medical intensive care unit: impact on the incidence of ventilator-associated pneumonia caused by antibiotic-resistant gram-negative bacteria. Am J Respir Crit Care Med 2000;162:837–43.

118. Bergstrom CT, Lo M, Lipsitch M. Ecological theory suggests that antimicrobial cycling will not reduce antimicrobial resistance in hospitals. Proc Natl Acad Sci U S A 2004;101:13285–90.

119. Bonhoeffer S, Lipsitch M, Levin BR. Evaluating treatment protocols to prevent antibiotic resistance. Proc Natl Acad Sci U S A 1997;94:12106–11.

120. Lipsitch M, Bergstrom CT, Levin BR. The epidemiology of antibiotic resistance in hospitals: paradoxes and prescriptions. Proc Natl Acad Sci U S A 2000;97: 1938–43.

121. Raymond DP, Pelletier SJ, Crabtree TD, et al. Impact of a rotating empiric antibiotic schedule on infectious mortality in an intensive care unit. Crit Care Med 2001;29:1101–8.

122. Hughes MG, Evans HL, Chong TW, et al. Effect of an intensive care unit rotating empiric antibiotic schedule on the development of hospital-acquired infections on the non-intensive care unit ward. Crit Care Med 2004;32:53–60.

123. Allegranzi B, Gottin L, Bonora S, et al. Antibiotic rotation in intensive care units: its usefulness should be demonstrated without pitfalls. Crit Care Med 2002;30: 2170–1.

124. Paterson DL, Rice LB. Empirical antibiotic choice for the seriously ill patient: are minimization of selection of resistant organisms and maximization of individual outcome mutually exclusive? Clin Infect Dis 2003;36:1006–12.

125. Evans HL, Hughes MG, Chong TW, et al. Comparison of dual- versus single-antibiotic rotation strategies in an intensive care unit. Surg Infect 2002;3:45 [abstract].

126. Evans HL, Milburn ML, Hughes MG, et al. Nature of gram-negative rod antibiotic resistance during antibiotic rotation. Surg Infect 2005;6:223–31.

127. Martinez JA, Nicolas JM, Marco F, et al. Comparison of antimicrobial cycling and mixing strategies in two medical intensive care units. Crit Care Med 2006;34: 329–36.

128. Hedrick TL, Schulman AS, McElearney ST, et al. Outbreak of resistant *Pseudomonas aeruginosa* infections during a quarterly cycling antibiotic regimen. Surg Infect (Larchmt) 2008;9:139–52.

129. Warren DK, Hill HA, Merz LR, et al. Cycling empirical antimicrobial agents to prevent emergence of antimicrobial-resistant gram-negative bacteria among intensive care unit patients. Crit Care Med 2004;32:2450–6.

130. Barie PS, Hydo LJ, Shou J, et al. Influence of antibiotic therapy on mortality of critical surgical illness caused or complicated by infection. Surg Infect (Larchmt) 2005;6:41–54.

131. Bennett KM, Scarborough JE, Sharpe M, et al. Implementation of antibiotic 0rotation protocol improves antibiotic susceptibility profile in a surgical intensive care unit. J Trauma 2007;63:307–11.

132. Smith RL, Evans HL, Chong TW, et al. Reduction in rates of methicillin-resistant *Staphylococcus aureus* infection after introduction of quarterly linezolid-vancomycin cycling in a surgical intensive care unit. Surg Infect (Larchmt) 2008;9: 423–31.

A Systems Approach to the Prevention of Surgical Infections

Donald E. Fry, MD[a,b,c],*

KEYWORDS

- Surgical site infections • Postoperative urinary tract infection
- Catheter-associated bacteremia • Postoperative pneumonia
- *Clostridium difficile* enterocolitis

Infections continue to be the major source of morbidity and death following surgical care. These infections can be subdivided into those that occur at the surgical site (SSI) and those nosocomial infections remote from the surgical site, such as the lung and urinary tract. These infections are the consequence of the complex interaction of the bacterial colonization of the patient, the microbial species of the hospital environment, the breech of the sterile sanctity of selected body compartments by mechanical intervention, and the efficiency of the host defense. All are potentially preventable infections (PPIs).

The frequency, severity, and the economic cost of infections that complicate surgical care have become an increased focus of attention within the lay media and even in the political process. Infections from "super bugs" such as methicillin-resistant *Staphylococcus aureus* and *Clostridium difficile* have drawn considerable public attention. The lay public and politicians are demanding accountability on the parts of hospitals and surgeons to address prevention. The frequency of medicolegal actions where infectious events after operations are the foundation claim gives testimony to the public sensitivity on this issue. The Surgical Infection Prevention (SIP) project, the Surgical Care Improvement Project (SCIP), and governmental legislation and policy positions have evolved where infection in the surgical patient is a major issue.

Prevention of surgical infections has been attempted through exhaustive educational methods. The peer-reviewed and commercial literature has an abundance of information about prevention of infection in surgical patients. Symposia and focused in-service programs have emphasized behavioral changes that are necessary for prevention. Hospital policy and procedures are replete with detailed methodologies on

[a] Michael Pine and Associates, 5020 South Lake Shore Drive, #304N, Chicago, IL 60615, USA
[b] Northwestern University Feinberg School of Medicine, Chicago, IL, USA
[c] University of New Mexico School of Medicine, Albuquerque, NM, USA
* Correspondence address: Michael Pine and Associates, 5020 S. Lake Shore Dr., #304N, Chicago, IL 60615.
E-mail address: dfry@consultmpa.com

Surg Clin N Am 89 (2009) 521–537
doi:10.1016/j.suc.2008.09.010
0039-6109/08/$ – see front matter © 2009 Elsevier Inc. All rights reserved.

the prevention of infections after operations. Signage that encourages infection control practices within the hospital, and alcohol-rub dispensers at the entrance to patient rooms are likewise evidence of methods to modify practices that affect the frequency of infection.

Whereas educational programs may have transient success, bad habits inevitably reemerge with the consequence being that infections continue to occur at an alarming frequency after operations. Sustained success in the reduction of surgical infections may well be the failure of effective systems initiatives. We do not have consistent diagnostic criteria to say when infection has occurred. We do not have practical and efficient ways of identifying the incidence of the infectious events. We do not have real-time reporting of outcomes so that quality monitoring and quality improvement efforts can be objectively measured. Furthermore, there are no consequences for failed prevention because we do not know whether trends are improving, declining, or hopefully at least staying the same.

It will be the premise of this article that our hospitals and health care delivery units have as their principal responsibility the development of systems to provide accurate, reliable, and accountable methods for the identification of adverse infectious events that can and should be outcomes that are progressively declining in our patients. Accurate systems are necessary to measure the adverse outcome attributable to infection. Accountable systems are necessary to define the costs of complications in care. Systems are necessary to provide feedback information to fuel improvement. Systems are necessary to monitor the results of interventions to improve care. Systems must link rewards to quality outcomes and not just compliance with processes.

SURVEILLANCE AND COST OF POTENTIALLY PREVENTABLE INFECTIONS

In surgical care, infectious complications are identified as binomial events, ie, they either occurred or they did not occur. However, infections in the surgical patient can have highly variable degrees of severity. A wound infection may vary from a fairly innocent minimal amount of drainage from the inferior aspect of a midline wound, to severe fascial necrosis and abdominal evisceration. Pneumonia can be an area of extended atelectasis on a chest radiograph with very minimal symptoms, or it may be a catastrophic event resulting in ventilator dependence for the patient. This variability in the severity and consequences of infection has serious implications about the rigor of the surveillance process. In the following discussions about the costs of postoperative infections, it should be understood that there is a continuum of different severity of infections within each category, and that commonly data presented on the subject is referring to a heterogeneous mix.

Surgical Site Infection

The National Nosocomial Infections Surveillance (NNIS) program identified an overall SSI rate of 2.6% from its participating hospitals that voluntarily reported outcomes.[1] More recent reports have abandoned efforts to identify a national rate of SSI but rather have focused on the identification of reported rates by procedure and by NNIS risk category.[2] **Table 1** provides a summary of the SSIs reported to NNIS by participating hospitals from January 1992 through June 2004. The NNIS risk system adds one risk point for contaminated and dirty operations, one point for American Society of Anesthesiology scores of 3 or higher, and one point for operations that go beyond the 75th percentile (cut point) of that procedure in duration. Although not a complete risk adjustment of the risk factors in SSI, this NNIS risk score has been an easily used method

Table 1
The rate of surgical site infections by selected procedures as a function of the National Nosocomial Infections Surveillance risk category

Procedure	Risk Index 0	Risk Index 1	Risk Index 2	Risk Index 3
Coronary artery bypass graft: chest and donor site	0.49	3.17	5.16	NR
Colon resection	3.22	5.1	9.09	13.33
Gastric surgery	2.58	4.21	7.27	*
Small bowel surgery	4.77	5.9	7.52	NR
Herniorraphy	0.8	1.92	3.82	NR
Craniotomy	0	1.04	1.3	*
Cesarean section	2.17	3.19	5.38	*
Abdominal hysterectomy	0.91	1.96	4.21	*
Spinal fusion	0.68	2.16	4.78	*
Hip prosthesis	0.5	1.41	2.06	*
Knee prosthesis	0.66	1.09	2.04	*
Vascular surgery	0	1.54	4.79	*

The rate of infection is the rate reported by the median (50th percentile) reporting hospital.
Abbreviation: NR, not reported.
* Risk Index for groups 2 and 3 are merged together.

to stratify patients. **Table 1** identifies that different operations have different rates of SSI, and that the frequency increases as the risk score increases.

A large number of studies of different populations of patients have identified increased costs and prolonged hospitalizations, although the accuracy and variability of methodologies makes accurate cost accounting difficult.[3] Kirkland and colleagues[4] examined a large number of patients with SSIs from multiple, high-volume procedures to analyze the cost impact. They identified patients with SSIs and then identified control patients who were matched with respect to age, procedure, NNIS risk score, date of the operation, and the surgeon. They identified that SSIs in all categories studied resulted in 4- to 22-day increases in median length of hospital stay, and $4000 to $10,000 increases in total direct costs per case.

Zoutman and colleagues[5] similarly studied a diverse group of 108 patients with SSI following both clean and clean-contaminated operations. In 26 patients, the diagnosis was not made until after discharge and none of these patients required rehospitalization. In 22 patients, a total of 28 reoperations were required for management of the SSI. Among the 82 patients with inpatient care for SSI, a total of 10 extra hospital days were required at an extra cost of nearly $4000 per case. Similar studies from Scotland,[6] Denmark,[7] Finland,[8] and Spain[9] have underscored that SSIs from a mixed population of surgical patients leads to extended length of stay and increased hospital costs.

There are special circumstances that enhance the morbidity and the costs associated with surgical site infections. McGarry and colleagues[10] noted increased postoperative hospital days, increased hospital costs, and increased mortality rates among elderly patients with SSIs, especially when *Staphylococcus aureus* was the pathogen. Olsen and colleagues[11] identified an added risk to the frequency and cost of SSI in breast surgery for cancer as opposed to similar operations for benign indications. Infection of the sternal wound, particularly when associated with dehiscence and mediastinitis, is an especially severe SSI both in terms of cost and mortality rates.[12,13] While infections of total hip and joint prostheses are fortunately uncommon events, infection of the prosthesis entails extreme costs, potential amputations, and even deaths.[14–16] Vascular graft infections are yet another very morbid condition that may not be declared for many months after placement.[17] Delayed disruption of the arterial anastomosis and pseudoaneurysm are events that represent special complications in addition to the costs and lengthy hospitalization ordinarily associated with SSI.

Because the surveillance and identification of postdischarge SSIs is fraught with numerous difficulties, it is likely that the rate of SSIs for each procedure is greater than what has been reported. Kobayashi and colleagues[18] noted a 17% SSI rate for elective colorectal surgical patients when 30 days of postoperative surveillance was conducted, but only 5% SSI during the actual hospitalization. Reilly and colleagues[19] noted that operations with relatively short hospital length of stay, such as breast surgery and hysterectomy, were particularly underestimated without dedicated postdischarge surveillance. Avato and Lai[20] identified that 72% of SSIs following coronary artery bypass surgery were identified following discharge. Chest infections were more common during the hospitalization, and donor site infections were most common after discharge. Finally, Huotari and colleagues[21] noted that questionnaires were suboptimal in the identification of SSI following discharge and that direct follow-up observation was necessary.

When viewing the entire literature on the incidence and cost, it is apparent that the actual rate of SSI is highly variable depending on the intensity of the surveillance process, and that costs have principally been tabulated on the most severe of cases. Most cost studies have focused only on inpatient costs at the time of hospitalization for the index operation, and that little information is available to identify the cost profile of rehospitalization, postdischarge outpatient expenses, or long-term associated events such as ventral hernia. It can be said with confidence that reductions in the rate of SSIs will reduce health care costs.

Postoperative Pneumonia

Not unlike SSIs, postoperative pneumonia has a spectrum of severity. Some infections associated with atelectasis in favorable risk patients can be treated with pulmonary toilet and oral antibiotics, and may represent only a modest cost. Ventilator-associated pneumonia is a severe and life-threatening event that leads to prolonged hospitalization and considerable preventable expense.

Table 2 identifies the reported rates of ventilator-associated pneumonia of the surgical areas of the hospital in the National Healthcare Safety Network (NHSN),[22] which is an Internet-based surveillance system at the Centers for Disease Control and Prevention (CDC) that replaced NNIS in 2005.[23] From these data, it can be identified that 40% of specialty unit/intensive care unit days result in patients being on the ventilator. Ventilator-associated infection occurred about five times for every 1000 days of ventilator support.

Ventilator and surgical intensive care unit (SICU)-associated pneumonia is consistently found to increase length of stay, increase mortality rates, and increase health care costs. Khan and colleagues[24] studied more than 7000 noncardiac surgical patients over a 21-month period of time and identified a 3% incidence of postoperative pneumonia that resulted in a 75% increase in postoperative length of stay and a 55% increase in hospital costs. Thompson and colleagues[25] studied more than 600,000 intra-abdominal surgery patients from the National Inpatient Sample of the Health Care Cost and Utilization Project. They identified postoperative pneumonia significantly increased the mortality rate to 10.7% from 1.2% among patients without

Table 2
Frequency of ventilator-associated infections from hospital sites likely to be for postoperative surgical patients

Hospital Location	No. Cases	Days on Ventilator	Infections/1000 Ventilator Days	Location-specific Hospital Days	Percentage of Hospital Days on Ventilator
Burn unit	124	10,098	12.3	24,067	42%
Cardiothoracic surgery ICU	265	46,710	5.7	115,199	41%
Medical/Surgical ICU	674	220,076	3.1	598,328	37%
Surgical ICU	384	73,205	5.2	176,695	41%
Neurosurgery ICU	97	13,799	7.0	32,632	42%
Trauma ICU	329	32,297	10.2	56,251	57%
Total	1873	396,185	4.7	1,002,902	40%

Data from Edwards JR, Peterson KD, Andrus ML, et al. National Healthcare Safety Network (NHSN) report, data summary for 2006, issued June 2007. Am J Infect Control 2007;35:290–301.

pneumonia. The postoperative length of stay was increased by 11 days and hospital charges were increased by 75%. Collins and colleagues[26] identified postoperative pneumonia as a major contributor to increased length of stay, particularly following elective colon and aortic aneurysm surgery in a Veterans Administration study, and Penel and colleagues[27] identified a 17-day increase in length of stay and a 19,000 euro increased cost for postoperative pneumonia in head and neck cancer patients. Multidrug-resistant bacteria (eg, *Acinetobacter baumannii*) in pneumonia have been identified with a 13-day excess length of stay and greater than $60,000 excess hospital charges in SICU patients.[28] Hyperglycemia was identified with increased rates of postoperative pneumonia in cardiac surgical patients with increase length of stay and costs.[29]

Urinary Tract Infection (UTI)

Catheter-associated urinary tract infections (CA-UTI) are bacteriologically common events in postoperative patients, but whether they are clinically relevant infections in many cases remains unclear. Using the traditional criteria of a positive urine culture of more than 10^5 organisms/mL of urine, this author reported 20 years ago that positive cultures from the urine commonly were not the cause of the patients' fever or leukocytosis, and that many of the patients cleared the bacteriuria either without antibiotics or with antibiotics to which the cultured organism was resistant.[30] Recently, Golob and colleagues[31] identified that positive urine cultures were not responsible for the fever and leukocytosis seen in trauma patients. It should be emphasized that the traditional culture threshold for establishing a diagnosis of UTI was established by Kass[32] 50 years ago but in community-acquired cystitis. The extrapolation of a very useful diagnostic method in community-acquired cystitis to the CA-UTI of an SICU patient is accepted but not necessarily proven.

Table 3 summarizes the CA-UTIs that were reported by NHSN for 2006 by hospital location for surgical patients. About 80% of SICU days had the presence of the urinary catheter. Positive cultures were obtained in about four patients for every 1000 days of SICU stay. Nearly 40% of positive cultures were considered to be asymptomatic. The morbidity and economic consequences of the CA-UTI appear to be modest at best. Laupland and colleagues[33] studied over 4000 ICU patients and concluded that

Table 3
Frequency of nosocomial urinary catheter–associated infections among reported patients from hospital sites likely to be for postoperative surgical patients

Hospital Location	No. Cases	Days with Catheter	Infections/1000 Catheter Days	Location Specific Hospital Days	Percentage of Hospital Days with Catheter
Burn unit	96	12,860	7.5	18,704	69%
Cardiothoracic surgery ICU	262	70,221	3.7	87,976	80%
Medical/Surgical ICU	1147	353,531	3.2	495,863	71%
Surgical ICU	509	126,887	4.0	155,557	82%
Neurosurgery ICU	171	26,253	6.5	31,530	83%
Trauma ICU	283	51,027	5.5	56,166	91%
Medical/Surgical Ward	87	23,416	3.7	102,014	23%
Total	2555	664,195	3.8	1,020,014	65%

Data from Edwards JR, Peterson KD, Andrus ML, et al. National Healthcare Safety Network (NHSN) report, data summary for 2006, issued June 2007. Am J Infect Control 2007;35:290–301.

CA-UTI could not be established as an independent variable in contributing to postoperative deaths. Clec'h and colleagues[34] similarly found no contribution of the CA-UTI to death in ICU patients. Tambyah and colleagues[35] studied the direct costs associated with CA-UTI in 235 patients with positive cultures, most of which were asymptomatic and only one of which was associated with bacteremia. Attributable costs from the CA-UTI were $589 per patient. In a multi-hospital study of hospital-acquired infections, Anderson and colleagues[36] found attributable cost estimates of $25,000 for each ventilator-associated pneumonia, $23,000 for nosocomial blood stream infections, and over $10,000 for SSIs, but only $758 was identified for each CA-UTI.

The magnitude of morbidity and cost of CA-UTI remains unclear at this point. It is likely that significant infections do occur, but that many cultures are done simply as a routine after a period of catheterization and are not cost-effective in the management of the patient.[37] Further refinements in the diagnosis and assessment of the economic impact of the infections that are presumed to occur with urinary bladder catheterization are necessary.

Intravascular Device Bacteremia

Bacteremia from indwelling lines and catheters in surgical patients represents a complication that is most commonly associated with central lines. While much of this discussion will focus on those bacteremic events from central lines, it should be emphasized that peripheral catheters, arterial lines, pacemaker wires, and any other device that represents access from the external environment into the intravascular compartment can be a portal of entry.[38]

Table 4 details the national sample of central line–associated blood stream infections (CL-BSI) occurring at sites in the hospital for surgical patients in 2006. These nosocomial infections appear to occur less frequently than ventilator-associated pneumonia for CA-UTI when indexed to days at risk for the device used, with a rate of 2.5 cases per 1000 central line days. Infections are most commonly with hospital-acquired bacteria such as methicillin-resistant *Staphylococcus aureus,* multidrug-resistant gram-negative bacteria, and fungal species. Surgical patients have been identified as having higher rates of these infections.[39] Metastatic infections to remote sites (eg, heart valves) is yet an additional adverse consequence.

Table 4
Frequency of central line–associated blood stream infections among reported patients from hospital sites likely to be for postoperative surgical patients

Hospital Location	No. Cases	Days with Central Line	Infections/1000 Line Days	Location Specific Hospital Days	Percentage of Hospital Days with Line
Burn unit	127	18,612	6.8	29,007	64%
Cardiothoracic surgery ICU	150	92,484	1.6	127,333	73%
Medical/Surgical ICU	735	327,053	2.2	631,306	52%
Surgical ICU	378	137,484	2.7	222,459	62%
Neurosurgery ICU	75	21,412	3.5	44,364	48%
Trauma ICU	182	39,635	4.6	61,176	65%
Medical/Surgical Ward	58	38,340	1.5	163,510	23%
Total	1705	674,725	2.5	1,279,155	53%

Data from Edwards JR, Peterson KD, Andrus ML, et al. National Healthcare Safety Network (NHSN) report, data summary for 2006, issued June 2007. Am J Infect Control 2007;35:290–301.

The morbidity and economic consequences of CL-BSI are quite significant. In 1994, Pittet and colleagues[40] studied catheter-associated bloodstream infections in surgical patients. A total of 86 patients with matched controls demonstrated a 35% increase (actual rate = 50%) in mortality rate, a 16-day increase in hospitalization, and an average of $40,000 of cost attributable to the infection. Warren and colleagues[41] studied 41 patients with catheter-associated bloodstream infections and found direct attributable increased length of stay of 7.5 days and increased costs of nearly $12,000. Mortality rate was 51% for the bloodstream infection group compared with 28% in the matched control patients. Shannon and colleagues[42] studied 54 of these cases among intensive and coronary care patients. CL-BSI was associated with a mean hospital stay of 34 days and a 41% mortality rate. Each patient had a 43% increase in hospital costs with operational hospital losses computed at more than $26,000 per case.

Despite efforts to reduce the frequency of catheter and central line–associated bloodstream infections, the recognized rate of these infections has not changed. Considerable efforts have been made to reduce infections by maximal barrier precautions and infection control practices during central line placement.[43] It is likely that infections occur more frequently than observed since positive blood cultures in critically ill patients may inconsistently recover the pathogen because of concomitant antibiotic therapy and because of the episodic nature of the bacteremia from the intravascular device.

Clostridium difficile Enterocolitis

Enterocolitis secondary to *Clostridium difficile* is increasing in severity and frequency in US hospitals. While methicillin-resistant *Staphylococcus aureus* has become a serious infectious complication in SSIs, postoperative pneumonia, and intravascular device infections, the frequency of *C difficile* among hospitalized patients is pursuing an ominously similar growth rate (**Fig. 1**). The trends of the past 6 years would indicate that an incidence of *C difficile* (CD) infection is approaching 1% of all hospitalizations.

In 1998,[44] Spencer reviewed the literature at that time and found a highly variable cost profile for CD infection, noting that greater expense and prolonged length of stay tended to be associated with increasing age of the patient. An expense of £4000 and 20 days of extended hospitalization was identified in that English study.

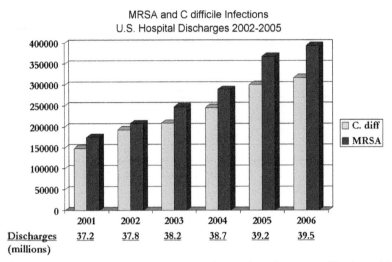

MRSA and C difficile Infections
U.S. Hospital Discharges 2002-2005

Discharges (millions): 2001 — 37.2, 2002 — 37.8, 2003 — 38.2, 2004 — 38.7, 2005 — 39.2, 2006 — 39.5

Fig. 1. The progressive increase in the primary and secondary diagnoses of both methicillin-resistant *Staphylococcus aureus* (MRSA) and *Clostridium difficile* infections in the United States over the past 6 years. (*Data from* Agency for Health Care Research and Quality, National Inpatient Sample; HCUPnet. Available at: http://hcupnet.ahrq.gov/.)

Miller and colleagues[45] studied 269 CD infections and found prolonged hospitalization, a greater than 1% mortality rate directly attributable to the infection, and a 7% readmission rate for hospital-acquired infection. They identified an added cost for readmission of about $13,000 (Canadian) per case. Kyne and colleagues[46] prospectively studied patients developing CD infection during hospitalizations for the treatment of other site infections and found nearly a 4-day extension of hospitalization and increased hospital costs of nearly $3700. Vonberg and colleagues[47] used a 3:1 ratio of matched controls for 45 CD patients in Germany and identified an increased cost of over €7000 per infected patient and had a median prolonged hospitalization of an additional 7 days. Zerey and colleagues[48] used a large administrative claims database and studied over 8000 CD infections occurring in patients after a general surgical procedure. They found CD infection resulted in a 16-day increase in hospitalization, and higher total hospital charges of $77,000. CD infection was an independent predictor of increased postoperative death rate (odds ratio = 3.37).

GOVERNMENT INITIATIVES

From the preceding discussion, it is apparent that infections in the surgical patient are extracting a large measure of morbidity and economic cost. Despite a constant amount of discussion about better prevention strategies in the literature, rates of infections continue with only modest improvement and the economic costs of infectious complications continue. It could only be anticipated that government intervention into the situation would evolve.

The Surgical Infection Prevention (SIP) project was initially launched as a joint effort between the CDC and the Centers for Medicare and Medicaid Services (CMS) to reduce preventable SSIs. The strategy was simply to get clinicians and hospitals to consistently apply the processes and methods that have been shown to prevent SSIs. National experts were convened representing the surgical society stakeholders.

Evidence-based performance measures were drafted. Data were accumulated that documented that compliance was a problem with established principles.[49] Papers were published.[50,51] Educational collaboratives were organized at the state level through the Quality Improvement Organizations (QIOs) of CMS, and a concerted effort was made to bring compliance to the nationally derived performance measures. The 1-year follow-up to this effort has demonstrated measurable improvement in compliance, but more importantly, evidence of improved rates of SSIs.[52]

The SIP project has now transitioned to the Surgical Care Improvement Project (SCIP).[53] With SCIP, the number of performance measures has been increased from the three measures governing systemic preventive antibiotic use to include removal of hair at the surgical site, glycemic control in open heart surgery, and temperature control during colon surgery. Additional "bundles" were added to the prevention of SSIs, which include deep venous thrombophlebitis (DVT)/pulmonary embolism prevention, prevention of postoperative cardiac events, and the prevention of postoperative pneumonia. It is likely that additional process measures will be added. Some discussion is focusing on reporting of outcome measures to include rates of SSI and DVT/pulmonary embolism.

Federal legislation entered into the arena of health care performance measures in 2003 with the Medicare Modernization Act.[54] Although best known for the creation of Part D of Medicare for prescription drug benefits, this legislation introduced 10 performance measures covering acute myocardial infarction, congestive heart failure, and community-acquired pneumonia that hospitals were to start reporting to CMS. The performance of the hospital was to be "voluntarily" reported or the hospital would sustain a 0.4% penalty in their annual Medicare payment update. Compliance with the reporting requirement was robust.

This led to the Deficit Reduction Act of 2005 that expanded the number of measures to be reported to 21 and the penalty for nonreporting was increased to 2% of the annual Medicare update payment.[55] Included in this legislation were the three original performance measures for the use of preventive antibiotics in surgery by SIP and SCIP. The number of measures that are being reported is increasing, and the results are publicly posted.[56] As of October 1, 2008, the number of National Hospital Performance Measures to be reported will be over 40. In addition to the three performance measures for the use of preventive antibiotics, additional measures for the prevention of surgical site infection will include proper hair removal at the surgical site, glycemic control in cardiac surgery, and normothermia in colorectal surgery.[57] It can only be anticipated that the number of measures will increase, and that there will be a progressive transition to outcomes reporting in addition to the reporting of process measures.

Yet another important part of the Deficit Reduction Act of 2005 was that the Secretary of Health and Human Services was directed to begin phasing out Medicare payments for complications of care. **Box 1**[58] lists the eight conditions that are scheduled to not receive supplemental payments by CMS beginning October 1, 2008. In addition, nine additional conditions are listed that are proposed for nonpayment beginning in 2009. Hospital-acquired infections in surgical patients represent a major component of the complications for which payments are to be denied.

These prior legislative actions have been directed at hospital reporting. The Tax Relief and Health Care Act–Medicare Improvements and Extension Act of 2006 have now introduced expectations of physician reporting of quality measures.[59] This act created the Physician Quality Reporting Initiative (PQRI) that was begun in 2007. Some 74 quality measures were to be reported on a voluntary basis by a claims-based submission method. About 100,000 (about 16%) of eligible physicians participated in the initial 6-month reporting period, and nearly 57,000 received the 1.5% bonus ($36

Box 1
The diagnoses for which CMS will not make supplemental payments effective October 1, 2008 (List A), and those additional diagnoses that are similarly proposed for nonpayment status in 2009 (List B)

List A

- Catheter-associated urinary tract infections
- Pressure ulcers (decubitus ulcers)
- Vascular catheter-associated infections
- Mediastinitis after coronary artery bypass graft surgery
- Fractures, dislocations, and other hospital-acquired injuries
- Objects left in during surgery
- Air embolisms
- Blood incompatibilities

List B

- Elective surgical site infections

  Total knee replacement

  Lap gastric bypass/lap gastroenterostomy

  Ligation and stripping of varicose veins

- Legionnaires' disease
- Extreme blood sugar derangement
- Iatrogenic pneumothorax
- Delirium
- Ventilator-associated pneumonia
- Deep vein thrombosis/pulmonary embolism
- *Staphylococcus aureus* septicemia
- *Clostridium difficile*-associated infection

---

million)[60] for correctly reporting the information. The program was extended into 2008 with the number of final quality measures for reporting being expanded to 119. The 1.5% Medicare bonus for correctly reporting the information was extended into 2008. However, for 2009 the number of measures is further expanded and measures are being aggregated into "measures groups" for reporting.[61] It is likely that the number of measures will continue to grow, but it is uncertain whether "voluntary" reporting will continue or whether mandatory participation for payment will become the standard.

A SYSTEMS APPROACH

From the foregoing discussion, it should be apparent that infections that are associated with surgical care are an all-to-frequent event. The biggest testimony to the inadequacy of our professional response is the fact that the federal government is passing legislation that requires the reporting of hospital events down to the level of hair removal at the surgical site before the incision is made, and refusal of payment for specific complications. It can only be anticipated that if the practicing community does not take the leadership in new directions of infection control, then the federal government will.

Are the problems of infection control because providers are unwilling or unable to execute the necessary behaviors? Or are there systems within our hospitals and ambulatory surgical facilities that are defective? Can a better organizational structure for the identification and evaluation of infectious events result in improvement? While blaming the "system" for failures can be a form of denial of personal responsibility, a systems approach can provide significant value when implemented in an environment where clinicians are dedicated to improvement.

A systems approach requires the understanding of the complexity of the health care environment where surgical care is delivered. There are many people and many clinical services that are involved in each case. Each component of this interaction views that they are doing their specific part in the care of the patient in a precise and accurate fashion, and yet bad outcomes are still the result. The answer to many of the outcome dilemmas of the present environment rests with the complex interactions of the component parts, and not whether individuals performed their specific tasks correctly. The complexity is beyond detailed policies and procedures. The number of different interactions between people and departments are so large that it becomes very difficult to design an analytic process for correct and proper behavior. A more efficient system is required to identify the adverse events in the health care environment, and an effective process by which adverse events can be evaluated. We must take a chapter from the industrial quality control book and design systems to measure what our results are, apply continuous quality improvement strategies based on the analysis of defective outcomes, and carefully measure the impact of our interventions.

Information Technology

Information technology in health care within the United States is grossly deficient compared with other industries. Indeed, the penetration of information technology in health care in the United States lags far behind other world health care systems.[61] Paper documentation continues unabated in our hospitals and in our physician offices. Handwritten prescriptions continue as a source of medical error despite the electronic capacity to solve this issue, and has now resulted in yet another government program to give 2% Medicare bonuses to physicians that use electronic prescribing.[62]

While much of the discussion about information technology has appropriately revolved around electronic medical records, a real shortfall in the system is real-time outcome measures of care. In no area is this deficiency felt more acutely than in infection control and surveillance. A major impediment to a meaningful continuous improvement strategy is that each of our hospitals really does not know what the results of care happen to be, and what the "significant" infection rates happen to be. Without a continuous and real-time monitoring system for all adverse outcomes, a meaningful strategy for evaluation and corrective interventions cannot happen. Without a functional scoreboard, how can the players know whether they are winning or losing the game?

In the earlier discussion of individual infections, it was identified that rates of infection are reported very differently by different sources, and that it is clear that the severity of infectious complications occurs across a very broad continuum. SSIs may be trivial or catastrophic. Pneumonia may be a limited consolidation on chest x-ray or may be a ventilator-dependent disaster with a high mortality rate. CA-UTI may not be an infection at all. Hiring surveillance personnel proves to be expensive, commonly results in the recognition of events that are of little or any consequence, and does not have an effective means of tracking postdischarge events.

A unifying concept of an *adverse surgical event* is needed. It is proposed that an adverse surgical event occurs when one of three clearly measurable events occurs: (1) patient death, (2) excess postoperative length of stay, and (3) readmission or re-intervention following discharge for events related to the index surgical episode of care. Overall adverse outcomes can be tracked over time for the institution and for each provider. Identified adverse events then have focused review and the basis for the outcome is determined. Events can then be classified into complication categories (eg, infection, cardiovascular, anesthesia, technical error) for critical evaluation.

The critical foundation for the unifying concept of the adverse surgical event is tracking the entire episode of care. Postdischarge deaths and re-admissions need to be traceable. Current systems do not have this capacity. This means that the "system" for a true paradigm of quality and identification of outcomes needs to be one where hospitals, physicians, and insurers have an electronic-linked network that captures the full outcomes of an appropriate temporal interval following discharge (eg, 90 days). While many seasoned veterans of the health care wars over the years will say that this is not achievable, it must happen to get an accurate measure of outcomes. Without postdischarge information, which is very recoverable from the administrative claims of the insurer, a true cost and quality profile of the episode of care cannot be identified.

The control chart has been a method endorsed by the Joint Commission for the Accreditation of Hospital Organizations (JCAHO) for quality improvement in hospitals.[63] The XmR control chart is a method that allows the real-time identification of cases that are risk-adjusted, length-of-stay outliers for purposes of defining an important parameter of the adverse surgical event. The expected risk-adjusted length of stay (from a risk equation) is subtracted from the observed length of stay (O − E), and sequential cases are mapped as identified in **Fig. 2**. The absolute differences between each temporally paired O − E observation is calculated, and an average moving range (XmR) is

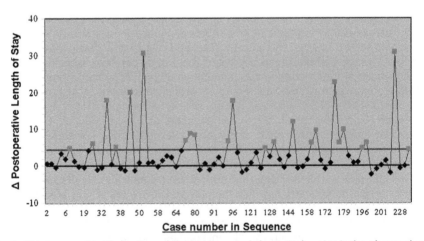

Fig. 2. This is a graphic illustration of the XmR control chart. Each point is the observed minus the predicted postoperative length of stay (vertical axis) for each patient in the sequence (horizontal axis). The lower line running parallel to the horizontal axis represents the absolute mean of differences between each sequential observation in the series. The upper parallel line represents the upper threshold or 2.66 times the absolute mean. Those absolute differences that exceed the upper threshold are outliers, and represent adverse outcomes for that hospital admission.

determined as the mean of all absolute differences. An upper threshold of 2.66 times the XmR defines the threshold of a length-of-stay outlier. This threshold can be determined from a prior year's experience, and outlier events can be determined for each patient at the conclusion of each hospitalization. The only reason for articulating the detail of the control chart is to demonstrate that effective information technology systems allow sophisticated methods to be designed to capture adverse surgical events and to set the stage for analysis and formulation of focused corrective strategies. Good information systems and honest coding practices allow hybrid databases to be designed that can integrate clinical information with administrative claims to provide outcomes and cost data to drive behavioral change.[64,65] The foundation for a valid systems initiative to address the prevention of infection is to have comprehensive information technology that can provide a current and accurate measure of clinical outcomes.

Analysis of Adverse Outcomes

Complexity surrounding adverse events is because the patient becomes the focal point for multiple interactions in the hospital. When attempting to define the trends of adverse events, or the analysis of a single particularly severe event, then it becomes important to have all of the players in the complex interaction involved in the process. Involvement gives them a stake in the ownership of the process and its results. The review of adverse events needs to be a free-standing group (The Surgical Infection Control Committee), independent of the traditional educational conferences used for teaching purposes. When infectious events are extracting a toll of millions of dollars of preventable cost within a hospital, not to mention pain and suffering, then a committed group(s) to be actively involved in this process is essential. In large facilities, separate review groups may be desirable by specialty. The group for a given large program (eg, cardiac surgery, total joint surgery) would have surgical representatives, nursing, anesthesiology, pharmacy, administration, and a standing infectious disease consultant.

The spirit of the deliberations should be for improvement for future outcomes, and not assignment of blame or fault. In analyses that the author has done, the surgical adverse outcome rates (ie, deaths plus length-of-stay outliers) will approach 10% for elective cardiac surgery and colon resections.[66] There will be plenty of events that will inevitably involve all members of the surgical staff. Priorities in the process will require establishing those events that occur most commonly, or have the greatest patient or economic impact.

When examining groups of adverse outcome cases of a common type, it is important to not be satisfied with a single event being responsible for the outcomes in question. C difficile infection may appropriately be linked to antibiotic use practices, but the source of the spore and issues of hand hygiene will clearly deserve attention as well. Infectious events across a number of patients will commonly have a number of causes. Outlier events are not just an opportunity to address the specific case, but represent a chance to impact the baseline rate of that complication.

The data generated by capturing adverse events and the efforts to initiate corrective action should be disseminated to the interested parties in the hospital. The Hawthorne effect is real and has been identified in health care as well as in industry. When it is understood that adverse events are being actively surveyed and reviewed, there will be an obligatory improvement. Sustained improvement will require a continued distribution about actions to be taken, behavioral practices to be modified, and dissemination of the current level of performance indexed to prior time intervals.

In summary, this discussion offers the premise that the systems approach for prevention of surgical infections requires a systems commitment. That commitment is to both improved information technology and to multidisciplinary representation for the analysis and interpretation of variables responsible for infection. A systems commitment does not mean an increased volume of policies and procedures, but a commitment of resources and people to obtain the evidence about outcomes, and a commitment to interventions to change results. While many will argue that the costs of this proposal are excessive, the reality is that the costs of infection in the surgical patient are already too great. Significant improvement in outcomes will justify the investment in prevention.

REFERENCES

1. Mangram AJ, Horan TC, Pearson ML, et al. Guideline for prevention of surgical site infection, 1999. Infect Control Hosp Epidemiol 1999;20:247–78.
2. Centers for Disease Control and Prevention. National Nosocomial Infections Surveillance (NNIS) system report, data summary from January 1992 through June 2004, issued October 2004. Am J Infect Control 2004;32:470–85.
3. Yasunaga H, Ide H, Imamura T, et al. Accuracy of economic studies on surgical site infection. J Hosp Infect 2007;65:102–7.
4. Kirkland KB, Briggs JP, Trivette SL, et al. The impact of surgical-site infections in the 1990s: attributable mortality, excess length of hospitalization, and extra costs. Infect Control Hosp Epidemiol 1999;20:725–30.
5. Zoutman D, McDonald S, Vethanayagan D. Total and attributable costs of surgical-wound infections at a Canadian tertiary-care center. Infect Control Hosp Epidemiol 1998;19:254–9.
6. Reilly J, Twaddle S, McIntosh J, et al. An economic analysis of surgical wound infection. J Hosp Infect 2001;49:245–9.
7. Poulsen KB, Bremmelgaard A, Sorensen AI, et al. Estimated costs of postoperative wound infections: a case-control study of marginal hospital and social security costs. Epidemiol Infect 1994;113:283–95.
8. Hyryla ML, Sintonen H. The use of health services in the management of wound infection. J Hosp Infect 1994;26:1–14.
9. Fernandez AM, Herruzo Cabrera R, Gomez-Sancha F, et al. Economical saving due to prophylaxis in the prevention of surgical wound infection. Eur J Epidemiol 1996;12:455–9.
10. McGarry SA, Engemann JJ, Schmader K, et al. Surgical-site infection due to Staphylococcus aureus among elderly patients: mortality, duration of hospitalization, and cost. Infect Control Hosp Epidemiol 2004;25:461–7.
11. Olsen MA, Chu-Ongsakul S, Brandt K, et al. Hospital-associated costs due to surgical site infection after breast surgery. Arch Surg 2008;143:53–60.
12. Hollenbeak CS, Murphy DM, Koenig S, et al. The clinical and economic impact of deep chest surgical site infections following coronary artery bypass graft surgery. Chest 2000;118:397–402.
13. Hollenbeak CS, Murphy D, Dunagan WC, et al. Nonrandom selection and the attributable cost of surgical-site infections. Infect Control Hosp Epidemiol 2002;23: 177–82.
14. Whitehouse JD, Friedman D, Kirkland KB, et al. The impact of surgical-site infections following orthopedic surgery at a community hospital and a university hospital: adverse quality of life, excess length of stay, and extra cost. Infect Control Hosp Epidemiol 2002;23:183–9.

15. Sculco TP. The economic impact of infected total joint arthroplasty. Instr Course Lect 1993;42:349–51.
16. Hebert CK, Rodrek W, Levy RS, et al. Cost of treating an infected total knee replacement. Clin Orthop 1996;331:140–5.
17. Fry DE, Marek JM, Langsfeld M. Infection in the ischemic lower extremity. Surg Clin North Am 1998;78:465–79.
18. Kobayashi M, Mohri Y, Inoue Y, et al. Continuous follow-up of surgical site infections for 30 days after colorectal surgery. World J Surg 2008;32:1142–6.
19. Reilly J, Allardice G, Bruce J, et al. Procedure-specific surgical site infection rates and postdischarge surveillance in Scotland. Infect Control Hosp Epidemiol 2006; 27:1318–23.
20. Avato JL, Lai KK. Impact of postdischarge surveillance on surgical-site infection rates for coronary artery bypass procedures. Infect Control Hosp Epidemiol 2002;23:364–7.
21. Huotari K, Lyytikainen O, and the hospital infection surveillance team. Impact of postdischarge surveillance on the rate of surgical site infection after orthopedic surgery. Infect Control Hosp Epidemiol 2006;27:1324–9.
22. Edwards JR, Peterson KD, Andrus ML, et al. National healthcare safety network (NHSN) report, data summary for 2006, issued June 2007. Am J Infect Control 2007;35:290–301.
23. Centers for Disease Control and Prevention. National healthcare safety network (NHSN). Available at: http://www.cdc.gov/ncidod/dhqp/nhsn.html. July 15, 2008.
24. Khan NA, Quan H, Bugar JM, et al. Association of postoperative complications with hospital costs and length of stay in a tertiary care center. J Gen Intern Med 2006;21:177–80.
25. Thompson DA, Makary MA, Dorman T, et al. Clinical and economic outcomes of hospital acquired pneumonia in intra-abdominal surgery patients. Ann Surg 2006;243:547–52.
26. Collins TC, Daley J, Henderson WH, et al. Risk factors for prolonged length of stay after major elective surgery. Ann Surg 1999;230:251–9.
27. Penel N, Lefebvre J-L, Cazin JL, et al. Additional direct medical costs associated with nosocomial infections after head and neck cancer surgery: a hospital-perspective analysis. Int J Oral Maxillofac Surg 2008;37:135–9.
28. Young LS, Sabel AL, Price CS. Epidemiologic, clinical, and economic evaluation of an outbreak of clonal multidrug-resistant Acinetobacter baumannii infection in a surgical intensive care unit. Infect Control Hosp Epidemiol 2007;28: 1247–54.
29. Estrada CA, Young JA, Nifong LW, et al. Outcomes and perioperative hyperglycemia in patients with or without diabetes mellitus undergoing coronary artery bypass grafting. Ann Thorac Surg 2003;75:1392–9.
30. Asher EF, Oliver BG, Fry DE. Urinary tract infections in the surgical patient. Am Surg 1988;54:466–9.
31. Golob JF Jr, Claridge JA, Sando MJ, et al. Fever and leukocytosis in critically ill trauma patients: its not the urine. Surg Infect (Larchmt) 2008;9:49–56.
32. Kass EH. Bacteriuria and the diagnosis of infection of the urinary tract. Arch Intern Med 1957;100:709–14.
33. Laupland KB, Bagshaw SM, Gregson DB, et al. Intensive care unit-acquired urinary tract infections in a regional critical care system. Crit Care 2005;9:R60–5.
34. Clec'h C, Schwebel C, Français M, et al. Does catheter-associated urinary tract infection increase mortality in critically ill patients? Infect Control Hosp Epidemiol 2007;28:1367–73.

35. Tambyah PA, Knasinski V, Maki DG. The direct costs of nosocomial catheter-associated urinary tract infection in the era of managed care. Infect Control Hosp Epidemiol 2002;23:27–31.
36. Anderson DJ, Kirkland KB, Kaye KS, et al. Underresourced hospital infection control and prevention programs: penny wise and pound foolish? Infect Control Hosp Epidemiol 2007;28:767–73.
37. Horowitz E, Dekel A, Yogev Y, et al. Urine cultures at removal of indwelling catheter after elective gynecologic surgery: is it necessary? Acta Obstet Gynecol Scand 2004;83:1003–4.
38. Fry DE, Fry RV, Borzotta AP. Nosocomial blood-borne infection secondary to intravascular devices. Am J Surg 1994;167:268–72.
39. Sreeramoju PV, Tolentino J, Garcia-Houchins S, et al. Predictive factors for the development of central line-associated bloodstream infection due to gram-negative bacteria in intensive care unit patients after surgery. Infect Control Hosp Epidemiol 2008;29:51–6.
40. Pittet D, Tarara D, Wenzel RP. Nosocomial bloodstream infection in critically ill patients. Excess length of stay, extra costs, and attributable mortality. JAMA 1994; 272:1598–601.
41. Warren DK, Quadir WW, Hollenbeak CS, et al. Attributable cost of catheter-associated bloodstream infections among intensive care patients in a non-teaching hospital. Crit Care Med 2006;34:2084–9.
42. Shannon RP, Patel B, Cummins D, et al. Economics of central line-associated bloodstream infections. Am J Med Qual 2006;21(Suppl):7S–16S.
43. Centers for Disease Control and Prevention. Guidelines for the prevention of intravascular catheter-related infections. MMWR Recomm Rep 2002;51(RR-10): 1–36.
44. Spencer RC. Clinical impact and associated costs of Clostridium difficile-associated disease. J Antimicrob Chemother 1998;41(Suppl C):5–12.
45. Miller MA, Hyland M, Ofner-Agostini M, et al. Morbidity, mortality, and healthcare burden of nosocomial Clostridium difficile-associated diarrhea in Canadian hospitals. Infect Control Hosp Epidemiol 2002;23:137–40.
46. Kyne L, Hamel MB, Polavaram R, et al. Health care costs and mortality associated with nosocomial diarrhea due to Clostridium difficile. Clin Infect Dis 2002; 34:346–53.
47. Vonberg R-P, Reichardt C, Behnke M, et al. Costs of nosocomial Clostridium difficile-associated diarrhea. J Hosp Infect 2008;70:15–20.
48. Zerey M, Paton BL, Lincourt AE, et al. The burden of Clostridium difficile in surgical patients in the United States. Surg Infect 2007;8:557–66.
49. Bratzler DW, Houck PM, Richards C, et al. Use of antimicrobial prophylaxis for major surgery: baseline results from the National Surgical Infection Prevention Project. Arch Surg 2005;140(2):174–82.
50. Bratzler DW, Houck PM. Antimicrobial prophylaxis for surgery: an advisory statement from the National Surgical Infection Prevention Project. Am J Surg 2005; 189(4):395–404.
51. Bratzler DW, Houck PM. Antimicrobial prophylaxis for surgery: an advisory statement from the national surgical infection prevention project. Clin Infect Dis 2004; 38:1706–15.
52. Dellinger EP, Hausmann SM, Bratzler DW, et al. Hospitals collaborate to decrease surgical site infections. Am J Surg 2005;190:9–15.
53. MedQic SCIP Project Information. Available at: www.medqic.org/scip. Accessed July 15, 2008.

54. Centers for Medicaid and Medicare Services. Medicare modernization update. Available at: http://www.cms.hhs.gov/MMAUpdate/. Accessed July 15, 2008.
55. Deficit Reduction Act of 2005. Available at: http://thomas.loc.gov/cgi-bin/query/ C?c109:./temp/~c109clnOHx. Accessed July 15, 2008.
56. Centers for Medicare and Medicaid Service. Hospital compare. Available at: http://www.hospitalcompare.hhs.gov. Accessed July 15, 2008.
57. Medicare Quality Improvement Community. Hospitals: surgical care improvement project. Available at: http://www.medqic.org/hospitals/measures. Accessed July 15, 2008.
58. Centers for Medicare and Medicaid Services. CMS proposes additions to list of hospital-acquired conditions for fiscal year 2009. Available at: http://www.cms. hhs.gov/apps/media/press/factsheet.asp. Accessed July 15, 2008.
59. Federal Register. Physician Quality Reporting Initiative (PQRI). Federal Register July 7, 2008;73:38558–75.
60. Centers for Medicare and Medicaid Services. Press release: Medicare quality reporting initiative pays over $36 million to participating physicians from the 2007 PQRI reporting period. July 15, 2008. Available at: http://www.cms.hhs. gov/apps/media/press/release.asp. Accessed July 15, 2008.
61. The Commonwealth Fund on a high performance health system: Why not the best/Results from the national scorecard on U.S. health system performance. Available at: http://www.cmwf.org/usr_doc/site_docs/pdfs/national_scorecard_ 2008_ex2.pdf. Accessed July 15, 2008.
62. Kornblum J. Writing is on the wall for doctors' e-prescriptions. Available at: http://www.usatoday.com/new/health/2008-07-28-eprescribe_N.htm.   Accessed July 28, 2008.
63. Lee K, McGreevey C. Using control charts to assess performance measurement data. Jt Comm J Qual Improv 2002;28:90–101.
64. Pine M, Jordan HS, Elixhauser A, et al. Enhancement of claims data to improve risk adjustment of hospital mortality. JAMA 2007;297:71–6.
65. Fry DE, Pine M, Jordan HS, et al. Combining administrative and clinical data to stratify surgical risk. Ann Surg 2007;246:875–85.
66. Fry DE, Pine M, Jones BL, et al. Adverse outcomes in surgery: redefinition of post-operative complications. Presented at the 32nd Annual Meeting of the Association of VA Surgeons. Dallas (TX), May 4–6, 2008.

Future Diagnostic and Therapeutic Approaches in Surgical Infections

Barbara Haas, MD[a,b,*], Avery B. Nathens, MD, PhD, MPH[a,b]

KEYWORDS

• Surgical infections • Microbiology • Antibiotics • Vaccines

Infections in surgical patients remain a significant cause of morbidity and mortality despite advances made in source control, antimicrobial therapy, and adjunctive therapies. Although there is much focus on optimizing the use of currently available therapy and the translation of evidence into practice,[1–5] there are a wide variety of innovations that might prove to be critical assets in the battle between microbes and their human host.

These innovations come at a critical time. The ability to support acute organ failure through advances in critical care or chronic organ failure through transplantation and immunosuppression is being challenged by the threat of increasing antimicrobial resistance. As a result, many have emphasized the urgent need for novel strategies either to prevent or treat infections caused by multidrug-resistant organisms.[6–10]

A number of diagnostic and therapeutic modalities currently in experimental phases of development have the potential not only to improve patient outcomes, but also to provide novel approaches to bypassing microbial resistance mechanisms, and represent potentially sustainable strategies in slowing the current rate of antimicrobial resistance. These innovative approaches include new and rapid diagnostic tests that could limit exposure to broad-spectrum antimicrobials through quicker diagnosis and more timely de-escalation; novel microbial targets to reduce pathogenicity; vaccine approaches to infection prevention; and prognostic markers to identify those at highest risk.

[a] Department of Surgery, University of Toronto, 100 College Street, Toronto, Ontario, M5G 1L5, Canada
[b] Division of General Surgery, St. Michael's Hospital, 30 Bond Street, Toronto, Ontario, M5B 1W8, Canada
* Corresponding author. St. Michael's Hospital, Queen Wing, 3N-073, 30 Bond Street, Toronto, Ontario M5B 1W8, Canada.
E-mail address: barbara.haas@utoronto.ca (B. Haas).

Surg Clin N Am 89 (2009) 539–554
doi:10.1016/j.suc.2008.09.013
0039-6109/08/$ – see front matter © 2009 Elsevier Inc. All rights reserved.

surgical.theclinics.com

NOVEL APPROACHES TO DIAGNOSTIC ASSESSMENT

Antibiotic exposure is the principal driving force behind emerging resistance.[6] Many antimicrobial guidelines emphasize the need to avoid the use of antimicrobials in clinical settings where they are unlikely to be of benefit, to narrow the spectrum when possible, and to reduce the duration of exposure.[11–13] These goals are counter to those that might be in the best interest of the patient, as early empiric broad-spectrum therapy has been associated with a survival benefit.[14–16]

The current approach to antimicrobial prescribing is in conflict with what might be ideal practice because of currently used microbial diagnostics. Conventional culture and microbial identification techniques typically require almost 72 hours for pathogens to be identified, speciated, and susceptibility patterns established.[8] During this time of diagnostic uncertainty, the patient, particularly the critically ill patient, is treated with broad-spectrum antibiotics, with de-escalation of therapy delayed until a definitive diagnosis is made. Moreover, conventional cultures may not identify the offending pathogen. This is particularly true of fastidious or slow-growing organisms, which include not only unusual pathogens, but also many fungal pathogens and a number of commonly encountered bacteria.[17] In addition, cultures taken after the initiation of antimicrobial therapy may have low yield, despite the presence of clinically important infection.[18]

The need to balance efforts to minimize the use of antimicrobials and to treat the patient adequately during a period of diagnostic uncertainty has led to the development of novel diagnostic strategies for the detection of pathogenic organisms based on advances in genomics and molecular biology.

Rapid Diagnostic Assessment

Traditionally, patient specimens are collected and then cultured in automated systems that detect the presence of any bacterial or fungal growth. If a culture "flags" positive, the pathogen is examined by means of Gram staining, which offers some diagnostic clues as to the nature of the microorganism, and is then further cultured and examined by various biochemical assays. Antibiotic susceptibilities are also examined during this period. New diagnostic assays use a variety of molecular diagnostic techniques to accelerate the diagnosis. The most common techniques include fluorescent in situ hybridization (FISH), polymerase chain reaction (PCR) amplification of unique genetic sequences, and microarray-based technology.

FISH relies on the use of a suspension of molecular probes that bind to a marker specific to a particular pathogen (eg, a highly specific ribosomal RNA). The probes have a detection system comprised of fluorescent markers that can be visualized by microscopy. PCR relies on the exponential amplification of microbial genetic material through an automated system; only a particular segment of genetic information is targeted by the assay, which ensures that if no pathogen with the genetic sequence is present in the sample, no amplification occurs. The amplified product is then detected, either directly or indirectly, through the presence of an automated detection system. Finally, microarray technology refers to the practice of fixing a large number of highly specific probes onto a stable medium, thereby enabling analysis of a large number of DNA or RNA sequences in an automated fashion. Each of these techniques has a large number of variations, and they are frequently used in tandem.

Culture-Based Assays

The majority of newer diagnostic assays use specimens derived from microbial cultures after specimen collection, as opposed to immediae analysis of specimens obtained from the patient. Identifying pathogens from culture-positive specimens has a number of potential advantages. It ensures that only cultures with live bacteria result in a positive test. It also ensures that the appropriate molecular probes are used through preliminary information obtained through Gram staining and early culture.[19] An excess number of probes in a single reaction can lead to a greater chance of a false-positive assay, and the information obtained through Gram staining and culture can help tailor the choice of probes, limit costs, and increase the chance of a valid result.

A wide range of assays aiming to identify pathogens from positive blood cultures have been designed. Although some are designed to detect only one or two specific pathogens, many have been developed to assess for the presence of a wide spectrum of organisms. As an example of the diagnostic utility of some of these assays, Oliveira and coworkers[20] developed a FISH assay to detect *Staphylococcus aureus* from a positive blood culture specimen. Results diverged from conventional culture results in less than 1% of cases, and results were available within 2.5 hours of a positive culture. Marlowe and coworkers[21] described a DNA probe matrix designed to identify a variety of gram-positive, gram-negative, and fungal pathogens within 1 hour of positive culture. The assay demonstrated less than 2% discordance with conventional cultures.

There is considerable variability, however, in accuracy across the reported studies. For example, a FISH assay designed to detect a wide range of pathogens identified species in only 81% of cases with positive conventional cultures. This loss of sensitivity was caused by an inadequate breadth of gram-negative probes, illustrating some of the inherent limitations of the high specificity of molecular diagnostic techniques.[22] Specifically, there must be a probe present for all potential organisms. Other assays designed to detect a wide range of pathogens, by FISH or amplification methods, have reported similar difficulties in identifying all clinically encountered pathogens to the species level.[23–26] These assays are not quite ready for widespread use in the clinical setting.

Other Uses for Molecular Diagnostic Strategies

There are several other potential applications for molecular diagnostic strategies that might prove valuable in the future. In part, these applications provide greater hope for success because they focus on particular organisms or clinical problems rather than casting a wide diagnostic net. For example, molecular diagnostic assays have proved to be useful in the rapid detection of antibiotic resistance genes. Several assays have been developed that can detect the presence of multiple genes concurrently in a matter of hours.[27–31] One study examined an oligonucleotide microarray that could, through PCR amplification, detect 90 different antibiotic resistance genes in gram-positive bacteria.[32] Another assay used microarray analysis to detect 61 different resistance genes from different species of bacteria, and to identify instances of horizontal gene transfer.[33] Nevertheless, the practical limitation of this approach is the constant evolution of new resistance genes, or their transfer to new pathogens, which requires a continuous updating of available assays.

Where the molecular diagnostic approach does seem to offer an advantage is in the rapid detection of methicillin-resistant *S aureus* (MRSA), a phenotype generally conferred by the mecA gene in *S aureus*.[34] *S aureus* is the most common blood-borne pathogen and the most important pathogen in the postoperative period.[35,36] Further, the increasing prevalence of MRSA has altered the approach to both prevention and treatment of suspected infections caused by *S aureus*.[36,37] New diagnostic assays might simplify the approach to the identification and treatment of staphylococcal infections. For example, the preliminary Gram stain of a blood culture result might be "gram-positive cocci in clusters." Most commonly, this result might represent a clinically insignificant contaminant with coagulase-negative staphylococci, or a bacteremia caused by methicillin-sensitive S aureus or MRSA. Several groups have developed PCR and microarray-based assays that discriminate between S aureus and coagulase-negative staphylococci with 100% reliability within hours of a positive culture.[38–41] More importantly, although genomic analysis does not always correlate precisely with phenotypic resistance patterns, multiple groups have described PCR-based assays with an accuracy of greater than 95% for the detection of MRSA in mixed cultures.[39,42–44]

The clinical utility of rapid diagnosis of S aureus bacteremia and identification of MRSA has been demonstrated in a number of studies. In a retrospective study where PCR was performed on specimens derived from patients with a positive conventional blood culture, the PCR result, if available, would have better directed therapy in a significant proportion of patients through a significant reduction in the use of vancomycin.[39] In other studies comparing conventional and molecular diagnostic methods, rapid results regarding MRSA status would have changed therapy in over 25% of patients.[42,45] PCR detection of MRSA directly from patients' specimens has not only been shown to decrease MRSA infection rates, but has been shown to be cost-effective in the clinical setting.[46]

Like MRSA detection, postoperative fungemia represents another clinical domain in which new diagnostic techniques could prove to be invaluable. Fungal organisms are frequently difficult to detect and are associated with significant morbidity and mortality. Further, it might take as long as 4 to 5 days to reliably declare a blood culture negative for fungal pathogens. Novel diagnostic strategies using PCR or FISH have shown tremendous promise in the rapid detection of these pathogens.[47–55] For example, Lau and coworkers[56] reported a PCR-based assay capable of detecting 11 species of fungus from positive blood cultures. This assay correctly identified all cultures that contained pathogens targeted by the assay with great accuracy in as little as 4 hours. Another assay using FISH to detect Candida albicans from positive blood cultures even demonstrated improved sensitivity compared with conventional methods.[57]

These fungal assays vary considerably in their complexity and costs, but many are likely to be cost-effective given the changing face of fungal infections. The widespread use of fluconazole has been associated with the emergence of resistant fungi including non-albicans Candida and non-fumigatus Aspergillus.[8] As a result, caspofungin or other more costly antifungals might be required as empiric therapy in certain clinical settings.[58] Rapid detection systems for fungal pathogens might allow for more rapid de-escalation and overall cost savings.[59,60]

Specimen-Based Assays

The primary disadvantage of the previously described molecular diagnostic techniques is their reliance on a period of in vitro culture of the organism. With the advent of newer diagnostic techniques that might directly detect pathogens in specimens without the need for prior culture, there is the potential for further reducing the time to diagnosis. PCR-based assays designed to detect S aureus and Enterococcus faecalis directly from blood samples have been developed.[61] Of greater use might be a recently described multiplex PCR assay that detects the presence of multiple gram-negative, gram-positive, and fungal organisms in blood samples, and which provides results within 7 hours of specimen collection.[62,63] Most specimen-based assays have sensitivities in the range of 65% to 75%, however, particularly with clinical specimens, too low to be of clinical use.[61–64] This lower sensitivity is likely caused by the presence of other compounds that interfere with the sensitive reactions on which these diagnostic tests rely. Although these assays hold promise, there are significant technical limitations that need to be overcome.

Pathogen Profiling

In addition to providing conventional information faster, molecular diagnostics are improving to the point that they will soon provide a new class of diagnostic information. Specifically, it will likely be possible to generate a more comprehensive, genetically based profile of the organism to better estimate the potential for pathogenicity or contribution to the clinical picture. This pathogen profiling provides information regarding the organism of interest, including the presence of resistance genes and virulence factors, and acknowledges the tremendous within-species and temporal variability in gene expression.[65] With the data accruing over time, this information could be linked to the probability of a clinically relevant phenotypic behavior and could be used to guide clinical decision-making. This approach would provide not only information about the pathogen's present phenotype (potentially in a more timely manner), but also might provide insight into the likely future behavior of the pathogen in vivo. For example, pathogen profiling has been used to guide use, dose, and duration of antiviral therapy in the context of hepatitis C infection.[65] Pathogen profiling has also been applied to the evaluation of a wide range of pathogens, including *Escherichia coli*, *Pseudomonas aeruginosa*, and *S aureus* strains, and to their virulence factors.[66,67] With further experience it might soon be possible to determine whether an organism is a colonizer or a pathogen and its propensity for the development of antimicrobial resistance. The rapid transmission of this information to the clinician might have direct impact on the approach to any identified organism.

NOVEL APPROACHES TO THERAPEUTICS

The discovery of effective and relatively nontoxic antimicrobial agents from environmental sources has historically led to a focus on natural sources of new antibacterial and antifungal agents.[68] Few antimicrobials are purely synthetic in origin, and potential antimicrobials are typically identified by screening candidate compounds against live pathogens. Compounds identified by this method target molecular processes required by the organism for survival or for propagation. By definition, this approach has led to antimicrobials that stimulate bacterial evolution by making high mutation rates more adaptive, and leads to resistance.[69,70]

A proposed alternative is the targeting of so-called "virulence factors," bacterial products that play a causal role in the manifestations of disease either by enabling the steps that lead to infection, or by causing disease symptoms (eg, secreted toxins),[69,71] but which are not essential to the pathogen's survival. It is thought that such antimicrobials, which may cause less selection pressure, would be less likely to lead to the rapid emergence of resistance.[69]

Although antimicrobial strategies targeted at virulence factors are as varied as the potential mechanisms of virulence, the greatest future success might lie in targeting bacterial quorum-sensing pathways. Quorum-sensing, which is the mechanism by which bacterial populations modify their gene expression in response to changes in the density of surrounding organisms, is closely linked to pathogenic behavior in many bacterial species. This behavior includes host invasion; surface adhesion; intercellular signaling; evasion of host defenses; and modification of the host environment (eg, toxins).[71,72] This strategy holds tremendous promise for therapy and might also play an important role in limiting the surface adhesion and biofilm formation that is a necessary first step in infections of surgical implants.

Quorum-sensing seems to be so critical to bacterial pathogenicity that therapies against this target may be highly effective. For example, inhibition of the quorum-sensing cascade in a murine model of S aureus infection blocked abscess formation. Further, this effect was evident with only transient blockade of the quorum-sensing cascade in the earliest phases of infection.[73] RNAIII-inhibiting peptide (RIP), which inhibits quorum-sensing in S aureus without decreasing bacterial cell counts, has been found to be potentially useful in a number of models. When administered as an antibiotic lock therapy to animals in a model of catheter-related bacteremia, catheter colonization was reduced after injection of S aureus directly into the catheter, and completely eliminated when RIP was used in combination with antibiotics.[74] In a murine model of polyethylene terephthalate (Dacron) graft infection, presoaking the graft with RIP decreased the growth of S aureus by a thousand-fold.[75,76] Further, a compound that is a nonpeptide analogue of RIP, and occurs naturally in the bark of witch hazel, interfered with bacterial adhesion and biofilm formation in an in vitro model, and demonstrated a dose-dependent inhibition of graft colonization in a murine model.[77] Finally, quorum-sensing has been targeted through the generation of monoclonal antibodies against AIP-4, which is involved in the quorum-sensing system of S aureus. Passive immunization with these antibodies resulted in increased survival in a murine model of S aureus intraperitoneal sepsis.[78]

Quorum-sensing mechanisms have also been well documented and extensively studied in another common hospital-acquired pathogen, P aeruginosa. It has been demonstrated, for example, that azithromycin interferes in quorum-sensing pathways of P aeruginosa, and may be potentially beneficial in patient populations susceptible to chronic infections by this pathogen.[79] The therapeutic potential of targeting quorum-sensing is also evident in another experimental approach, involving immunization against a pseudomonal autoinducer. This increased survival in a murine model of P aeruginosa pulmonary infection, but resulted in no change in bacterial cell counts.[80] This suggests that the observed decrease in mortality was caused by prevention of bacterial pathogenicity, rather than by growth inhibition. Targeting quorum-sensing pathways is not universally beneficial, however, and there seems to be dose-related effects that might even be harmful. The complex nature of quorum-sensing has been highlighted in this species in experiments demonstrating that subtherapeutic doses of other common agents, such as tetracycline, tobramycin, and ciprofloxacin, paradoxically induced genes associated with biofilm formation, and that subtherapeutic doses of tobramycin promote motility.[81,82]

Based on evidence to date, therapies targeted at bacterial virulence factors potentially offer a highly attractive combination: decreased pathogenicity without interference in cell replication, and a decreased likelihood of creating a strong selective pressure for resistance. Although the described therapies have not been evaluated in clinical trials, therapies aimed at virulence factors may be highly promising novel antimicrobials.

INFECTION PREVENTION THROUGH VACCINATION

Vaccines have likely been, historically, the most effective medical intervention for the prevention of infection. The advent of pathogen profiling and a broader understanding of the relationship between organism and host have led to a more sophisticated approach to vaccine development. Many of the pathogens commonly seen in surgical practice, such as S aureus and group A streptococci (GAS), have not been, until recently, preventable through vaccine strategies. A major obstacle in the development of effective vaccines against these pathogens is the high degree of variability of their surface antigens. The large number of resultant serotypes, the number of which is further increased by bacterial phase variation, makes creating a vaccine that results in universal resistance against the pathogen challenging.[83,84]

There are efforts underway to develop vaccines effective in preventing infections caused by S aureus given the burden of disease caused by this organism. Animal experiments and clinical trials have met with mixed results. A vaccine based on the S aureus capsular polysaccharide types 5 and 8, which account for 93% of clinical isolates, was evaluated in a large cohort of patients with end-stage renal disease.[85,86] The vaccine did not reduce the incidence of S aureus bacteremia over the year of observation; however, additional analyses suggest that periodic boosters might improve the vaccine's efficacy.

In a more recent study, animals were vaccinated with a nontoxic peptide similar in structure to alpha hemolysin, a cytotoxin produced by S aureus, which resulted in the production of an antibody directed against the active peptide. This antibody proved protective in a murine model of S aureus pneumonia.[87] S aureus quorum-sensing has also been used as a vaccine target. For example, immunization against a bacterial product involved in staphylococcal quorum-sensing resulted in increased survival in a murine model of intraperitoneal S aureus sepsis.[88]

GAS is a highly virulent organism, and like S aureus is of considerable surgical importance given its role in severe skin and soft tissue infections. As a result, many investigators have focused on developing effective vaccines directed against this organism or its virulence factors. The M protein of GAS, of which there are at least 100 variants, is responsible for specific immunity against this pathogen. In addition, antibodies directed against the M protein cross-react with certain human antigens. Taken together, these two factors significantly complicate the development of a safe and effective vaccine.[89,90] Recent analyses, however, have identified regions of the M protein that are both highly antigenic and specific to GAS. This has resulted in the construction of a polyvalent vaccine that has undergone phase I studies in humans.[90] It is estimated the vaccine could prevent up to 50% cases of invasive disease in adults, and an equal proportion of GAS-related deaths.[89]

Some of the challenges associated with identifying a universal vaccine target for species with highly variable antigens have recently been simplified with novel genomics-based approaches. "Reverse vaccinology" refers to the process of screening genomic sequences for regions that are likely to represent potential vaccine targets, such as cell membrane proteins that are conserved across species subtypes.[83] This approach has been used to identify potential vaccine targets for Streptococcus pneumoniae,[91] GAS,[92] and Neisseria meningitidis.[93,94] This approach has also been used to create a potential S aureus vaccine, which in preliminary studies has been demonstrated to provide protective immunity against S aureus from human clinical isolates in a murine model.[95]

Another innovative methodology in vaccine development is the use of the so-called "antigenome" approach to vaccine target identification.[96] This approach uses antibodies collected from convalescent patients to screen antigen expression libraries. In this way, only genes that produce antigens to which patients produce antibodies are selected for further study. This limits the number of targets studied, and identifies targets that are actually expressed in vivo. The antigenome strategy has, for example, been successfully used in S aureus vaccine development where it has been proved efficacious in murine models.[97] More importantly, this vaccine generated a strong immunologic response in primates despite pre-existing antibodies, suggesting that the vaccine could be used as a nosocomial vaccine. Similar approaches have been used by other groups for S aureus and for S pneumoniae.[96,98,99]

Infection control through vaccination holds great promise. Although the described therapies require many years of evaluation, a vaccine that might confer a moderate degree of protection could have significant effects on the burden of disease without the selection pressures associated with antimicrobial therapy. The challenge will then be to target those at highest risk for infections, a daunting task given our relatively primitive understanding of host-microbial interactions.

ADVANCES IN UNDERSTANDING HOST-MICROBIAL INTERACTIONS

The wide variation in outcomes following infection emphasizes the multiple factors that play a role in dictating the host's response to a microbial challenge. The host's response to infection might very well play a greater role in outcome than either the clinical context or the implicated pathogen. The observation that individuals differ in their susceptibility to infection over and above the known clinical risk factors has been well documented.[100] Recent advances in high throughput genomics may allow identification of high-risk individuals by virtue of their genotypes. Specifically, several single nucleotide polymorphisms, which represent minor genetic variations that occur in a small proportion of the population, have been associated with adverse outcomes related to infection.[100,101]

A systematic review of genes investigated for polymorphisms linked to the response to infection identified 76 studies examining 51 different genetic polymorphisms.[102] Genes investigated to date relate to those previously implicated in the host response to infection, including genes associated with cytokine production, the coagulation cascade, and signal transduction.[103,104] As the associated technology becomes increasingly rapid and affordable, however, it will likely become possible to scan the genome for genes associated with susceptibility to infectious disease without prior knowledge of their function.[100]

Polymorphisms related to tumor necrosis factor (TNF)-α and the Toll-like receptor (TLR) family have been among the more extensively studied given the current understanding of the role of these proteins in the manifestations of infection. TNF-α is a proinflammatory mediator that is produced in response to a wide range of stimuli, and that has been implicated in a number of inflammatory diseases, including sepsis.[101] The prevalence of the TNF2 polymorphism has been found to be significantly higher among patients with septic shock than the general population,[105,106] and has been found to be an independent predictor of death among patients with septic shock.[105] Among surgical patients, TNF-α polymorphisms have been associated with adverse outcomes among patients with postoperative septic shock.[107]

TNF-α polymorphisms have also been associated with surgical site or other nosocomial infections, suggesting it might be possible to identify those predisposed to infection and to better target preventive measures. In a study of patients undergoing esophagectomy, there was an association between TNF-α polymorphisms and subsequent infection.[108] The relationships are not simple, however, as the polymorphisms associated with infection in this study were found to confer protection in others.[105,106] Polymorphisms of the TNF-α gene have also been associated with increased susceptibility to sepsis following severe burns and trauma.[109–111]

Similar associations have been identified when polymorphisms pertaining to the TLR receptor family have been evaluated. These receptors are key in recognizing bacterial cell wall components and initiating the inflammatory cascade.[112] The TLR4 mutation has been associated with increased susceptibility to gram-negative infection among ICU patients[113] and in patients with major burns.[109] Others have demonstrated an association between a polymorphism at the TLR2 gene and increased susceptibility to gram-positive and fungal infection among patients with septic shock.[114,115]

Although this line of investigation might yield promise in identifying those at highest risk for infection, and those who might benefit from novel interventions, many of these results are inconsistent across studies.[108,116–122] The inconsistent findings might be caused by differences in methodology, small sample size, confounding through cosegregation of genetic loci, or gene interactions that are only poorly understood.[100,102,112]

It is anticipated that over time these investigations will yield considerable insights into risk factors (and prognosis) related to infection. These association studies must be performed using large populations of patients representing diverse ethnic and racial backgrounds, however, to ensure the findings are generalizable to the population at large, and they must consider the complex interactions between genetic polymorphisms at multiple gene loci.[103,123,124] If these methodologic issues can be overcome, the clinical benefits would be tremendous. Additionally, these studies would then allow for evaluation of new pathways that play a role in the development or manifestations of infection, and provide new avenues of study for targeted interventions. These novel interventions would be directed against the host response or host-microbial interactions, and would not be encumbered by the adverse selection pressures associated with antimicrobial therapy.

SUMMARY

Innovations in the field of infection hold significant promise in the way surgical infections are prevented, diagnosed, and treated. Diagnostics will allow for more rapid assessment of the causal pathogen and the likelihood of any particular organism contributing to the manifestations of disease. Treatment strategies will focus not on adding further selection pressures, but on compromising microbial virulence factors to render them innocuous. We are still in the early phases of experimenting with vaccine strategies for infection prevention in this clinical setting, but newer techniques might allow the development of effective vaccines for common nosocomial pathogens. Finally, the ability to identify patients at highest risk for infection through analyses of genetic polymorphism provides an opportunity to better understand host-microbial interactions and to target novel interventions.

REFERENCES

1. Bratzler DW, Houck PM. Antimicrobial prophylaxis for surgery: an advisory statement from the National Surgical Infection Prevention Project. Am J Surg 2005;189(4):395–404.
2. Bratzler DW, Hunt DR. The surgical infection prevention and surgical care improvement projects: national initiatives to improve outcomes for patients having surgery. Clin Infect Dis 2006;43(3):322–30.
3. Dellit TH, Owens RC, McGowan JE Jr, et al. Infectious diseases society of America and the society for healthcare epidemiology of America guidelines for developing an institutional program to enhance antimicrobial stewardship. Clin Infect Dis 2007;44(2):159–77.
4. Warren DK, Yokoe DS, Climo MW, et al. Preventing catheter-associated bloodstream infections: a survey of policies for insertion and care of central venous catheters from hospitals in the prevention epicenter program. Infect Control Hosp Epidemiol 2006;27(1):8–13.

5. Wu JH, Howard DH, McGowan JE Jr, et al. Adherence to Infectious Diseases Society of America guidelines for empiric therapy for patients with community-acquired pneumonia in a commercially insured cohort. Clin Ther 2006;28(9): 1451–61.

6. Livermore DM. Minimising antibiotic resistance. Lancet Infect Dis 2005;5(7): 450–9.

7. Hedrick TL, Smith PW, Gazoni LM, et al. The appropriate use of antibiotics in surgery: a review of surgical infections. Curr Probl Surg 2007;44(10):635–75.

8. Monk BC, Goffeau A. Outwitting multidrug resistance to antifungals. Science 2008;321(5887):367–9.

9. Siegel JD, Rhinehart E, Jackson M, et al. Management of multidrug-resistant organisms in health care settings, 2006. Am J Infect Control 2007;35(10 Suppl 2): S165–93.

10. Spellberg B, Guidos R, Gilbert D, et al. The epidemic of antibiotic-resistant infections: a call to action for the medical community from the Infectious Diseases Society of America. Clin Infect Dis 2008;46(2):155–64.

11. Shlaes DM, Gerding DN, John JF Jr, et al. Society for healthcare epidemiology of America and infectious diseases society of America esistance: guidelines for the prevention of antimicrobial resistance in hospitals. Clin Infect Dis 1997;25(3): 584–99.

12. Mazuski JE, Sawyer RG, Nathens AB, et al. The Surgical Infection Society guidelines on antimicrobial therapy for intra-abdominal infections: an executive summary. Fall. Surg Infect (Larchmt) 2002;3(3):161–73.

13. American Thoracic Society; Infectious Diseases Society of America. Guidelines for the management of adults with hospital-acquired, ventilator-associated, and healthcare-associated pneumonia. Am J Respir Crit Care Med 2005;171(4): 388–416.

14. Kumar A, Roberts D, Wood KE, et al. Duration of hypotension before initiation of effective antimicrobial therapy is the critical determinant of survival in human septic shock. Crit Care Med 2006;34(6):1589–96.

15. Garey KW, Rege M, Pai MP, et al. Time to initiation of fluconazole therapy impacts mortality in patients with candidemia: a multi-institutional study. Clin Infect Dis 2006;43(1):25–31.

16. Ibrahim EH, Sherman G, Ward S, et al. The influence of inadequate antimicrobial treatment of bloodstream infections on patient outcomes in the ICU setting. Chest 2000;118(1):146–55.

17. Peters RP, van Agtmael MA, Danner SA, et al. New developments in the diagnosis of bloodstream infections. Lancet Infect Dis 2004;4(12):751–60.

18. Grace CJ, Lieberman J, Pierce K, et al. Usefulness of blood culture for hospitalized patients who are receiving antibiotic therapy. Clin Infect Dis 2001;32(11): 1651–5.

19. Procop GW. Molecular diagnostics for the detection and characterization of microbial pathogens. Clin Infect Dis 2007;45(Suppl 2):S99–111.

20. Oliveira K, Brecher SM, Durbin A, et al. Direct identification of Staphylococcus aureus from positive blood culture bottles. J Clin Microbiol 2003;41(2):889–91.

21. Marlowe EM, Hogan JJ, Hindler JF, et al. Application of an rRNA probe matrix for rapid identification of bacteria and fungi from routine blood cultures. J Clin Microbiol 2003;41(11):5127–33.

22. Peters RP, van Agtmael MA, Simoons-Smit AM, et al. Rapid identification of pathogens in blood cultures with a modified fluorescence in situ hybridization assay. J Clin Microbiol 2006;44(11):4186–8.

23. Peters RP, Savelkoul PH, Simoons-Smit AM, et al. Faster identification of pathogens in positive blood cultures by fluorescence in situ hybridization in routine practice. J Clin Microbiol 2006;44(1):119–23.
24. Kempf VA, Trebesius K, Autenrieth IB. Fluorescent in situ hybridization allows rapid identification of microorganisms in blood cultures. J Clin Microbiol 2000; 38(2):830–8.
25. Anthony RM, Brown TJ, French GL. Rapid diagnosis of bacteremia by universal amplification of 23S ribosomal DNA followed by hybridization to an oligonucleotide array. J Clin Microbiol 2000;38(2):781–8.
26. Jansen GJ, Mooibroek M, Idema J, et al. Rapid identification of bacteria in blood cultures by using fluorescently labeled oligonucleotide probes. J Clin Microbiol 2000;38(2):814–7.
27. Strommenger B, Kettlitz C, Werner G, et al. Multiplex PCR assay for simultaneous detection of nine clinically relevant antibiotic resistance genes in *Staphylococcus aureus*. J Clin Microbiol 2003;41(9):4089–94.
28. Grimm V, Ezaki S, Susa M, et al. Use of DNA microarrays for rapid genotyping of TEM beta-lactamases that confer resistance. J Clin Microbiol 2004;42(8): 3766–74.
29. Lee Y, Lee CS, Kim YJ, et al. Development of DNA chip for the simultaneous detection of various beta-lactam antibiotic-resistant genes. Mol Cell 2002; 14(2):192–7.
30. Volokhov D, Chizhikov V, Chumakov K, et al. Microarray analysis of erythromycin resistance determinants. J Appl Microbiol 2003;95(4):787–98.
31. Batchelor M, Hopkins KL, Liebana E, et al. Development of a miniaturised microarray-based assay for the rapid identification of antimicrobial resistance genes in gram-negative bacteria. Int J Antimicrob Agents 2008;31(5):440–51.
32. Perreten V, Vorlet-Fawer L, Slickers P, et al. Microarray-based detection of 90 antibiotic resistance genes of gram-positive bacteria. J Clin Microbiol 2005;43(5):2291–302.
33. Frye JG, Jesse T, Long F, et al. DNA microarray detection of antimicrobial resistance genes in diverse bacteria. Int J Antimicrob Agents 2006;27(2):138–51.
34. de Lencastre H, Oliveira D, Tomasz A. Antibiotic resistant *Staphylococcus aureus*: a paradigm of adaptive power. Curr Opin Microbiol 2007;10(5):428–35.
35. van Rijen MM, Kluytmans JA. New approaches to prevention of staphylococcal infection in surgery. Curr Opin Infect Dis 2008;21(4):380–4.
36. Wisplinghoff H, Bischoff T, Tallent SM, et al. Nosocomial bloodstream infections in US hospitals: analysis of 24,179 cases from a prospective nationwide surveillance study. Clin Infect Dis 2004;39(3):309–17.
37. Zhanel GG, Decorby M, Nichol KA, et al. Antimicrobial susceptibility of 3931 organisms isolated from intensive care units in Canada: Canadian National Intensive Care Unit Study, 2005/2006. Diagn Microbiol Infect Dis 2008;62(1):67–80.
38. Zhu LX, Zhang ZW, Wang C, et al. Use of a DNA microarray for simultaneous detection of antibiotic resistance genes among staphylococcal clinical isolates. J Clin Microbiol 2007;45(11):3514–21.
39. Ruimy R, Dos-Santos M, Raskine L, et al. Accuracy and potential usefulness of triplex real-time PCR for improving antibiotic treatment of patients with blood cultures showing clustered gram-positive cocci on direct smears. J Clin Microbiol 2008;46(6):2045–51.
40. Palomares C, Torres MJ, Torres A, et al. Rapid detection and identification of *Staphylococcus aureus* from blood culture specimens using real-time fluorescence PCR. Diagn Microbiol Infect Dis 2003;45(3):183–9.

41. Shrestha NK, Tuohy MJ, Hall GS, et al. Rapid identification of *Staphylococcus aureus* and the mecA gene from BacT/ALERT blood culture bottles by using the LightCycler system. J Clin Microbiol 2002;40(7):2659–61.
42. Tan TY, Corden S, Barnes R, et al. Rapid identification of methicillin-resistant *Staphylococcus aureus* from positive blood cultures by real-time fluorescence PCR. J Clin Microbiol 2001;39(12):4529–31.
43. Maes N, Magdalena J, Rottiers S, et al. Evaluation of a triplex PCR assay to discriminate *Staphylococcus aureus* from coagulase-negative staphylococci and determine methicillin resistance from blood cultures. J Clin Microbiol 2002;40(4):1514–7.
44. Thomas LC, Gidding HF, Ginn AN, et al. Development of a real-time *Staphylococcus aureus* and MRSA (SAM-) PCR for routine blood culture. J Microbiol Methods 2007;68(2):296–302.
45. Hallin M, Maes N, Byl B, et al. Clinical impact of a PCR assay for identification of *Staphylococcus aureus* and determination of methicillin resistance directly from blood cultures. J Clin Microbiol 2003;41(8):3942–4.
46. Harbarth S, Masuet-Aumatell C, Schrenzel J, et al. Evaluation of rapid screening and pre-emptive contact isolation for detecting and controlling methicillin-resistant *Staphylococcus aureus* in critical care: an interventional cohort study. Crit Care 2006;10(1):R25.
47. Elie CM, Lott TJ, Reiss E, et al. Rapid identification of *Candida* species with species-specific DNA probes. J Clin Microbiol 1998;36(11):3260–5.
48. Carvalho A, Costa-De-Oliveira S, Martins ML, et al. Multiplex PCR identification of eight clinically relevant *Candida* species. Med Mycol 2007;45(7):619–27.
49. Li YL, Leaw SN, Chen JH, et al. Rapid identification of yeasts commonly found in positive blood cultures by amplification of the internal transcribed spacer regions 1 and 2. Eur J Clin Microbiol Infect Dis 2003;22(11):693–6.
50. Innings A, Ullberg M, Johansson A, et al. Multiplex real-time PCR targeting the RNase P RNA gene for detection and identification of *Candida* species in blood. J Clin Microbiol 2007;45(3):874–80.
51. Pryce TM, Palladino S, Price DM, et al. Rapid identification of fungal pathogens in BacT/ALERT, BACTEC, and BBL MGIT media using polymerase chain reaction and DNA sequencing of the internal transcribed spacer regions. Diagn Microbiol Infect Dis 2006;54(4):289–97.
52. Selvarangan R, Bui U, Limaye AP, et al. Rapid identification of commonly encountered *Candida* species directly from blood culture bottles. J Clin Microbiol 2003;41(12):5660–4.
53. Rigby S, Procop GW, Haase G, et al. Fluorescence in situ hybridization with peptide nucleic acid probes for rapid identification of *Candida albicans* directly from blood culture bottles. J Clin Microbiol 2002;40(6):2182–6.
54. Shepard JR, Addison RM, Alexander BD, et al. Multicenter evaluation of the *Candida albicans/Candida glabrata* peptide nucleic acid fluorescent in situ hybridization method for simultaneous dual-color identification of *C. albicans* and *C. glabrata* directly from blood culture bottles. J Clin Microbiol 2008; 46(1):50–5.
55. Metwally L, Hogg G, Coyle PV, et al. Rapid differentiation between fluconazole-sensitive and -resistant species of *Candida* directly from positive blood-culture bottles by real-time PCR. J Med Microbiol 2007;56(Pt 7):964–70.
56. Lau A, Sorrell T, Chen S, et al. Multiplex-tandem PCR: a novel platform for the rapid detection and identification of fungal pathogens from blood culture specimens. J Clin Microbiol 2008;46:3021–7.

57. Wilson DA, Joyce MJ, Hall LS, et al. Multicenter evaluation of a *Candida albicans* peptide nucleic acid fluorescent in situ hybridization probe for characterization of yeast isolates from blood cultures. J Clin Microbiol 2005;43(6):2909–12.
58. Pappas PG, Rex JH, Sobel JD, et al. Guidelines for treatment of candidiasis. Clin Infect Dis 2004;38(2):161–89.
59. Alexander BD, Ashley ED, Reller LB, et al. Cost savings with implementation of PNA FISH testing for identification of *Candida albicans* in blood cultures. Diagn Microbiol Infect Dis 2006;54(4):277–82.
60. Forrest GN, Mankes K, Jabra-Rizk MA, et al. Peptide nucleic acid fluorescence in situ hybridization-based identification of *Candida albicans* and its impact on mortality and antifungal therapy costs. J Clin Microbiol 2006;44(9):3381–3.
61. Peters RP, van Agtmael MA, Gierveld S, et al. Quantitative detection of *Staphylococcus aureus* and *Enterococcus faecalis* DNA in blood to diagnose bacteremia in patients in the intensive care unit. J Clin Microbiol 2007;45(11):3641–6.
62. Louie RF, Tang Z, Albertson TE, et al. Multiplex polymerase chain reaction detection enhancement of bacteremia and fungemia. Crit Care Med 2008;36(5): 1487–92.
63. Lehmann LE, Hunfeld KP, Emrich T, et al. A multiplex real-time PCR assay for rapid detection and differentiation of 25 bacterial and fungal pathogens from whole blood samples. Med Microbiol Immunol 2008;197(3):313–24.
64. Wiesinger-Mayr H, Vierlinger K, Pichler R, et al. Identification of human pathogens isolated from blood using microarray hybridisation and signal pattern recognition. BMC Microbiol 2007;7:78.
65. Sintchenko V, Iredell JR, Gilbert GL. Pathogen profiling for disease management and surveillance. Nat Rev Microbiol 2007;5(6):464–70.
66. Bekal S, Brousseau R, Masson L, et al. Rapid identification of *Escherichia coli* pathotypes by virulence gene detection with DNA microarrays. J Clin Microbiol 2003;41(5):2113–25.
67. Cleven BE, Palka-Santini M, Gielen J, et al. Identification and characterization of bacterial pathogens causing bloodstream infections by DNA microarray. J Clin Microbiol 2006;44(7):2389–97.
68. Wright GD. The antibiotic resistome: the nexus of chemical and genetic diversity. Nat Rev Microbiol 2007;5(3):175–86.
69. Cegelski L, Marshall GR, Eldridge GR, et al. The biology and future prospects of antivirulence therapies. Nat Rev Microbiol 2008;6(1):17–27.
70. Denamur E, Matic I. Evolution of mutation rates in bacteria. Mol Microbiol 2006; 60(4):820–7.
71. Wu HJ, Wang AH, Jennings MP. Discovery of virulence factors of pathogenic bacteria. Curr Opin Chem Biol 2008;12(1):93–101.
72. March JC, Bentley WE. Quorum sensing and bacterial cross-talk in biotechnology. Curr Opin Biotechnol 2004;15(5):495–502.
73. Wright III JS, Jin R, Novick RP. Transient interference with staphylococcal quorum sensing blocks abscess formation. Proc Natl Acad Sci U S A 2005; 102(5):1691–6.
74. Cirioni O, Giacometti A, Ghiselli R, et al. RNAIII-inhibiting peptide significantly reduces bacterial load and enhances the effect of antibiotics in the treatment of central venous catheter-associated Staphylococcus aureus infections. J Infect Dis 2006;193(2):180–6.
75. Giacometti A, Cirioni O, Gov Y, et al. RNA III inhibiting peptide inhibits in vivo biofilm formation by drug-resistant *Staphylococcus aureus*. Antimicrobial Agents Chemother 2003;47(6):1979–83.

76. Cirioni O, Giacometti A, Ghiselli R, et al. Prophylactic efficacy of topical temporin A and RNAIII-inhibiting peptide in a subcutaneous rat pouch model of graft infection attributable to staphylococci with intermediate resistance to glycopeptides. Circulation 2003;108(6):767–71.
77. Kiran MD, Adikesavan NV, Cirioni O, et al. Discovery of a quorum-sensing inhibitor of drug-resistant staphylococcal infections by structure-based virtual screening. Mol Pharmacol 2008;73(5):1578–86.
78. Park J, Jagasia R, Kaufmann GF, et al. Infection control by antibody disruption of bacterial quorum sensing signaling. Chem Biol 2007;14(10):1119–27.
79. Nalca Y, Jansch L, Bredenbruch F, et al. Quorum-sensing antagonistic activities of azithromycin in *Pseudomonas aeruginosa* PAO1: a global approach. Antimicrobial Agents Chemother 2006;50(5):1680–8.
80. Miyairi S, Tateda K, Fuse ET, et al. Immunization with 3-oxododecanoyl-L-homoserine lactone-protein conjugate protects mice from lethal *Pseudomonas aeruginosa* lung infection. J Med Microbiol 2006;55(Pt 10):1381–7.
81. Linares JF, Gustafsson I, Baquero F, et al. Antibiotics as intermicrobial signaling agents instead of weapons. Proc Natl Acad Sci U S A 2006;103(51): 19484–9.
82. Hoffman LR, D'Argenio DA, MacCoss MJ, et al. Aminoglycoside antibiotics induce bacterial biofilm formation. Nature 2005;436(7054):1171–5.
83. Zagursky RJ, Anderson AS. Application of genomics in bacterial vaccine discovery: a decade in review. Curr Opin Pharmacol 2008, in press.
84. Nagy G, Emody L, Pal T. Strategies for the development of vaccines conferring broad-spectrum protection. Int J Med Microbiol 2008;298(5–6):379–95.
85. Fattom A, Fuller S, Propst M, et al. Safety and immunogenicity of a booster dose of *Staphylococcus aureus* types 5 and 8 capsular polysaccharide conjugate vaccine (StaphVAX) in hemodialysis patients. Vaccine 2004;23(5):656–63.
86. Shinefield H, Black S, Fattom A, et al. Use of a *Staphylococcus aureus* conjugate vaccine in patients receiving hemodialysis. N Engl J Med 2002;346(7):491–6.
87. Bubeck Wardenburg J, Schneewind O. Vaccine protection against *Staphylococcus aureus* pneumonia. J Exp Med 2008;205(2):287–94.
88. Yang G, Gao Y, Dong J, et al. A novel peptide isolated from phage library to substitute a complex system for a vaccine against staphylococci infection. Vaccine 2006;24(8):1117–23.
89. O'Loughlin RE, Roberson A, Cieslak PR, et al. The epidemiology of invasive group A streptococcal infection and potential vaccine implications: United States, 2000–2004. Clin Infect Dis 2007;45(7):853–62.
90. McNeil SA, Halperin SA, Langley JM, et al. Safety and immunogenicity of 26-valent group a streptococcus vaccine in healthy adult volunteers. Clin Infect Dis 2005;41(8):1114–22.
91. Wizemann TM, Heinrichs JH, Adamou JE, et al. Use of a whole genome approach to identify vaccine molecules affording protection against *Streptococcus pneumoniae* infection. Infect Immun 2001;69(3):1593–8.
92. McMillan DJ, Batzloff MR, Browning CL, et al. Identification and assessment of new vaccine candidates for group A streptococcal infections. Vaccine 2004; 22(21–22):2783–90.
93. Pizza M, Scarlato V, Masignani V, et al. Identification of vaccine candidates against serogroup B meningococcus by whole-genome sequencing. Science 2000;287(5459)):1816–20.
94. Giuliani MM, Adu-Bobie J, Comanducci M, et al. A universal vaccine for serogroup B meningococcus. Proc Natl Acad Sci U S A 2006;103(29):10834–9.

95. Stranger-Jones YK, Bae T, Schneewind O. Vaccine assembly from surface proteins of *Staphylococcus aureus*. Proc Natl Acad Sci U S A 2006;103(45): 16942-7.
96. Giefing C, Meinke AL, Hanner M, et al. Discovery of a novel class of highly conserved vaccine antigens using genomic scale antigenic fingerprinting of pneumococcus with human antibodies. J Exp Med 2008;205(1):117-31.
97. Kuklin NA, Clark DJ, Secore S, et al. A novel *Staphylococcus aureus* vaccine: iron surface determinant B induces rapid antibody responses in rhesus macaques and specific increased survival in a murine *S aureus* sepsis model. Infect Immun 2006;74(4):2215-23.
98. Etz H, Minh DB, Henics T, et al. Identification of in vivo expressed vaccine candidate antigens from *Staphylococcus aureus*. Proc Natl Acad Sci U S A 2002;99(10):6573-8.
99. Beghetto E, Gargano N, Ricci S, et al. Discovery of novel *Streptococcus pneumoniae* antigens by screening a whole-genome lambda-display library. FEMS Microbiol Lett 2006;262(1):14-21.
100. Cooke GS, Hill AV. Genetics of susceptibility to human infectious disease. Nat Rev Genet 2001;2(12):967-77.
101. Cariou A, Chiche JD, Charpentier J, et al. The era of genomics: impact on sepsis clinical trial design. Crit Care Med 2002;30(5 Suppl):S341-8.
102. Clark MF, Baudouin SV. A systematic review of the quality of genetic association studies in human sepsis. Intensive Care Med 2006;32(11):1706-12.
103. Stuber F, Klaschik S, Lehmann LE, et al. Cytokine promoter polymorphisms in severe sepsis. Clin Infect Dis 2005;41(Suppl 7):S416-20.
104. Holmes CL, Russell JA, Walley KR. Genetic polymorphisms in sepsis and septic shock: role in prognosis and potential for therapy. Chest 2003;124(3):1103-15.
105. Mira JP, Cariou A, Grall F, et al. Association of TNF2, a TNF-alpha promoter polymorphism, with septic shock susceptibility and mortality: a multicenter study. J Am Med Assoc 1999;282(6):561-8.
106. Reid CL, Perrey C, Pravica V, et al. Genetic variation in proinflammatory and anti-inflammatory cytokine production in multiple organ dysfunction syndrome. Crit Care Med 2002;30(10):2216-21.
107. Tang GJ, Huang SL, Yien HW, et al. Tumor necrosis factor gene polymorphism and septic shock in surgical infection. Crit Care Med 2000;28(8):2733-6.
108. Azim K, McManus R, Brophy K, et al. Genetic polymorphisms and the risk of infection following esophagectomy: positive association with TNF-alpha gene -308 genotype. Ann Surg 2007;246(1):122-8.
109. Barber RC, Aragaki CC, Rivera-Chavez FA, et al. TLR4 and TNF-alpha polymorphisms are associated with an increased risk for severe sepsis following burn injury. J Med Genet 2004;41(11):808-13.
110. Menges T, Konig IR, Hossain H, et al. Sepsis syndrome and death in trauma patients are associated with variation in the gene encoding tumor necrosis factor. Crit Care Med 2008;36(5):1456-62, e1451-6.
111. O'Keefe GE, Hybki DL, Munford RS. The G->A single nucleotide polymorphism at the -308 position in the tumor necrosis factor-alpha promoter increases the risk for severe sepsis after trauma. J Trauma 2002;52(5):817-25 [discussion: 825-6].
112. Lin MT, Albertson TE. Genomic polymorphisms in sepsis. Crit Care Med 2004; 32(2):569-79.
113. Agnese DM, Calvano JE, Hahm SJ, et al. Human toll-like receptor 4 mutations but not CD14 polymorphisms are associated with an increased risk of gram-negative infections. J Infect Dis 2002;186(10):1522-5.

114. Lorenz E, Mira JP, Cornish KL, et al. A novel polymorphism in the toll-like receptor 2 gene and its potential association with staphylococcal infection. Infect Immun 2000;68(11):6398–401.

115. Woehrle T, Du W, Goetz A, et al. Pathogen specific cytokine release reveals an effect of TLR2 Arg753Gln during *Candida* sepsis in humans. Cytokines 2008; 41(3):322–9.

116. Jessen KM, Lindboe SB, Petersen AL, et al. CD14 and TLR4 polymorphisms are not associated with disease severity or outcome from gram negative sepsis. BMC Infect Dis 2007;7:108.

117. Moore CE, Segal S, Berendt AR, et al. Lack of association between Toll-like receptor 2 polymorphisms and susceptibility to severe disease caused by *Staphylococcus aureus*. Clin Diagn Lab Immunol 2004;11(6):1194–7.

118. Majetschak M, Obertacke U, Schade FU, et al. Tumor necrosis factor gene polymorphisms, leukocyte function, and sepsis susceptibility in blunt trauma patients. Clin Diagn Lab Immunol 2002;9(6):1205–11.

119. Calvano JE, Um JY, Agnese DM, et al. Influence of the TNF-alpha and TNF-beta polymorphisms upon infectious risk and outcome in surgical intensive care patients. Surg Infect (Larchmt) Summer 2003;4(2):163–9.

120. Gordon AC, Lagan AL, Aganna E, et al. TNF and TNFR polymorphisms in severe sepsis and septic shock: a prospective multicentre study. Genes Immun 2004; 5(8):631–40.

121. Allen A, Obaro S, Bojang K, et al. Variation in Toll-like receptor 4 and susceptibility to group A meningococcal meningitis in Gambian children. Pediatr Infect Dis J 2003;22(11):1018–9.

122. Feterowski C, Emmanuilidis K, Miethke T, et al. Effects of functional Toll-like receptor-4 mutations on the immune response to human and experimental sepsis. Immunology 2003;109(3):426–31.

123. Gordon A, Knight JC, Hinds CJ. Genes and sepsis: how tight is the fit? Crit Care Med 2008;36(5):1652–4.

124. Arcaroli J, Fessler MB, Abraham E. Genetic polymorphisms and sepsis. Shock 2005;24(4):300–12.

Index

Note: Page numbers of article titles are in **boldface** type.

Surg Clin N Am 89 (2009) 555–561
doi:10.1016/S0039-6109(09)00025-5
0039-6109/09/$ – see front matter © 2009 Elsevier Inc. All rights reserved.

surgical.theclinics.com

Printed and bound by CPI Group (UK) Ltd, Croydon, CR0 4YY

03/10/2024

01040450-0010